Series Editor: Richard Riegelman

Essentials of
Public Health
Biology

*Biologic Mechanisms of Disease
and Global Perspectives*

ESSENTIAL PUBLIC HEALTH

Loretta DiPietro, PhD, MPH

Professor

Exercise and Nutrition
Sciences

Milken Institute of
Public Health

The George Washington
University

Washington, DC

Julie A. DeLoia, PhD

Dean

Jefferson College of
Health Sciences

Roanoke, Virginia

Victor K. Barbiero

Adjunct Professor

Department of
Global Health

Milken Institute of
Public Health

The George Washington
University

Washington, DC

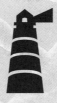

JONES & BARTLETT
LEARNING

World Headquarters
Jones & Bartlett Learning
5 Wall Street
Burlington, MA 01803
978-443-5000
info@jblearning.com
www.jblearning.com

Jones & Bartlett Learning books and products are available through most bookstores and online booksellers. To contact Jones & Bartlett Learning directly, call 800-832-0034, fax 978-443-8000, or visit our website, www.jblearning.com.

Substantial discounts on bulk quantities of Jones & Bartlett Learning publications are available to corporations, professional associations, and other qualified organizations. For details and specific discount information, contact the special sales department at Jones & Bartlett Learning via the above contact information or send an email to specialsales@jblearning.com.

09993-5

Production Credits

VP, Product Management: David D. Cella
Director of Product Management: Michael Brown
Product Specialist: Danielle Bessette
Production Editor: Vanessa Richards
Senior Marketing Manager: Sophie Fleck Teague
Manufacturing and Inventory Control Supervisor: Amy Bacus
Composition: codeMantra U.S. LLC

Cover Design: Michael O'Donnell
Rights & Media Specialist: Merideth Tumasz
Media Development Editor: Shannon Sheehan
Cover Image (Title Page, Part Opener, Chapter Opener):
 © vitstudio/Shutterstock
Printing and Binding: Edwards Brothers Malloy
Cover Printing: Edwards Brothers Malloy

Library of Congress Cataloging-in-Publication Data

Names: DiPietro, Loretta, author. | DeLoia, Julie, author. | Barbiero, Victor, author.
Title: Essentials of public health biology. Biologic mechanisms of disease and global perspectives / Loretta DiPietro, Julie DeLoia, Victor Barbiero.
Other titles: Biologic mechanisms of disease and global perspectives | Essential public health.
Description: Burlington, Massachusetts: Jones & Bartlett Learning, 2018. | Series: Essential public health | Includes bibliographical references and index.
Identifiers: LCCN 2017056636 | ISBN 9781284077919 (paperback)
Subjects: | MESH: Public Health | Communicable Diseases | Noncommunicable Diseases | Global Health
Classification: LCC RA425 | NLM WA 100 | DDC 362.1—dc23
LC record available at https://lccn.loc.gov/2017056636

6048

Printed in the United States of America
22 21 20 19 18   10 9 8 7 6 5 4 3 2 1

Contents

Chapter 6   Epigenetics in Human Health and Disease 63

Julie A. DeLoia

SECTION 2   Applications to Current Public Health Issues   73

Chapter 7   A Public Health View of Cancer . . . 75

Julie A. DeLoia

Chapter 8   Nutrition and Public Health 85

Kim Robien

Chapter 9   Overfeeding, Disuse, and Cardiometabolic Outcomes 99

Loretta DiPietro

Chapter 10   Maternal Biology 109

Madeline Bundy

Chapter 17   HIV/AIDS 207

Victor K. Barbiero

Prologue

Public health biology provides a critical foundation for the study of public health. In recent years, it has become increasingly clear that public health students at all levels need to understand the biologic basis for public health. New developments in genetics, immunology, and brain function require a basic understanding of biology. New preventive, diagnostic, and therapeutic technologies cannot be successfully applied without such an understanding of underlying biology.

Essentials of Public Health Biology starts by introducing students to basic concepts of cellular biology, immunology, and physiology, which are key to appreciating the connections between biology and public health. The authors build on these concepts to discuss the biologic aspects of important public health problems from communicable and noncommunicable diseases to aging, nutrition, environmental exposures, and injuries.

Essentials of Public Health Biology is unique in its focus on populations. It emphasizes the population as well as the individual implications of biology. The population perspective is key to understanding the biology of epidemic disease and immunizations as well as issues of environmental risk. The text does not assume that students have had previous biology courses. It starts with the fundamentals and leads the students to appreciate the implications of the biology for public health.

The lead authors of the text have worked together to offer on-site as well on online course work emphasizing public health biology. Their diverse disciplinary backgrounds and complementary areas of interest provide a strong basis for a comprehensive text. The authors utilize graphics, case studies, and in-depth examples to provide an engaging curriculum well designed for use as a textbook.

The text is organized into two sections beginning with fundamental concepts and followed by extensive applications to current public health issues. This step-by-step approach should help students understand and apply biology to current and future public health issues. The text provides the basis for course work that addresses the Council on Education for Public Health expectations for accreditation as well as preparing students for the certifying examination in public health.

The text's emphasis on basic concepts and applications to current public health issues should serve students well for many years to come. I'm very pleased that *Essentials of Public Health Biology* is part of the Essential Public Health series.

Richard Riegelman, MD, MPH, PhD
Series Editor—Essential Public Health

Contributors

Benjamin Aronson
Master's Candidate
Milken Institute School of Public Health
The George Washington University
Washington, DC

Madeline Bundy, MPH, MSN, CNM, WHNP-BC
Certified Nurse Midwife
Centro Internacional de Maternidad
Atlanta, GA

Sean D. Cleary, PhD, MPH
Associate Professor
Milken Institute School of Public Health
The George Washington University
Washington, DC

Mary Pat McKay
Chief Medical Officer
National Transportation Safety Board
Washington, DC

Pamela Poe, PhD, MPH, CHES
Director, Graduate Certificate in Health Education
    and Communication
Visiting Assistant Professor
University of the Sciences
Philadelphia, PA

Kim Robien, PhD, RD, CSO, FAND
Associate Professor
Milken Institute School of Public Health
The George Washington University
Washington, DC

Amy E. Seitz
Epidemic Intelligence Service Officer
National Center for Health Statistics
Centers for Disease Control and Prevention
Washington, DC

Carol A. Smith, MS
Former Assistant Professor and Education
    Coordinator
Clinical Laboratory Science Program
The George Washington University
Washington, DC

Reviewers

Richard Baumgartner, PhD
Professor & Chair
Department of Epidemiology & Population Health
University of Louisville - School of Public Health and
  Information Sciences
Louisville, KY

Gretchen De Silva, PhD, MPH
Assistant Clinical Professor
University of Maryland School of Public Health
College Park, MD

Dale A. Dickinson, PhD
Assistant Professor and Graduate Program Director
University of Alabama at Birmingham
Birmingham, AL

Michael Grantham, PhD
Assistant Research Professor
University of Maryland School of Public Health
College Park, MD

Alexis N. LaCrue, PhD
Instructor
University of South Florida
Tampa, FL

Travis Knuckles, PhD, DABT
Research Assistant Professor
West Virginia University
Morgantown, WV

Steven E. Seifried, PhD
Associate Professor, Adjunct Professor
University of Hawaii School of Public Health
Kailua, HI

Julie Smith-Gagen, PhD, MPH
Associate Professor
University of Nevada
Reno, NV

Introduction

Essentials of Public Health Biology is designed as an introductory text for undergraduates and as part of the Master of Public Health core that aims to (1) provide an overview of current knowledge about the biologic mechanisms of diseases that are major causes of death and disability in both developed and developing countries; (2) understand and interpret the reciprocal relationships of genetic, environmental, and behavioral determinants of health and disease within an ecologic context; and (3) provide opportunities to analyze, discuss, and communicate biologic principles of disease across the biologic and the public health spectra.

▶ The Public Health Core Competencies Addressed by This Text

After using this textbook, students will be able to:

1. Apply fundamental biologic concepts of the disease process as they relate to important communicable and noncommunicable diseases that are observed globally in public health.

2. Integrate these fundamental concepts with regard to their relation to exposures and disease outcomes across the public health spectrum.

3. Identify the role of host and environmental factors in determining susceptibility and resistance to disease.

4. Explain the multidisciplinary nature of contemporary public health issues and the role that various professionals play in addressing these issues.

5. Summarize the social, legal, ethical, economic, and political context of contemporary public health problems.

—Richard Riegelman, MD, MPH, PhD
Series Editor—Essential Public Health

Overview of Public Health Biology

Loretta DiPietro, Julie A. DeLoia, and
Victor K. Barbiero

▶ Introduction

The World Health Organization defines public health as "the art and science of preventing disease, prolonging life and promoting health through the organized efforts of society."[1] This includes all organized public or private measures to prevent disease, promote health, and prolong life at the population level. Public health efforts intend to provide physical, social, and political conditions that can empower people to gain control over the determinants of their own health. One obvious goal of public health is disease prevention and control—an effort that demands collaboration among scientists in several different disciplines. Sound public health practice requires knowledge and understanding of health- and disease-related terminology, concepts and processes spanning the biologic spectrum (cell, tissue, organ, system, and whole-body levels). The purpose of this textbook is to help students understand fundamental concepts of the disease process as they relate to important communicable and noncommunicable diseases that are observed globally. Moreover, students will apply these fundamental biologic concepts to exposures and disease outcomes across the public health spectrum in order to recognize optimal time points and strategies for successful intervention.

▶ Basic Principles of Challenge and Homeostasis

Stress is a common and adaptive component of our interaction with the environment, and the human body has evolved over the millennia to adapt to various environmental stressors. A stressor can be defined as any type of challenge to the body's basal function. This challenge will result in an increased demand on physiologic function and a consequent disruption in *homeostasis*. In order to regain homeostasis, the body needs to adapt to the particular challenge by undergoing either transient or long-term adjustments. For example, simply standing up from a chair and walking across the room is a challenge to basal function and requires a series of adjustments in heart rate and blood pressure to ensure adequate blood flow to working muscles and to the brain to support even this minimal activity.

Cellular and tissue functions are controlled within narrow limits, and therefore, to maintain homeostatic control, the human body must be able to detect deviations in the internal environment. Once detected, the body must then be able to control the appropriate factors responsible for adjusting these deviations back to the basal state. For instance, when core body temperature drops too low, a number of alterations will occur automatically. Blood flow will shift away from the skin toward the central organs (resulting in "goose bumps" on the skin surface) and rapid, involuntary muscle contractions (shivering) will begin to generate heat. "Negative feedback" occurs when a deviation in a controlled function triggers a response that opposes that deviation, thereby restoring function in the opposite direction back to normal (**FIGURE 1**).

In public health, we can identify myriad exposures that challenge, perturb, or stress basal function. These can be beneficial exposures, like exercise and work activity, or they can be harmful, such as exposure to cigarette smoking or toxic chemicals. Our ability to respond and adjust to these challenges in a timely and appropriate manner relies on both the *plasticity* and *resiliency* of our physiology. Plasticity (or compliance) refers to the amount of expansion and recoil that occurs in certain types of tissues or organs in response to increased physiologic demands. In cardiovascular function, for instance, plasticity is a reflection of both the structure and functional properties of

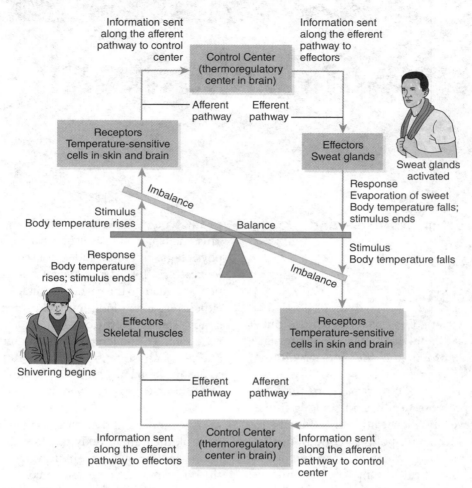

FIGURE 1 Homestasis and Temperature Control

the circulatory system. Resiliency (or *allostasis*) refers to the timely ability to regain normal homeostatic function following a given environmental challenge through the activation of neural, neuroendocrine, and neuroendocrine immune responses. Indeed, a near-collision in an automobile can double heart rate within 3 to 5 seconds and blood pressure within 10 to 15 seconds. Normally, heart rate and blood pressure would return to resting levels several minutes after the "threat" has disappeared, thereby indicating resiliency. In some people, however, this *fight-or-flight* response is exaggerated beyond the level of threat and remains long after the threat has dissipated. This exaggerated response also may occur in reaction to multiple other threats, such as occupational, financial, or interpersonal stressors. The *allostatic load* refers to the accumulated physiologic burden (wear and tear) to repeated cycles of allostasis. When the allostatic load is greater than the body's ability to compensate, errors or injuries will occur in the cells, tissues, organs, systems, or whole body, thereby initiating and promoting the disease process.

▶ The Natural History of Disease in Public Health

The natural history of disease refers to the manner in which a disease progresses in the absence of any medical or public health intervention. Public health practitioners rely on available knowledge about the stages, mechanisms, and causes of disease to determine the most appropriate time and manner to intervene. The goal of any intervention is to alter the natural history of a disease in a favorable way—either by preventing it entirely, delaying its onset, or by reversing it.

A disease develops over time and can be divided into three stages: pre-disease, latency, and symptomatic. The pre-disease stage precedes any pathologic process and is the ideal time to intervene, as stopping the disease before it causes damage may be the most cost-effective path. Early efforts to prevent exposures to harmful factors and thus prevent the disease process from even starting are termed *primary prevention*. When the disease process has begun but the person is not yet symptomatic is called the latency stage—or incubation period. In order to prevent the progression to the next stage, screening and early treatment may be necessary. This level of early detection and treatment is referred to as *secondary prevention*. Once disease symptoms become evident (symptomatic stage), efforts to slow or even reverse the progression of disease are called *tertiary prevention*. Examples of tertiary prevention include cardiac or physical rehabilitation and bariatric surgery.

▶ Models of Disease Transmission

Public health divides disease into those that are communicable (e.g., influenza, measles, polio, human immunodeficiency virus/acquired immune deficiency syndrome) and those that are noncommunicable (e.g., heart disease, cancer, diabetes). The *etiology* of most diseases involves an interactive triad of factors: the agent, the host, and the environment. For many communicable diseases, a fourth factor is added: the vector or vehicle.

An *agent of disease* is a necessary initiator of that disease; for instance, without the agent, there is no disease. Biologic agents include bacteria, viruses, allergens, toxins, and even foods (those high in trans fats, for example); chemical agents include toxins such as lead, arsenic, or asbestos; physical agents include radiation, uncontrolled mechanical energy (the factor in vehicular injuries and bullet wounds), heat, cold, micro-gravity, and a chronic positive energy balance (the agent of obesity). *Host factors* are those traits that affect one's susceptibility to the disease agent. Host resistance is influenced by genotype, age, sex, immune

response, and behavior. Several host factors can work synergistically to influence resistance or susceptibility to disease. For example, frail, older people often are undernourished and have other comorbid conditions, thereby making them particularly susceptible to diseases like influenza. The *environment* influences the probability of contact between the agent and the host. Poor sanitation, poverty, laws pertaining to firearm access, the political environment, urban design, and crowded schools are all examples of environmental factors that influence disease causation. Vectors of disease are those factors that transmit or spread the disease among populations. These can include insects, animals, and water; however, the definition also could apply more broadly to people (drug dealers) or objects (contaminated needles, elevators, guns). To be an effective transmitter of disease, the vector must have a specific relationship to the agent, the host, and the environment. For example, the vector in malaria transmission is the *Anopheles* mosquito, which carries the agent for malaria (e.g., *Plasmodium vivax*) in its salivary glands. When the mosquito feeds on human blood, this parasite is transferred to the host. The warm, humid climate of central Africa is a particularly friendly environment for this species of mosquito, thereby enhancing the contact between humans, mosquitos, and the parasite in that geographic area.

More recent epidemiologic models of noncommunicable disease transmission embrace a multifactorial model of causation, which describes the interactions among a variety of agent, host, and environmental factors. The sufficient–component model (**FIGURE 2**) illustrates how different combinations of various risk factors may work together to

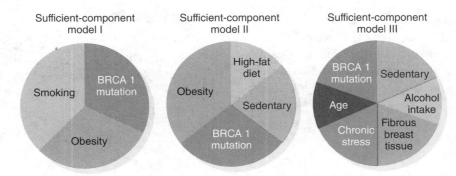

In these examples, the necessary component in breast cancer etiology (i.e., present in every model) is the BRCA 1 gene mutation. In Model I, co-existing risk factors of obesity and cigarette smoking create a sufficient set of components to initiate the disease onset. Models II and III illustrate how combinations of other risk factors may work together to create sufficient sets of components to initiate the disease onset or progression. Public health efforts are directed toward keeping various "pieces of the puzzle" from completing a set.

FIGURE 2 Sufficient-Component Model

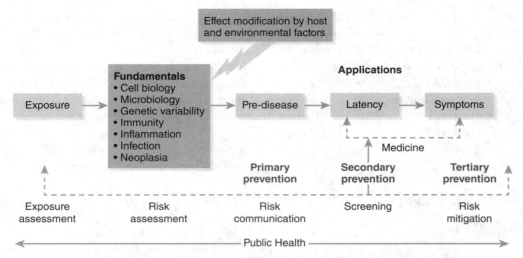

FIGURE 3 Paradigm for Relating Foundation Topics to Pervasive Health Issues Across the Biologic and Public Health Spectra

cause certain diseases. This model emphasizes that while a given risk factor may be a *necessary* component for a particular disease, in many cases that one factor may not be *sufficient* by itself to result in the disease. Rather, this necessary factor must be accompanied by a particular combination of other risk factors, and when a sufficient set of components is in place, disease onset occurs. Public health efforts can be directed toward blocking other risk components (e.g., hypertension, smoking, obesity) from completing the "sufficient set." Efforts and resources are best directed toward risk components that are easily modifiable either by behavior change, medication, or by policy.

▶ The Paradigm

As stated previously, the overarching goal of this textbook is to help students understand and apply fundamental biologic concepts of the disease process as they relate to globally observed communicable and noncommunicable diseases. Within the biologic

spectrum, we discuss cell anatomy and physiology, microbiology, immunity, inflammation, and genetic variation because they are the fundamental elements of human disease. We next apply these fundamental concepts and functions across the disease spectrum (pre-disease, latency, symptomatic) to illustrate how public health can affect the natural course of disease in the most cost-effective manner. The public health spectrum refers to primary, secondary, and tertiary levels of intervention with regard to disease prevention and management, but it involves the prevention and management of risk exposures as well. Indeed, sound public health practice requires that the disciplines of exposure assessment, risk assessment, risk communication, and risk mitigation work together to protect the health of the population (**FIGURE 3**).

▶ Reference

1. World Health Organization. Public health services. Available at http://www.euro.who.int/en/health-topics/Health-systems/public-health-services. Accessed November 27, 2017.

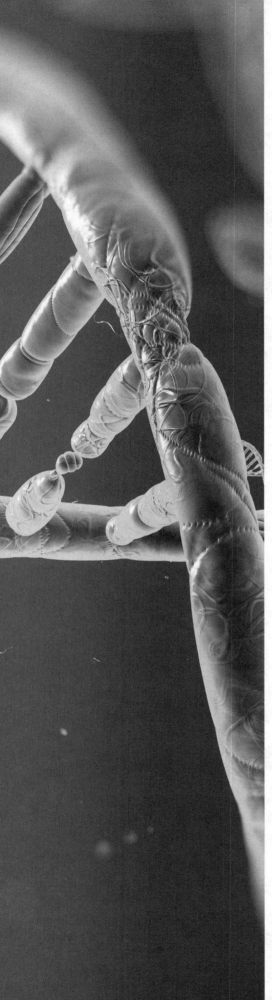

SECTION 1

Fundamental Concepts

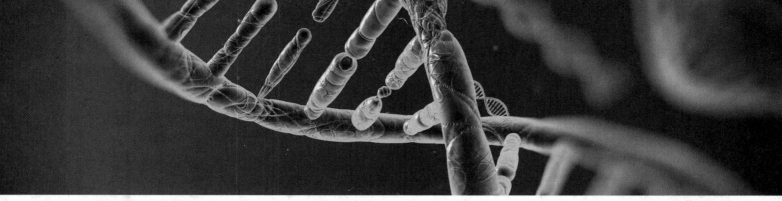

CHAPTER 1

Risk Assessment, Communication, and Management

Loretta DiPietro and Pamela Poe

LEARNING OBJECTIVES

By the end of this chapter, the student will be able to:

- Define the four components of risk analysis
- Identify various hazards encountered in everyday life
- Discuss examples of risk estimates
- Justify the importance of risk and health communications to risk management
- Examine the factors that affect risk perception
- Identify examples of risk management
- Summarize the importance of risk analysis to risk management

CHAPTER OUTLINE

▶ Introduction

The field of **risk analysis** and its elements of risk assessment, communication, and management is a multidisciplinary area of public health that comprises teams of basic and applied laboratory scientists, epidemiologists, medical and public health practitioners, lawyers, economists, and managers. Risk assessment concerns itself with defining the health risks associated with various biologic, chemical, thermal, or mechanical hazards. Risk assessment involves the quantification of exposure, biologic dose, and human response in order to determine the impact that a given hazard may have on the health and well-being of a given population. Risk communication is how we can best quantify and characterize the likelihood that a given hazard will cause harm. Risk assessment and communication are important to risk management with regard to the balance between the prevalence of a hazard, the magnitude of the risk, and the economic consequences of managing it (**FIGURE 1-1**). Although most of what we understand about risk analysis comes from the environmental health literature,[1] many of its elements can be applied to all aspects of public health concerned with the health effects of behavioral, environmental, societal, or political exposures.

▶ Risk Assessment

A **hazard** is any agent (biologic, chemical, thermal, mechanical, psychosocial) that has the potential to do harm. Examples of a hazard include a loaded handgun, a pesticide, a hot iron, an environmental pollutant, workplace stress, or even a bag of French fries. It is important to note that these agents cannot cause harm without human interaction. **Hazard identification**

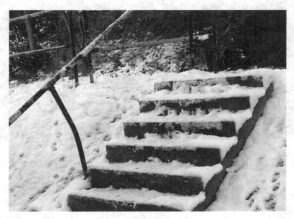

© Scott Latham/Shutterstock

is a component of risk assessment that determines whether or not a given agent actually causes an adverse effect on biologic tissue, based on laboratory and field studies of the interaction between the agent and the host. An adverse effect can be an event as simple as a transient impairment in lipid metabolism to something as discrete and dramatic as mortality.

Dose–response assessment, another component, determines the relationship between increasing (or decreasing) amounts of the hazard *at the site of the target tissues or organs* (the biologic burden) and increasing (or decreasing) levels of response (e.g., illness, perception of well-being, mortality, physical fitness, or body weight). Studies of potentially harmful exposures are conducted and usually rely on laboratory-based experiments with animal models. The field of toxicology has a notable history with regard to assisting industry and the government with setting standards or limits on potentially toxic substances in the air, water, food, or even cosmetics. The lethal dose$_{50}$ (LD$_{50}$) and the exposure dose$_{50}$ (ED$_{50}$) refer to the dose of a given hazard necessary to result in mortality or illness, respectively, among 50% of

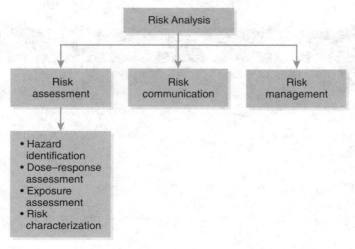

FIGURE 1-1 The Components of Risk Analysis in Public Health

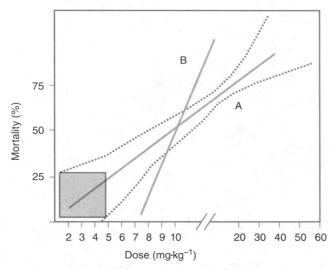

FIGURE 1-2 Accuracy in a Dose–Response Curve

the animals studied. The validity and the precision of dose–response experiments will affect the accuracy of the dose–response curve, and accuracy is often compromised at the lowest doses. **FIGURE 1-2** displays the dose–response curves for two substances, A and B. The dotted line on either side of the curve reflects the confidence band around the estimates. As the term implies, the confidence band is an indicator

of the precision or reliability of the estimate, and as observed in the figure, the confidence band is widest at very low and very high doses. This has important implications for people because standard limits for human beings are generally set at the lowest levels possible from data statistically extrapolated from these animal studies (**FIGURE 1-3**).

Another important issue regarding toxicology studies using animal models is the translation (or generalizability) of those findings to human beings. Differences in dose delivery (infusion of a substance subcutaneously or intravenously vs. breathing or absorption through skin among humans), similarity of the animal model to the human system under study, and posture (four legs vs. two legs!) are examples of such concerns. On the other hand, dose–response assessments in people are often hampered by the **heterogeneity of response** among humans. That is, host factors such as age, sex, body mass, disease status, and even hydration status will affect the biologic burden assumed by an individual and thus, the response to a uniform exposure. This explains why some people can tolerate a pint of beer with no consequence, while someone else might become incapacitated.

Exposure assessment, a third component of risk assessment, determines the level or prominence of a

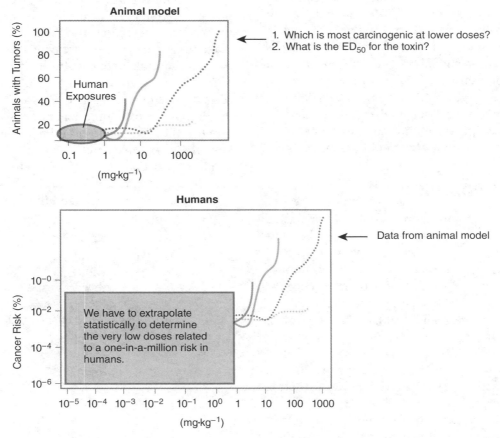

FIGURE 1-3 Extrapolation from Animal to Human Needs

given hazard experienced within a population under different conditions, based on studies performed in the field (rather than the laboratory). Objective measurement and characterization of air or water quality; the level of pesticides or other contaminants in produce; the clustering of fast food chains on a city block; or the number of handguns owned in a community are examples of exposure assessment. Exposure assessment takes into account the *source* of exposure, the *level* of exposure, and *how* the exposure is absorbed by the body. The quality of the exposure assessment data determines the accuracy of the risk assessment, and therefore precise measurement is extremely important. Many areas of public health have shifted from a reliance on self-reported exposure assessments to the use of objective monitors (personal air monitors, physical activity monitors, or geographic information systems) and the collection of biomarkers that reflect transient or chronic exposures (e.g., urinary cotinine, blood alcohol, glycated hemoglobin levels).

The final aspect of risk assessment is **risk characterization**, which involves one or more estimates of risk. A risk estimate is any measure of association between a given exposure and the likelihood of a disease outcome. Risk estimates are derived from statistical modeling and can be expressed as a correlation coefficient (least valid), a regression estimate, a simple proportion, or as a relative risk (the risk of disease or harm in the exposed group compared with the risk in the unexposed group). Importantly, any estimate of risk is always accompanied by confidence intervals or bands. Biologic plausibility, the predisposing of exposure to disease onset, the consistent observation of a dose–response relationship, and the magnitude of the risk estimate are important indicators that a hazard is indeed a risk to human health and function.

▶ Risk Communication

The accurate communication of the risk associated with a given hazard is often hampered by the public's misunderstanding and misperception of risk. As stated previously, risk can be characterized in numerous ways; however, the terms "odds of occurrence" or "cumulative incidence" have little meaning to the lay population. Therefore, public health practitioners often put risk in terms that are meaningful to people, such as "years of life lost" or "disability days." When communicating the risk of various toxic exposures to children, "years of productive life lost" is a very powerful metric.

Many times, risk is expressed as a 1:1 million risk (a **micromort**),[2] so that various exposures or behaviors can be compared with regard to their actual danger. For example, **FIGURE 1-4** shows the number of

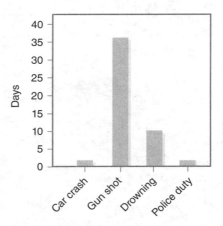

FIGURE 1-4 Time (Days) to Accumulate a 1:1 Million Risk of Death
Data from Wilson R. Analyzing the risks of daily life. *Technol Rev.* 1979;81:40-46.

days it would take to accumulate a 1:1 million of risk dying according to different methods. As indicated (and contrary to what most people believe), the risk of death is highest from a car crash or police duty, because either of these risks takes the fewest number of days to reach a 1:1 million chance. Examples of lifestyle activities related to a 1:1 million risk of death are drinking Miami tap water for one year, smoking 2 cigarettes, or traveling 10 miles by bicycle.[3]

Inherent in effective risk communication is people's perception of risk. People face numerous risks as part of their interaction with the environment, and we make trade-offs between one type of risk and another based on several factors. At the end of the day, choice and control remain key elements of how people perceive the magnitude of a given risk and whether or not they are willing to assume it. For example, driving a car is one of the riskiest choices we make on a daily basis; however, few people perceive it that way. On the other hand, some people refuse to fly in airplanes (which is actually safer than driving a car) primarily because someone else is in control and the consequences of a mistake could be disastrous.

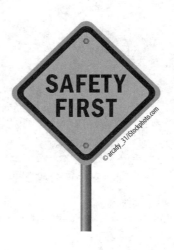

▶ Health Communication

Health communication is the use of communication strategies to inform and influence individual and community decisions that promote health and prevent disease, and is now recognized as a necessary element of public health.[4] **Health literacy** refers to how well individuals understand health communication messages in order to make appropriate health decisions. Health literacy is important to consider as part of health communication, as the targeting of messages to appropriate levels is an essential ingredient to constructing successful health (and risk) communication campaigns.

The first national assessment of health literacy was developed by several federal agencies and included in a national literacy test in 2003. This test examined three types of health literacy skills and included these aspects of health literacy in the Health Literacy Component of the 2003 National Assessment of Adult Literacy[5]:

- *Clinical type*: addressed aspects of the interaction process between doctors and patients, diagnosis and treatments, and clinical protocols, such as medication and following health regimens.
- *Prevention type*: addressed the actions people take to maintain health, such as physical activity, nutrition, knowing when to seek medical care, and health screenings.
- *Navigation of the healthcare system type*: assessed understanding of insurance procedures, healthcare system details, and patient rights or responsibilities under existing laws.[6]

Ultimately, the test findings suggested that relatively few Americans possess the health literacy skills needed to make accurate assessments and to understand the messages coming from health campaigns. If health literacy concerns are taken into account when health communication messages are constructed, it will likely result in much more successful communication if tailored to the abilities of the intended targets for the campaign. The Office of Disease Prevention and Health Promotion has developed a National Action Plan to Improve Health Literacy, incorporating seven goals to improve the health literacy levels in the United States.[7]

Other aspects of health literacy include *numeracy*, which is the ability to understand and work with numbers; *computer literacy*, that is, the ease with which consumers can access health information online (also known as e-health literacy); and *media literacy*, the ability to critically analyze media health messages including pictures, words, symbols and moving images.[8] Public health relies on health communication to relay in a timely manner important information about (1) prevention, (2) risk, and (3) crises such as disease outbreaks or natural disasters. The most important aspect of risk communication, and in particular crisis communication, is to begin with a structured plan based upon what is known, what is not yet known, and the specific information that needs to be communicated to a target audience in a manner that matches their level of health literacy.

As communication technology continues to evolve, public health practitioners must consider both proven health communication techniques and the need for innovative strategies. New ways to promote health messages will continue to evolve, as the public's use of advanced technologies changes in the social marketplace of ideas. At times, this evolution may create divisions between more and less savvy media consumers. If so, it is important to consider the best ways to define and reach each segment of the public (see **BOX 1-1**).

Health marketing is a term developed for use by the Centers for Disease Control and Prevention and is commonly referred to as **social marketing** in studies on health campaign strategies. Health marketing includes "creating, communicating, and delivering health information and interventions"[9] and uses a

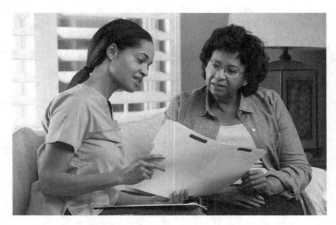

© Monkey Business Images Ltd/Monkey Business/Getty Images Plus

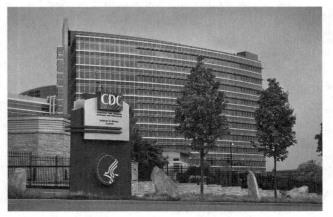

CDC/James Gathany

BOX 1-1 Health Communication in the New Media and the Digital Age

With the advent of interactive and new media, the rise of blogging, and other participatory media that narrowcast to specific audiences, public health professionals are facing a health communication landscape different from anything seen before. Public health information is now communicated via Twitter, LinkedIn, Facebook, Google Hangout, and other social media channels. At the same time, some audiences may not be able to take full advantage of the technological opportunities available to others. The changing media landscape raises a number of questions:

- Which communication strategies that have worked before continue to work as media technology evolves?
- Will audiences be best reached via traditional media or will they require interactive involvement and nontraditional media channels?
- How can public health messages be made to stand out in an increasingly saturated media environment?
- What targeting strategies will yield the most effective results for reaching the intended audiences and stakeholders?

customer-centered approach and scientific basis for developing and implementing these strategies to targeted audiences. This approach was founded on principles first used in the commercial sector and involves the use of marketing tactics that have traditionally been used to develop marketing and advertising campaigns. When applied to health-related strategic initiatives such as promoting health or preventing disease, the health marketing or social marketing approach has proved to be an effective strategy for understanding audiences, for developing, and for implementing public health campaigns. A communication strategy is a statement or document that expresses a planned process of assembling the components needed for an effective campaign. Elements of a communication strategy should include but are not limited to the following attributes: intended or target audiences, communication channels, key images, intended actions of audiences, benefits audiences will receive, and ways to convince audiences of these benefits.

▶ Risk Management

As stated, risk and health communication strategies are vital elements to our ability to mitigate (or manage) various hazards and their risks to human health.

Risk management refers to the strategies taken to eliminate risks or to lower them to acceptable levels (often determined by a government agency together with scientific and public input). Examples of risk management include: (1) making recommendations; (2) regulatory development; (3) licensing laws; (4) standard setting; (5) control measures; and (6) monitoring and surveillance.

In determining what actions might be necessary to eliminate or to reduce risk, the public health practitioner must juggle the weight of the scientific data; the availability of resources to assist in management; and the social, political, and economic consequences of either taking, or not taking, action. Indeed, the relationship between risk assessment and risk management is often problematic and the practitioner must balance *sound science* with effective and timely *public health practice* in dealing with uncertainty. With public health scientists, data are not considered to be "TRUE" unless the probability that the calculated risk estimate was due to chance falls below an alpha-level (P-value) of 0.05, with sufficient statistical power (beta: $1 - \beta \geq 0.80$) to avoid making a type II error (i.e., failing to reject the null hypothesis when it should be rejected). In contrast, the public health practitioner may not be able to wait for definitive science and often has to make important decisions with limited evidence; this is especially true in outbreak situations when quick decisions are necessary to save lives, such as with outbreaks of foodborne illnesses of high virulence. Consider, however, a situation in which there is a long developmental period between exposure to some type of hazard and the onset of disease, or one in which exposure affects subsequent generations. For example, suppose that a community's water supply has been polluted by a factory upstream for decades. The community reports several new cases of childhood leukemia that have occurred in the past several years that they believe might be linked to the water supply; however, the two environmental risk analysis studies that were performed yielded conflicting results. If the findings indicating a link between the water supply and childhood leukemia are indeed true, and the public health commissioner for that region shuts down the factory, then he or she might be perceived as a hero. On the other hand, if the commissioner shuts the factory down when there is no true link to disease, he or she may lose her job.

With regard to risk management, one constantly must weigh the costs of taking versus not taking action. In doing so, one must evaluate alternatives to the suspected hazard and whether those alternatives are accessible to the public. For instance, although eating organically grown fruits and vegetables and hormone-free meat is certainly an alternative to a fast-food, fat-dense diet, the higher cost and dearth of healthy foods often preclude their purchase among people living in low-resource communities. If the water in people's wells contains unacceptable levels of arsenic, is their alternative municipal water or bottled water? Do they have access to both? Another consideration is the cost-to-benefit ratio of taking action to reduce or manage risk. Reducing the level of air pollution by closing a factory will also result in job losses that may cripple a community economically. In the same manner, producing beef, chicken, and pork humanely and free of pesticides, antibiotics, and growth hormone will increase the costs of these items to the consumer. Also, if we increase the age for driver registration to 18 years in order to lower motor vehicle fatalities among new drivers, we may hinder the ability of a young person who lives in a rural area to have a part-time job.

▶ Why Do Risk Analysis?

Risk analysis allows us to determine the health and disease effects attributable to different types of exposures and activities. From this information, we can compare new versus existing technologies and strategies with regard to their effectiveness in controlling or mitigating risk (e.g., the effectiveness of air bags versus lowering the speed limit to 55 mph on automobile crash fatalities). Finally, the results from risk analyses allow public health practitioners and policy makers to set risk management priorities, which is especially important should budgets for public health infrastructure get cut (which they often are). As discussed previously, risk communication is essential to getting the public's acceptance of risk control programs and policies, and involves continued negation and consensus building between scientists, practitioners, and the public to answer the question, "How safe is safe enough"?

Key Terms

Dose–response assessment	Health communication	Risk analysis
Exposure assessment	Health literacy	Risk characterization
Hazard	Heterogeneity of response	Social marketing
Hazard identification	Micromort	

Discussion Questions

1. List four limitations with generalizing dose–response findings from animal studies to health effects in human beings.
2. What factors are important to communicating risk effectively to the public? How does the micromort metric enhance our ability to compare the risk associated with different exposures or behaviors?
3. What is exposure assessment and why is it so important to risk assessment and management? How has the use of objective monitoring improved the science of risk analysis?
4. Reflect on public health issues in your community and select several to consider in light of health communication strategies. Find a health issue or devise a fictional scenario that would be appropriate for each of these categories: prevention, risk, and crisis communication. Consider your target audiences and specific media channels for the issue you have selected. Which types of mass media access would be most relevant to the audiences you are trying to reach? How could you use the three types of research (formative, process, outcome) to monitor the effectiveness of your campaign?
5. Why is it so important to include input from the public when deciding on risk management strategies?

References

1. Friis RH. Environmental policy and regulation. In: Riegelman R, ed. *Essentials of Environmental Health*. Sudbury, MA: Jones and Bartlett Publishers; 2007:63-84.
2. Howard RA. On making life and death decisions. In: Schwing RC, Albers WA, eds. *Societal Risk Assessment: How Safe Is Safe Enough?* New York: Plenum Press; 1980:89-113.
3. Wilson R. Analyzing the risks of daily life. *Technol Rev.* 1979;81:40-46.
4. Office of Disease Prevention and Health Promotion. (n.d.). Healthy People 2020 Topics & Objectives: Health communication and health information technology. Washington, DC: U.S. Department of Health and Human Services. Available at https://www.healthypeople.gov/2020/topics-objectives/topic/health-communication-and-health-information-technology?_ga=2.243510082.696941203.1494178229-1307792197.1494177905. Accessed May 7, 2017.

5. Kutner M, Greenberg E, Jin Y, Paulsen C. *The Health Literacy of America's Adults: Results from the 2003 National Assessment of Adult Literacy*. U.S. Department of Education. Washington, DC: National Center for Education Statistics; 2006.

6. U.S. Department of Health and Human Services. *Communicating Health: Priorities and Strategies for Progress*. Washington, DC: U.S. Department of Health and Human Services; 2003.

7. U.S. Department of Health and Human Services, Office of Disease Prevention and Health Promotion. *National Action Plan to Improve Health Literacy*. Washington, DC: U.S. Department of Health and Human Services; 2010.

8. Bernhardt JM, Cameron KA. Accessing, understanding, and applying health communication messages: the challenge of health literacy. In: Thompson TL, Dorsey AM, Miller KI, Parrott R, eds. *Handbook of Health Communication*. Mahwah, NJ: Lawrence Erlbaum; 2003:583-605.

9. Centers for Disease Control and Prevention. Gateway to health communications & social marketing practice: What is health marketing? Available at https://www.cdc.gov/healthcommunication/toolstemplates/WhatIsHM.html. Updated February 2, 2011. Accessed May 7, 2017.

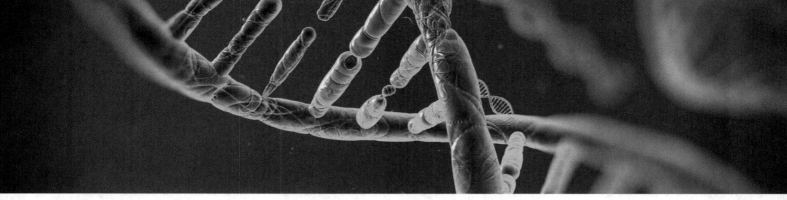

CHAPTER 2
Cell Properties and Function

Loretta DiPietro

LEARNING OBJECTIVES

By the end of this chapter, the student will be able to:

- Describe primary parts of the cell and their function
- Differentiate between basic and specialized cell functions
- Describe the basic principles of cellular homeostatic control
- Identify an example of a negative feedback loop in human physiology
- Explain the role of cell biology across the public health spectrum

CHAPTER OUTLINE

- Introduction
- Cell Basics
- Organelles
- Basic and Specialized Cell Functions
- Cell Organization
- Cell Exchanges

- Homeostasis
- **Case Report**
- **Key Terms**
- **Discussion Questions**
- **References**

▶ Introduction

Cells are the basic unit of life. Whether they exist as a single cell or a multicellular organism, all cells perform basic functions necessary to their own survival. Within each cell, chemical molecules are organized into a living unit. In turn, cells serve as building blocks for tissue, organ, and whole-body function. Cells are not visible to the human eye and not until the invention of the microscope in the mid-17th century were scientists able to detect them.

Modern-day advancements in light microscopes and later in electron microscopy (100 times more powerful than light microscopes) allowed scientists to understand the incredible complexity and diversity of the cell. Moreover, the internal structures of the cell were identified and the specific functions of these structural components became known (see **TABLE 2-1** for a summary of cell structures and function). Modern advances in cell physiology have enabled us to grow cells outside the body (*in vitro*) and have resulted in the related fields of cell engineering and genetics.

TABLE 2-1 Summary of Cell Structures and Functions

Cell Part	Structure	Function
Plasma membrane	Lipid-based and containing proteins	Selective barrier that controls transport in and out of cells
Nucleus	Double-layer membrane containing DNA and specialized proteins	Stores genetic material
Endoplasmic reticulum	A network of fluid-filled tubules and flattened sacs	Synthesizes proteins and transports materials through the cell
Golgi complex	Sets of flattened, curved sacs that are stacked in layers	Modifies, packages, and distributes newly synthesized proteins
Lysosomes	Membrane sacs containing hydrolytic enzymes	Digests and eliminates cellular waste
Peroxisomes	Membrane sacs containing oxidative enzymes	Detoxifies the cell
Mitochondria	Rod or oval-shaped bodies having a double outer membrane, a folded inner membrane (cristae), and an interior (matrix)	Major site for ATP (energy) production
Transport vesicles	Membrane-enclosed packages	Move molecules such as proteins from the rough endoplasmic reticulum to the Golgi complex
Vaults	Octagonal barrels	May transport either messenger RNA or ribosomal units from the nucleus to the cytoplasm

Reproduced from Sherwood L. *Human Physiology: From Cells to Systems*. 4th ed. Belmont, CA: Brooks/Cole; 2001:20-21.

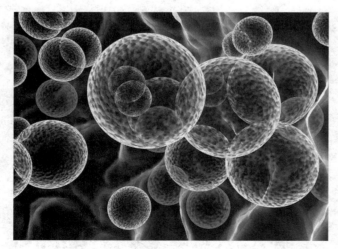

© Sebastian Tomus/Shutterstock

These advances have provided us with a greater ability to understand, prevent, and treat the major noncommunicable and communicable diseases affecting our global population.

▶ Cell Basics

Most cells have three major parts: the plasma (cell) membrane, the nucleus, and the cytoplasm (**FIGURE 2-1**). The cell membrane provides a selective barrier to the outside environment. The fluid contained inside the cell wall is known as intracellular fluid, whereas the fluid outside of the cell is referred to as extracellular fluid. The cell membrane controls all movement of molecules in and out of the cell. For example, the membrane allows nutrients to come in and waste products to go out, while it also serves to keep unwanted elements out of the cell.

The two primary structures on the inside of the cell are the nucleus and the cytoplasm. The cell **nucleus** is the largest single organized unit in the cell and it provides storage for the cell's genetic material—deoxyribonucleic acid (DNA). Nuclear DNA provides the blueprint for cell replication. It acts as the control center of the cell by directing synthesis of certain

The membrane-bounded organelles of an animal cell

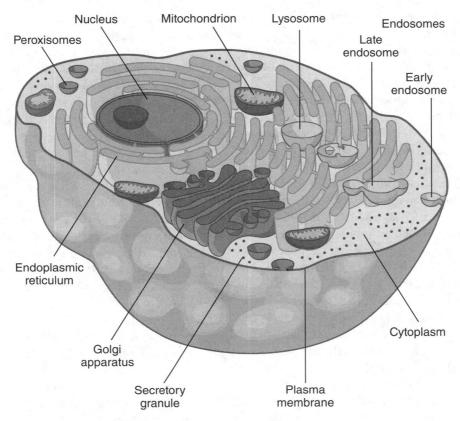

FIGURE 2-1 Animal Cell

proteins that determine the specificity of cell. Three types of ribonucleic acid (RNA) play a role in such protein synthesis: messenger RNA, ribosomal RNA, and transfer RNA. The genetic code for a specific protein is transcribed into messenger RNA, which then exits the nucleus and delivers the code to ribosomal RNA. The ribosomal RNA reads and translates the code into amino acid sequence and then transfer RNA delivers sequences within cytoplasm to designated site of protein production within the cell. In addition to providing the codes for protein synthesis, DNA also serves as a genetic blueprint during cell replication, thus ensuring that the cell produces additional cells identical to itself. In the reproductive cells, the DNA blueprint will pass along specific genetic characteristics to future offspring.

The cytoplasm is the portion of the cell interior that is not occupied by the nucleus. The cytoplasm comprises a complex gel-like mass called **cytosol**, within which are dispersed a variety of highly organized and distinct membrane-enclosed structures called **organelles**. Almost all cells contain six primary types of organelles: (1) the endoplasmic reticulum; (2) the Golgi complex; (3) lysosomes; (4) peroxisomes; (5) mitochondria; and

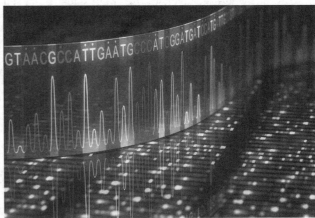

(6) vaults. Each type of organelle is a specialized internal compartment that contains specific types of chemicals for performing a particular cellular function. Organelles occupy about 50% of total cell volume. The remainder of the cytoplasm not occupied by organelles comprises cytosol. Cytosol is a semi-liquid mass laced with an intricate network of proteins—the **cytoskeleton**. This cytoskeleton is what gives the cell its shape, provides for its internal organization, and regulates its movements.

▶ Organelles

The **endoplasmic reticulum (ER)** is a protein-synthesizing factory. It has embedded ribosomes that synthesize proteins in addition to transporting materials throughout the cell. These membrane-bound and secreted proteins are made on ribosomes, which are found on the membrane of the rough ER. Most of these proteins mature in the Golgi apparatus before going to their final destination. Some proteins are sent for export to the exterior of the cell as secretory products (such as hormones or enzymes); other proteins are transported to sites within the cell for the construction of new cellular membranes or for other protein components of organelles. The smooth ER is a network of tiny interconnected tubules and contains no ribosomes. Its primary function is to transport materials throughout the cell. Some specialized cells have extensive smooth ER that performs additional functions. For example, some cells that specialize in lipid metabolism are abundant in smooth ER; in liver cells, the smooth ER has the capacity to detoxify harmful substances so that they can be eliminated more easily in the urine; and in muscle cells, the modified smooth ER (sarcoplasmic reticulum) stores calcium and plays an important role in muscle contractions.

The **Golgi complex** consists of sets of flattened, curved, membrane-enclosed sacs that are stacked in layers. The newly manufactured proteins coming from the ER travel through the layers of the Golgi stack to the cell membrane. During this transit, two important and inter-related functions take place: (1) the "raw" proteins are modified into their final form, and (2) the modified proteins are sorted and distributed to their final destination.

Lysosomes are membrane-enclosed sacs that contain hydrolytic acid. They are responsible for digesting and eliminating cellular waste products, such as bacteria, from the cell. Lysosomes can also re-package damaged cell parts, or extracellular materials that have been engulfed by the cell, into reusable cell parts. Each cell contains about 300 lysosomes, with each varying in size and shape depending on what they are digesting. **Peroxisomes** are also membrane-enclosed sacs that are smaller than lysosomes and contain several powerful oxidative enzymes. These enzymes use oxygen (O_2) to strip hydrogen from specific molecules. This reaction serves to detoxify various waste products produced within the cell, as well as foreign toxic compounds that have entered the cell, such as ethanol from alcoholic beverages.

The **mitochondrion** is the power plant of cell. Its role is to derive energy from ingested nutrients and convert that energy to a usable form. Adenosine triphosphate (ATP) is the common energy "currency" of the body and is made up of adenosine + 3 phosphate groups. The cells can use this ATP "currency" as payment for running the cellular machinery. When a high-energy bond (such as that binding the terminal phosphate to adenosine) splits, a substantial amount of energy is released. The number of mitochondria per cell varies (between 100–2,000) according to energy needs of the cell.

Food is digested and broken down into absorbable units that can be transported from the digestive tract lumen into the circulatory system. These molecules are then delivered to the cells and transported across the plasma membrane into the cytosol. The cytosol contains enzymes that are responsible for *glycolysis*—a chemical process that breaks down the glucose molecule into two pyruvic acid molecules to produce ATP. Glycolysis is not very efficient, however, with regard to energy extraction. Indeed, one molecule of glucose has a net yield of only two molecules of ATP, which is insufficient to support the energy needs of the body. This is where the mitochondria take over energy production.

Mitochondria are rod- or oval-shaped structures about the size of bacteria. Each mitochondrion is enclosed by a double membrane: a smooth outer membrane and an inner membrane that forms a series of folds called **cristae**. These cristae project into an inner cavity filled with a gel-like solution that is called the **matrix** (**FIGURE 2-2**). The pyruvic acid produced by glycolysis in the cytosol can be selectively transported into the mitochondrial matrix, where it is further broken down to form acetyl coenzyme A (acetyl CoA). Acetyl CoA then enters the *citric acid cycle* (also known as the Krebs cycle), where it goes through a cyclical series of eight separate biochemical reactions directed by the enzymes of the mitochondrial matrix to produce two more molecules of ATP from each glucose molecule. These two additional ATP molecules are still an inadequate yield; however, the citric acid cycle is an important step in preparing the hydrogen carrier molecules for their entry into the *electron transport chain*. The electron transport chain

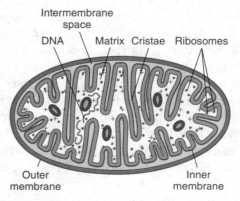

FIGURE 2-2 The Mitochondrion Inner Structures

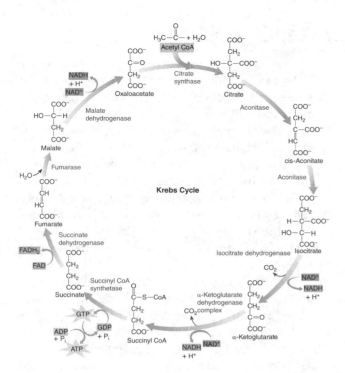

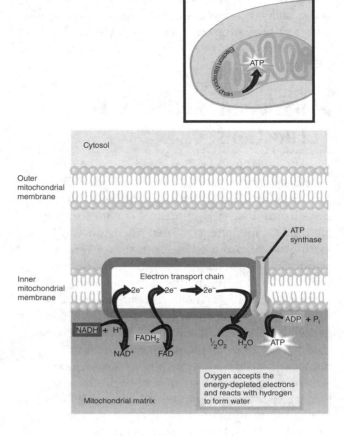

is essential for cellular respiration—the intracellular oxidation of nutrients—and occurs in the mitochondrial cristae. O_2 breathed in enters the mitochondria and combines with hydrogen ions to form water. As the electrons move through this chain, from high-energy to lower-energy levels, they release energy. Some of this energy is released as heat, but part of it is harnessed by the mitochondria to synthesize ATP.

The cell is a more efficient energy converter when O_2 is available. Under **anaerobic** (without O_2) conditions, the breakdown of glucose cannot go beyond glycolysis. Glycolysis happens in the cytosol as the breakdown of glucose into pyruvic acid. This breakdown produces a low yield of only two molecules of ATP per molecule of glucose. The remaining energy inside the glucose molecule is locked within the bonds

of the pyruvic acid molecule, which eventually are converted to lactic acid. In contrast, when sufficient O_2 is available (**aerobic** conditions), the citric acid cycle and the electron transport chain harness enough energy to yield 34 additional ATP molecules for a total yield of 36 per molecule of glucose (**FIGURE 2-3**).

Other organelles are **vaults**, which are octagonal barrel-shaped structures that apparently transport either messenger RNA or ribosomal units from the nucleus to the cytoplasm. **Transport vesicles** can move molecules such as proteins from the rough ER

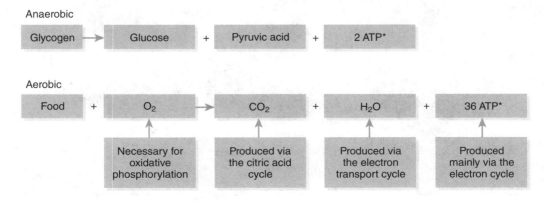

* Molecules of ATP produced per molecule of glucose

FIGURE 2-3 Energy Production

to the Golgi apparatus. These vesicles are primarily responsible for directing intracellular transportation and for regulating cellular movements. Transport vesicles also play a role in regulating cell growth and division.

▶ Basic and Specialized Cell Functions

All cells perform several basic and common functions, necessary for the survival of the cell itself. The basic functions include: (1) obtaining nutrients and O_2 from the surrounding environment; (2) converting nutrients and O_2 into energy, as described above; (3) eliminating waste products from such conversions; (4) synthesizing proteins for cell growth, structure, and function; (5) controlling the exchange of materials in and out of the cell; (6) moving materials around within the cell; (7) monitoring the environment surrounding the cell; and (8) reproducing, except in case of nerve or muscle cell loss from disease or trauma. The cells carry out these basic functions with remarkable similarity.

In multicellular organisms, each cell also performs a specialized function, which usually involves some modification of one of the basic cell functions. Examples of specialized functions include: (1) muscle cell contractions for movement; (2) elimination of waste by kidney cells; (3) the secretion of digestive enzymes by specialized glands in the digestive system; and (4) nerve cell messages to the brain in response to changes in the surrounding environment. An important concept here is that basic cell functions are important for the survival of the individual cell, while the specialized functions contribute to the survival of the system or whole body.

▶ Cell Organization

The body is organized progressively into four levels: cells, tissues, organs, and systems. Cells of similar structure and function comprise tissues. The body contains four different types of tissue: muscle, nervous, epithelial, and connective. Each type of tissue consists of cells having a single specialized function.

Muscle tissue is composed of cells specialized to contract and to generate force. The three types of muscle tissue are skeletal, cardiac, and smooth (**FIGURE 2-4**). Skeletal muscle is responsible for moving the skeleton. A single skeletal muscle cell, termed a muscle fiber, is elongated, cylinder-shaped, and contains multiple nuclei. These muscle fibers are *striated* (containing bands of fibers) and are under voluntary control. Because of the energy demands of muscle contractions and movement, muscle fibers contain more mitochondria compared with other types of cells. Cardiac (heart) muscle tissue is also striated. These cells appear branched, with one to three central nuclei. Cardiac tissue also has multiple nuclei to support the energy demands of the heart and circulatory system, but unlike skeletal muscle, it is not under voluntary control; rather, it is innervated by the autonomic nervous system. *Smooth muscle* is not striated, is arranged in sheets, and like cardiac muscle, it is not under voluntary control. Both smooth and skeletal muscle cells are elongated; however, smooth muscle cells are small, spindle-shaped, and contain a single nucleus. Most smooth muscle is found in the walls of hollow organs and tubes (e.g., stomach, uterus, small intestine). Smooth muscle is responsible for exerting pressure and moving contents forward through these structures (think of digestion or childbirth).

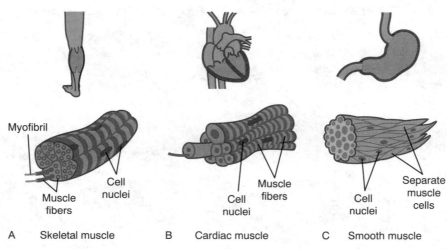

Myofibril

Muscle fibers

Cell nuclei

Muscle fibers

Cell nuclei

Cell nuclei

Separate muscle cells

A   Skeletal muscle   B   Cardiac muscle   C   Smooth muscle

FIGURE 2-4 Three Types of Muscle Tissue

Nervous tissue comprises cells (*neurons*) specialized for initiation and transmission of electrical impulses necessary to control the body. A typical neuron consists of three parts: the cell body, dendrites, and axon. The nucleus and organelles are stored in the cell body, from which numerous extensions, called dendrites, project. These dendrites are similar to antennae that reach out to receive signals from other nerve cells; they then carry these signals *toward* the cell body. The cell body and dendrites, therefore, comprise the *input zone* of the neuron because they receive and integrate incoming signals. In contrast, the axon is a long tubular extension that relays information *away from* the cell body toward cells in other parts of the body. The upper neck of the axon (closest to the cell body) is known as the axon hillock. The neuron's *trigger zone* is the axon hillock because it is the site where action potentials are triggered. These action potentials are carried from the axon hillock, along the axon toward the multiple branches of the axon terminals. The terminals then release chemical messages in communication with other cells (such as muscle). In that regard, the axon is the *conducting zone* (i.e., afferent) of the neuron, while the axon terminals are its *output zone* (i.e., efferent).

Damaged nervous tissue is quite difficult to regenerate, and this is especially true of central nervous tissue (brain and spinal cord) compared with peripheral nervous tissue. Nerve growth inhibitors, which appear during late fetal development in the myelin sheaths surrounding central nerve fibers, work to maintain the integrity of the central nervous system (CNS). While this growth-inhibiting action is advantageous for stabilizing the complex structure of the CNS, it is clearly a disadvantage when central nerve fibers are damaged (as in traumatic brain or spinal cord injuries), as these fibers may never regenerate.

Epithelial tissue is specialized for the exchange of materials between the cell and its environment and is organized into two types of structures: epithelial sheets and secretory glands. Epithelial sheets comprise cells that cover and line various body parts. The outer layer of skin is epithelial tissue, and so is the lining of the digestive tract. These sheets serve as boundaries between the body and the outside environment (as in skin), as well as between the body and the contents of certain cavities that communicate with the outside environment (e.g., the digestive tract). Only the transfer of certain materials is allowed between the regions separated by endothelial tissue, and the type and the extent of this controlled exchange will depend on the location and function of the epithelial tissue. For example, very few materials can be exchanged between the body and the outside environment through the skin. On the other hand, the epithelial tissue lining the digestive tract is specialized for the absorption of nutrients, and therefore it is quite permeable. *Secretory glands* are epithelial tissue specialized for secretion from the cell in response to a given signal, and these can be *exocrine* or *endocrine* glands. Exocrine glands secrete through ducts to the outside of the body, and salivary and sweat glands are examples of such. Endocrine glands release their secretions (hormones) into the blood. For example, the thyroid gland secretes thyroxin, which controls the body's metabolic rate.

Connective tissue contains cells specialized to connect, support, and anchor different body parts. It comprises loose connective tissue, which attaches epithelial tissue to underlying structures; tendons that attach skeletal muscle to bones; bone, which supports and protects the body; and blood, which transports various materials throughout the body.

Two or more types of tissue that perform similar functions make up an organ. Different organs are similarly organized into systems that perform related functions necessary for survival. For example, the circulatory system comprises the heart, blood vessels, and blood—all cooperating to deliver vital O_2, nutrients, waste, electrolytes, and hormones throughout the body. The body is divided arbitrarily into 11 major body systems: reproductive, digestive, nervous, respiratory, renal, musculoskeletal, integumentary, immune, endocrine, cardiac, and circulatory systems. A variety of intercoordinated and regulated systems then link together to form the whole body—a single, independently living human being.

▶ Cell Exchanges

Cells make vital exchanges with the external environment via the internal environment. This exchange is possible because of a liquid internal environment that is outside of the cell, but inside the body. This environment consists of *extracellular* fluid that contains both plasma and **interstitial fluid** (which surrounds the cells). Different systems also work to accomplish exchanges between the inside and outside environments. The digestive system delivers the nutrient from the foods we eat into the plasma through the process of absorption. The respiratory system transfers O_2 from the air we breathe into the plasma. The circulatory system then delivers these nutrients and O_2 throughout the body. Materials are exchanged between the plasma and interstitial fluid across the porous walls of the capillaries. The cells then make vital exchanges with the interstitial fluid to support its existence. In a similar manner, waste products generated by the cells are forced back into the interstitial fluid, picked up by plasma, and carried to the organ responsible for waste elimination from the internal to the external environment.

▶ Homeostasis

Homeostasis is necessary for each cell to survive, and each cell contributes to the homeostasis of an organized system. Homeostasis refers to the maintenance of a relatively stable internal environment. Regarding the cell, the chemical composition and physical state of its internal environment cannot deviate beyond a very narrow limit. In fact, when any factor begins to change the cell environment away from ideal conditions, a timely and appropriate countermeasure occurs to restore stability to the environment. The factors of the internal environment that must be homeostatically controlled are described.

1. *Concentrations of nutrients* – The cells need a constant supply of nutrients for the metabolic fuel necessary for energy production.
2. *O_2 and CO_2 concentrations* – CO_2 generation from energy production must be balanced with CO_2 removal by the lungs to maintain the proper acidity level (pH) in the cell.
3. *Concentrations of waste products* – The build-up of waste products from the various chemical reactions becomes toxic to the cell environment.
4. *Concentrations of water, salt, and other electrolytes* – The relative concentrations of sodium and water in the extracellular fluid determine how much water enters and leaves the cell, and thus these concentrations are regulated to ensure proper cell volume and function. Constant concentrations of other electrolytes, such as magnesium

and potassium, are also essential for muscle contractions.

5. *Temperature* – Cells function optimally within a narrow temperature range and therefore core body temperature must be carefully maintained.
6. *Volume and pressure* – An adequate plasma volume and pressure must be maintained to ensure the body-wide distribution of nutrients and others elements exchanged between the outside and inside environments.
7. **Redox** – The cellular balance of reducing (gain of electrons) and oxidizing (loss of electrons) equivalents (a molecule, atom, or ion) in response to environmental stressors.

The negative feedback loop is a common regulatory mechanism for maintaining homeostasis. To effectively maintain homeostatic control, the human body must be able to detect deviations in its internal environment. The body must then control those factors responsible for adjusting these deviations back to the basal state. Negative feedback occurs when a deviation in a controlled function (e.g., body temperature) triggers a response that opposes that deviation (e.g., shivering), thereby restoring function in the opposite direction back to normal (homeostasis).

Our discussion about cell physiology and function and the importance of maintaining homeostatic control at the cellular level is necessary as we begin to discuss elements of disease initiation and occurrence. When the body is stressed by harmful exposures and the perturbations to homeostatic control become greater than the body's ability to stabilize and regulate, there is injury to the cell and to tissue that, if not addressed, ends in organ system failure and death. Sound public health practice requires knowledge and understanding of health- and disease-related terminology, concepts and processes spanning the biologic spectrum (cell–tissue–organ–system–whole body levels) in order to mitigate the disease process at the earliest stage possible.

🔍 *CASE REPORT*

The Immortal Life of Henrietta Lacks[1-3]

Advances in the field of cellular physiology are attributable to the ability to grow cells outside of the body in what we call *in vitro* culture. In the 1950s, scientists attempted to culture human cells obtained from biopsies or surgical procedures. These attempts, however, were mostly unsuccessful. Then, an investigator at Johns Hopkins received a sample of cervical cancer cells from an African American woman named Henrietta Lacks. The culture was named HeLa and the cell line was fostered under culture, representing perhaps the earliest cell line grown successfully outside the body. Scientists around the globe were eager to have human cell lines available for research on the effects of various pathogens, drugs, and toxic

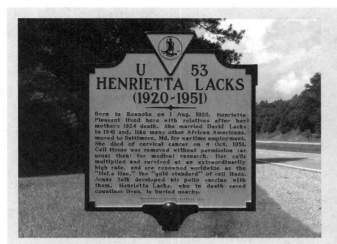

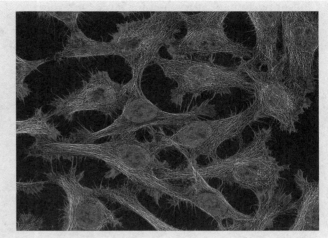

agents on human tissue. An early success of the HeLa cell line was its role in the development of the polio vaccine. Cell-culturing techniques improved, and cell lines were started from normal tissues like heart, kidney, and liver tissue. By the early 1960s, a central cell line repository was established in Washington, DC, and a multibillion-dollar industry was born.

Unfortunately, the success of the HeLa cells was short-lived, as beginning in 1966 scientists began to notice that their human cell lines were contaminated and taken over by HeLa cells. Over the next several years, it was confirmed that over three-quarters of the cell lines at the central repository were actually HeLa cells. Investigators who thought they were working with heart or kidney cells actually had been working with cervical cancer cells. This meant that hundreds of thousands of experiments performed in laboratories around the world were, in fact, invalid. This contamination continued well into the 1980s, resulting in enormous losses of money, resources, and in some cases, prestige for individual laboratories and scientists.

There is another very important twist to this story. Henrietta Lacks' physicians took her cervical cancer cells without asking her, and although these cells were used to launch a medical revolution, neither Henrietta Lacks or her family benefitted financially or otherwise. In fact, her family could not afford adequate health care. More than 20 years later, her children found out that her cells were still alive and became aware of the commercial use of them. What happened over the next 30 years helped to form our current practices of bioethics and informed consent.

1. If you were a scientist in the 1960s and learned that some of your most prestigious published work was invalid due to the contamination of your cell lines with HeLa cells, what would you do?
2. What claims do Henrietta Lacks' children have with regard to their mother's cells? With regard to the money made from those cells?
3. Discuss these issues in light of current public health views on social justice and healthcare disparity.

Key Terms

Aerobic	Golgi complex	Peroxisomes
Anaerobic	Interstitial fluid	Redox
Cristae	Lysosomes	Transport vesicles
Cytoskeleton	Matrix	Vaults
Cytosol	Mitochondrion	
Endoplasmic reticulum (ER)	Nucleus	

Discussion Questions

1. What happens when you try to hold your breath for more than one minute and why is this so? Similarly, what happens when you walk outside in the winter without a coat and why is this so? Are these voluntary or involuntary responses?

2. Hold a heavy object (such as a 5-lb. weight) straight out from your body for as long as you can. Describe what happens and why.

3. Why is it so difficult to regain speech after a stroke? Considering your answer, would you

support mandatory helmet laws for motorcyclists or children riding bikes or skateboards?

4. Give a biologic example of the negative feedback loop.

5. Why do we need to understand cell physiology in public health?

References

1. Sherwood L. *Human Physiology: From Cells to Systems.* 4th ed. Belmont, CA: Brooks/Cole; 2001:19.

2. Lamb NE, Manson AL, Horton-Szar D. *Crash Course: Cell Biology and Genetics.* St. Louis, MO: Mosby Inc.; 2007:3-12.

3. Skloot R. *The Immortal Life of Henrietta Lacks.* New York, NY: Crown Publishing Group; 2010.

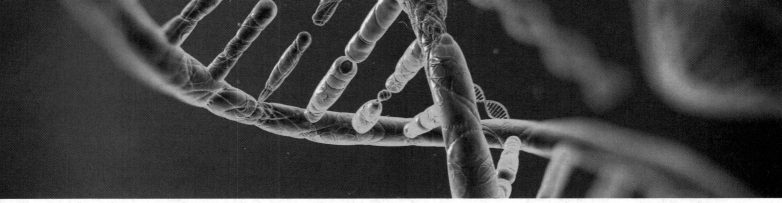

CHAPTER 3

Public Health Microbiology

Benjamin Aronson

LEARNING OBJECTIVES

By the end of this chapter, the student will be able to:

- Describe microbial defining characteristics
- Differentiate between harmful and beneficial microbes
- Describe characteristic structures, anatomy, and life cycle of bacteria
- List the different bacterial genetic strategies and their relevance to public health
- Explain what viruses are and their relevance to public health
- Understand principles of infectious disease epidemiology and its role in microbiology
- Describe some of the current challenges in public health microbiology

CHAPTER OUTLINE

▶ Introduction

The vast majority of life on earth is comprised of masses of microscopic organisms, invisible to the naked eye, called microbes. These invisible creatures, many of which can cause illness and death, pose a worldwide challenge to public health. Traditionally, there are five distinct kinds of microbes: **bacteria**, **viruses**, **protozoans**, **fungi**, and **unicellular algae**.

It should be emphasized early that most of the microbes in each group do *not* cause infection. In fact, most microbes are beneficial. Many are essential to the cycles of nature without which higher life forms, including humans, could not exist. In the language of public health, microbes that cause disease are referred to as **pathogens**.[1] This chapter will examine bacteria and viruses, discuss microbial disease, and end with a discussion on current challenges in public health microbiology.

▶ The Microbial World

To understand microbes, pathogenic or not, it is first necessary to appreciate a basic concept of biology, namely that cells are the basic unit of life. The *cell theory* postulates four major considerations[2]:

1. All **organisms** are composed of fundamental units called cells.
2. All organisms are unicellular (single cells) or multicellular (more than one cell).
3. All cells are fundamentally alike with regard to their structure and their metabolism.
4. Cells arise only from previously existing cells (i.e., "life begets life").

In essence, an understanding of cell theory is the basis for understanding the study of life, including microbial life. It is important to point out that cell theory does not apply to viruses, because viruses are not considered "alive" per se (to be discussed later).

What Is a Microbe?

The term *microbe*, or microorganism, is simply a term of convenience used to collectively describe biologic agents that in general are too small to be seen without the aid of a microscope, although there are some exceptions to this.[2] Microbiologists differentiate between microbial species via a number of different characteristics, including *metabolic diversity*, *oxygen requirements*, the type of *genetic information* used, and *cell type*.

Metabolic Diversity

In biology, we use certain characteristics to determine if something is biotic (living) or abiotic (nonliving). Recall that viruses are not considered living organisms. If viruses aren't "alive," what does *life* mean? In one way or another, all organisms exhibit certain characteristics, summarized in **TABLE 3-1**. To sustain life, organisms need to constantly replenish energy. All life needs energy to stay alive, whether it is a single cell or a component of a multicellular organism. For multicellular organisms, each cell contributes to the total energy requirement. A body's cells are always expending energy, even when not in motion.[2]

Organisms need to constantly replenish their energy stores. Through a complex series of biochemical reactions, cells metabolize **organic** compounds (proteins, fats, and carbohydrates) and release the energy stored in their chemical bonds into a biologically available, high-energy compound known as adenosine triphosphate.[2]

Organisms can be characterized by their method of metabolism. Most organisms, including most

TABLE 3-1 Characteristics of Life

Characteristic	Description
Cellular organization	The cell is the basic unit of life; organisms are unicellular or multicellular.
Energy production	Organisms require energy and a biochemical strategy to meet their energy requirement.
Reproduction	Organisms have the capacity to reproduce by asexual or sexual methods and in doing so pass on genetic material (DNA) to their progeny.
Irritability	Organisms respond to internal and external stimuli.
Growth and development	Organisms grow and develop in each new generation; specialization and differentiation occur in multicellular organisms.

microbes and humans, require organic compounds for energy. These organisms are called **heterotrophs**. Other microbes and plants are characterized as **autotrophs**. Autotrophs do not require organic compounds, but get their energy elsewhere. This is the case in **photosynthetic** autotrophs, which get their energy from the sun,[3] and **chemosynthetic** autotrophs, which derive energy form the metabolism of inorganic compounds. During this process, autotrophs produce organic compounds and oxygen (O_2). Thus, heterotrophs rely on autotrophs for energy (**FIGURE 3-1**).

Requirement for Oxygen

Organisms also exhibit diversity in their O_2 requirement. **Aerobes** (like humans) require O_2 for their metabolic activities. Some bacteria are **anaerobes** and do not require O_2[3]; other anaerobes, known as **obligate anaerobes**, are actually killed by O_2.[3] **Facultative anaerobes** are organisms that grow better in the presence of O_2 but can alter their metabolism, allowing them to grow in the absence of O_2. Understanding the O_2 requirements of microbial pathogens is essential in clinical microbiology for culturing (growing) and diagnosis.[2]

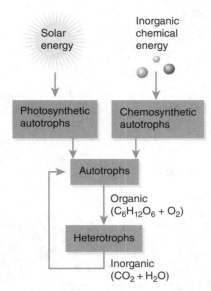

FIGURE 3-1 Flow Diagram Showing Heterotroph Dependence on Autotrophs and Different Energy Sources

Genetic Information

The organic molecule, deoxyribonucleic acid (DNA), stores the genetic information in cells. DNA generally exists in long chains, connected to a complementary chain. DNA in this form is referred to as double stranded DNA. DNA is like a blueprint or library for an organism's structure and function. It provides the code that gives an individual organism its defining features. A segment of DNA that codes for certain specific proteins and functions is known as a **gene**. The genetic code is responsible for heredity. We know that particular life forms give rise to the same life forms; that is, dandelions produce dandelions, humans produce humans, and *Escherichia coli* produces *Escherichia coli*. Each of these organisms has its characteristics embedded in DNA that confer its identity. DNA is transferred from parent to offspring by a variety of different reproductive strategies.[2]

Cell Type

In biology, there are two distinct classes of cells, referred to as **prokaryotes** and **eukaryotes**. Prokaryotic cells tend to have a simpler morphology than eukaryotic cells. For example, prokaryotes have no membrane around the nucleus. Rather, there is a DNA-rich nuclear area, called the **nucleoid**. Though the nucleoid serves as the carrier of genetic information, the DNA is not enclosed within a nuclear membrane. Thus, in prokaryotes, there is no true nucleus. Further, in prokaryotic cells, there are no membrane-bound organelles, in contrast with the cellular anatomy of eukaryotic cells. Prokaryotic and eukaryotic cells are compared in **TABLE 3-2** and **FIGURE 3-2**. All bacteria are prokaryotic, and all other microbes are eukaryotic. (Note that viruses are not cells, and are neither prokaryotic nor eukaryotic.[2])

TABLE 3-2 Comparison of Prokaryotic and Eukaryotic Cells

Characteristic	Prokaryotes	Eukaryotes
Life form	Bacteria, Archaea	All microbial cells (with the exception of bacteria, viruses, and prions) and all other cells
Nucleus	DNA chromosome but not enveloped by membrane	Chromosome present and enveloped by membrane
Cell size	About 1–10 μm	Over 100 μm
Chromosomes	Single circular DNA (two chromosomes in a few)	Multiple paired chromosomes present in nucleus
Cell division	Asexual binary fission; no "true" sexual reproduction	Cell division by mitosis; sexual reproduction by meiosis
Internal compartmentalization	No membrane-bound internal compartments	Organelles bound by membrane
Ribosomes	Smaller than eukaryotic cells and not membrane-bound	Membrane-bound and free

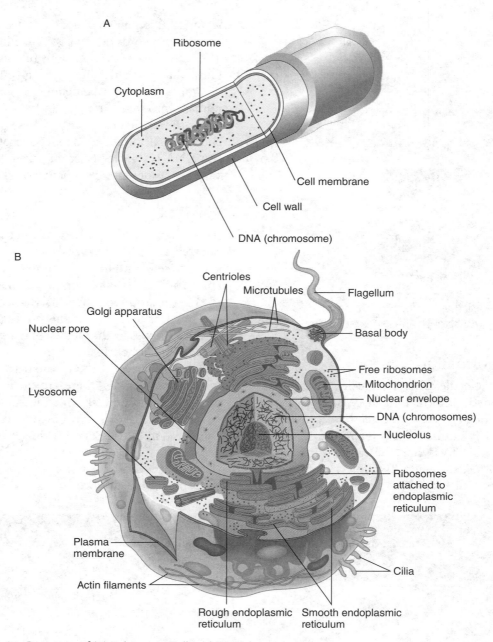

A

Ribosome

Cytoplasm

Cell membrane

Cell wall

DNA (chromosome)

B

Centrioles

Microtubules

Flagellum

Golgi apparatus

Nuclear pore

Basal body

Free ribosomes

Mitochondrion

Nuclear envelope

Lysosome

DNA (chromosomes)

Nucleolus

Ribosomes attached to endoplasmic reticulum

Plasma membrane

Cilia

Actin filaments

Rough endoplasmic reticulum   Smooth endoplasmic reticulum

FIGURE 3-2 Schematic Drawings of (A) Eukaryotic Cell and (B) Prokaryotic Cell

▶ The Beneficial Aspects of Microbes

Public health microbiology is mainly concerned with pathogenic microbes, as they are the invaders that cause human illness. Yet only a few microbes produce disease. In fact, not only are most microbes not harmful, but many are beneficial and essential to life on earth as we know it. Humans likely wouldn't be here if not for the billions of microbes with whom we share this planet. Microbes were the first inhabitants of Earth from which evolution to eukaryotic cells and multicellularity proceeded. Microbes are the largest component of Earth's biomass and are present in the most extreme habitats.[4]

Microbes are essential to the planet's ecosystem and are the foundation of the **biosphere**. Many act as **decomposers** or scavengers, cleaning and recycling the planet's dead matter. Bacteria are the foundations of **biogeochemical cycles** like carbon and nitrogen cycles. Although their direct role in these cycles cannot be seen, without microbes the cycles could not be completed and life would not be able to go on. With increasing technology, humans have the potential to interfere with and alter certain natural cycles.[4] Nonbiodegradable products, pollution, and human contributions to climate change are all ways in which humans can alter earth's environment.[5]

For centuries, cultures all over the world have been using microbes for their beneficial aspects long before people knew of a microbial world. One example of using microbes for human benefit is the production of distilled spirits (alcoholic beverages). Likewise, a variety of food products, including breads, yogurt, and cheeses, are the work of some helpful microbes. As knowledge of microbes and the proteins they produce in their metabolism has increased, their utility has expanded, resulting in an increasing array of fermented food and industrial products.[4]

Microbes are also powerful biologic research tools, due to the relative ease of culturing and obtaining them in large populations in a short period of time. Much of the evidence for DNA as the molecule of genetic material came from studies of viruses that infect bacteria (bacteriophages) and bacterial cells. The pharmaceutical industry needs microbes to produce many products, including antibiotics, vaccines, genetically engineered therapeutics, pesticides, and a large variety of other compounds to control or eliminate pathogens.[4]

Another use for microbes is bioremediation—the use of microorganisms to clean up polluted environments—which is on the rise; microbes played a role in reducing the impact of the Gulf Coast oil spill in April 2010. Microbes are also used in sewage treatment, where they consume and digest harmful contaminants, making the water in our rivers and lakes safer.

Because only a few microbes are disease producers and many are essential to our daily lives, it is important to recognize an essential objective of microbiologists is *not* to eradicate all microbes but to manage the pathogens' impact on human safety and the consequent burden of microbe-induced disease on public health.[4]

▶ Bacteria

Bacteria are a distinct group of prokaryotic microbes and likely represent the beginning of life on earth billions of years ago. These complex organisms have the potential to cause severe illness and even death.

Bacterial Cell Shapes and Patterns

Most bacteria are either rod-shaped, known as **bacilli** (singular, bacillus); spherical, known as **cocci** (singular, coccus); or spiral, known as **spirilla** (singular, spirillum), as shown in **FIGURE 3-3**. Some can also be spirochete (flexible spiral) or vibrio (comma-shaped). Bacterial cells also group themselves in different patterns.[6] They can exist alone in single-cell form, as is the case with most bacilli, or they can exist in chains, or even groups, characteristic of a number of cocci bacteria. For example, *Staphylococcus* species, like *Staphylococcus aureus,* exist in a cluster of cells clumped together,[7] while *Streptococcus* species, like *Streptococcus pneumoniae,* occur in longer chains.[8] Diplococci (two spheres) exist in pairs; this is the shape of *Neisseria gonorrhoeae,* the causative agent of the common sexually transmitted infection gonorrhea.[9] Similarly, tetrads are groupings of four. Other bacteria have been described as star-shaped, triangular, flat, or square. Microscopic determination of shape and pattern is often the first step in the identification of bacteria.[6]

Naming Bacteria

Bacterial names frequently identify important characteristics, so it is important to understand the naming convention.

All organisms, including bacteria, are named via the *binomial* system of nomenclature established by Carolus Linnaeus in 1735. The naming is as follows: organism names are Latinized, and each organism carries two names (binomial). The first name designates the **genus** and the second name designates the **species**. For example, humans are *Homo* (genus) *sapiens* (species). Note that the first letter of the genus is

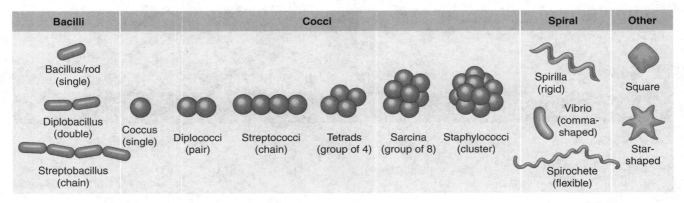

FIGURE 3-3 Bacterial Cell Shapes and Patterns

always capitalized, but the species name is not and that both names are italicized.[6]

Unfortunately for us, the meaning of a bacterial name is not always consistent. Some microbes are named in honor of the scientist responsible for first describing them such as *Rickettsia prowazekii*, the cause of epidemic typhus, which is named after Howard T. Ricketts and Stanislaus von Prowazek. Other names indicate the microbial characteristics like habitat, shape, associated disease, or a combination of these factors. For example, *Legionella pneumophila* is named after an outbreak of pneumonia at an American Legion conference in 1976.[6]

Bacteria can also be named based on their morphology. However, the use of these descriptive morphologic terms (e.g., *bacillus*) can lead to confusion, so it is important to be wary. For example, *Bacillus anthracis* is a member of the genus *Bacillus* (with a capital "B")

and morphologically is a bacillus (with a lowercase "b"). But *E. coli* is also a bacillus ("b") belonging to the genus *Escherichia* (that is what the "E" stands for). There are many other bacilli that do not belong to the genus *Bacillus* ("B"). So, all members of the genus *Bacillus* are bacilli, but not all bacilli are classified under *Bacillus*.[6]

Anatomy of the Bacterial Cell

To understand why bacteria can make us sick, we need to understand the anatomy of the typical bacterial cell. Bacteria, being prokaryotes, have key differences from animal cells and other microbes. The structures that compose these cells are outlined in **TABLE 3-3** and illustrated in **FIGURE 3-4**; note that some anatomic features are not common to all bacteria.[6] The general regions of the bacterial cell include the **envelope**, cytoplasm, and appendages.

TABLE 3-3 Anatomical Features of the Bacterial Cell

Structure	Function
Cell Envelope	
Capsule[a] (glycocalyx, slime layer)	Promotes virulence in some cases
Cell wall (with the exception of mycoplasmas)	Constrained structure that confers shape and provides tensile strength
Cell membrane	Controls movement of molecules into and out of cell; referred to as gatekeeper
Cytoplasm[b]	
Nucleoid	DNA-rich area not enclosed by a membrane
Plasmids[a]	Nonchromosomal DNA that confers properties, including antibiotic resistance
Spores[a]	Confers extreme resistance to environmental factors
Ribosome	Protein synthesis
Chromosome	Determinant of genetic traits
Inclusion bodies	Storage and reserve supply of nutrient materials
Appendages	
Flagella[a]	Motility
Pili[a]	Adhesion to surfaces, possible bridge for transfer of DNA

[a] Structure not found in all bacterial cells.
[b] Area within membrane; contains numerous organelles.

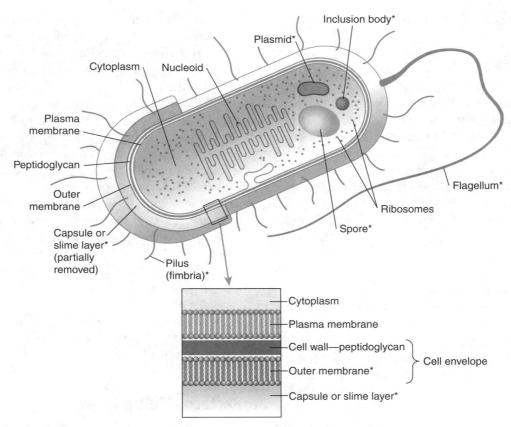

FIGURE 3-4 "Composite" Bacterial Cell

*Structures not present in all bacteria.

Envelope (The Capsule, Cell Wall, and Cell Membrane)

The **capsule** (or slime layer), if present, is an outer layer of a slime-like substance and is generally not integral to the life of the cell. However, in some species, the capsule can be a **virulence** factor. Virulence is a term that describes the capacity to produce disease.[6] Going down a layer, there is the **cell wall**, characteristic of all bacteria. The cell wall is a rigid, structural foundation responsible for the characteristic shape of the cell.[6] The cell wall prevents the cell membrane from swelling from the inward diffusion of water. If water were allowed to freely flow into the cell, the cell would lyse (burst). The cell wall is of high interest to the public health microbiologist, as a number of antibiotics (medicines used to kill bacteria) target the cell wall, including penicillin.

Bacterial cell walls are divided into two groups based on differences in the chemistry of their cell walls. One method of identification is the **Gram stain** procedure, which indicates if a bacterium is gram-positive or gram-negative. Gram-positive bacteria have a very thick cell wall and will turn a purplish color on a Gram stain test, while gram-negative bacteria have a thinner cell wall and will turn a pink color on a Gram stain test.[6] The staining procedure is an important first step in identifying the specific bacterial organism as the cause of infection. The *cell membrane* in bacteria is semipermeable and has a very similar role as an animal cell, which is mainly its nature of letting matter in and out of the cell. A key difference, however, in the bacterial cell membrane is that it is the site for energy-generating reactions. Bacterial cells do not have mitochondria (remember that prokaryotes do not have membrane-bound organelles and the mitochondria is indeed a membrane-bound organelle), so the site of energy production must occur somewhere else; in the case of bacteria, it is the cell membrane.[6]

Cytoplasm (Nucleoid, Plasmids, Spores)

The cytoplasm fills the inside of the cell (see Figure 3-4). Because the bacterial cell lacks a nuclear membrane (no membrane-bound organelles!), a DNA-rich area, known as the nucleoid, is present in the cytoplasm. Most bacterial cells contain a single chromosome, a threadlike structure consisting of DNA. In bacteria, the chromosome is present as a circular, double-stranded stretch of DNA. In eukaryotic cells, DNA is organized into "multiple" discrete linear bodies, the chromosomes.

(Humans, for example, have 23 pairs, or 46 chromosomes total.)

Bacteria also have smaller circular molecules of nonchromosomal DNA called **plasmids**. Plasmids can vary in the number of genes they have and range considerably in what they code for. Some plasmids carry genes that confer virulence. In addition, some plasmids are considered **infectious agents** because they can be transferred from one bacterial cell to another. Other plasmids carry genes that confer antibiotic resistance; these plasmids are referred to as *R (resistance) factors*.[6] The bacterial cytoplasm is also home to a number of ribosomes. Though different structurally, the ribosome, like in animal cells, is the site of protein synthesis.[3]

Appendages (Flagella and Pili)

Some bacteria contain **flagella** (singular: flagellum), which allow them to move (become motile) via a whip-tail action. There can be more than one flagellum on a cell, but the particular arrangement of flagella is consistent for those species that have flagella. Bacteria can control their movements toward or away from a chemical stimulus due to receptors present within the cell via a process called **chemotaxis**. Some bacteria travel toward an attractant (glucose) and away from repellents (acids).[6]

This ability to detect the smallest changes in environment is quite extraordinary and appears to play a role in the ability of some disease-producing bacteria to spread throughout the body and evade the immune system. For example, when *Salmonella* spp. (all species) are in low-nutrient environments, they have the ability to produce protective adherent layers called biofilms.[10] The formation of a biofilm as a response to bacterial environments poses a challenge to public health. Biofilms allow microbes to adhere to certain surfaces, introducing potential sites of infection. This can occur in medical devices like catheters and intravenous lines if they are not changed frequently, which can subsequently lead to infection.[11]

Similar to flagella are **pili**, which extrude through the cell wall and are present in many gram-negative species. They are shorter, straighter, and thinner than flagella. There may be only a single pilus or up to several hundred pili per cell. Pili can have many different functions in the bacterial cell.[6]

Bacterial Multiplication

The mechanism by which bacteria multiply is known as **binary fission**, which, simply put, means "splitting in two" (**FIGURE 3-5**). This process produces two

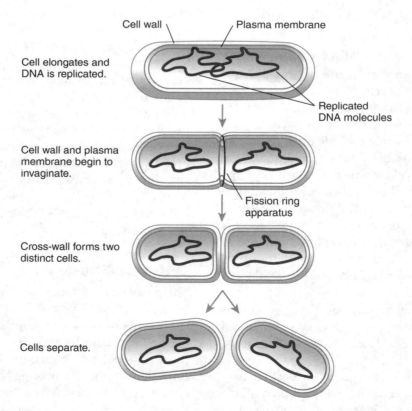

Cell wall   Plasma membrane

Cell elongates and DNA is replicated.

Replicated DNA molecules

Cell wall and plasma membrane begin to invaginate.

Fission ring apparatus

Cross-wall forms two distinct cells.

Cells separate.

FIGURE 3-5 Binary Fission

identical copies, or clones, of the original parent cell.[6] If left unchecked with unlimited resources, bacteria would multiply until they covered the planet. However, a number of factors control bacterial population size. For example, availability of resources, temperature, and competition with other organisms all prevent a population from getting too large. Bacterial populations, or **cultures**, typically exhibit a general sequence of events.

The first section of the curve is known as the *lag phase*. This phase represents the time where a bacterial species is adapting to the new environment, as would occur during initial infection. There may be an initial drop in bacterial number associated with this new environment. Once the bacteria have adapted to their new environment, they begin to divide rapidly in the *exponential (logarithmic) phase*, where there is an explosion of growth governed by the **generation time**—the time it takes a cell to undergo binary fission, producing two "new" cells. *E. coli*, for example, has a generation time of only 20 minutes, assuming optimal growth conditions. After each round of division, the culture doubles— hence the exponential growth. Eventually, however, in any environment, there is a population limit set by the conditions present. Whether it is due to lack of resources or some environmental change, adverse conditions set in, and binary fission slows down leading to the next phase, the *stationary phase*. At this point, there are just not enough resources to continue to grow the culture. Binary fission continues to occur but at a rate equal to the death rate, and thus, the culture reaches a plateau so that there is no net increase in numbers. Finally, the next phase, known as the *death phase*, occurs when the number of cells dying exceeds the rate of binary fission. It still may be possible to save the culture if a new, viable environment is introduced. Likewise, the bacteria can be transmitted to a new person to start the cycle anew.[6]

An understanding of this growth curve is valuable to public health. During a bacterial infection, most bacteria don't make it past the initial lag phase. However, for those that do, replication can occur very rapidly as a product of the generation time, which can lead to serious disease or even death. For example, due to its incredibly fast generation time, *E. coli* is the most common cause of urinary tract infection, even though it is rarely present in this area of the body. If *E. coli* is able to reach this environment, this rapid replication rate gives *E. coli* an infectious advantage.[12] Treatments, like antibiotics, complement our immune system in an effort to slow or interrupt the

logarithmic phase. These will hopefully then trigger the stationary phase and subsequent death phase.[6]

▶ Bacterial Genetics

Genetic diversity is essential for the success of a species and its ability to adapt over time to changing environments. Different organisms have developed different mechanisms to contribute to a species' overall genetic diversity.[3] Microbial diversity, particularly as related to bacteria, is the result of expression of gene **mutation** and gene recombination. The gene is the basic unit of heredity and is a segment of a chromosome consisting of tightly coiled DNA; most bacteria have a single chromosome. Sexual reproduction and mutation account for variation in eukaryotic life forms. Bacteria, however, are prokaryotes and reproduce asexually via binary fission.[13] As we just learned, this process creates two identical clones and is limited in the genetic diversity it can create. To account for this, bacteria have developed unique ways to add to their genetic diversity. Through a process called **horizontal gene transfer**, bacteria are able to exchange genetic information without reproducing. Conversely, **vertical gene transfer** occurs when genes are passed down subsequent generations, as is the case in sexual reproduction (**FIGURE 3-6**).[14] Bacteria engage in horizontal gene transfer through **transformation**, **transduction**, and **conjugation**. Both mutation and recombination by transformation, transduction, and conjugation are the mechanisms by which new genes and new combinations of genes arise in prokaryotic cells, accounting for their diversity.[13]

Mutations and Recombination

The specifics of mutation will not be discussed here; for now, it is important to know that a mutation is

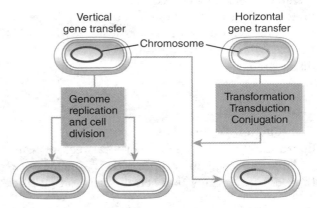

FIGURE 3-6 Horizontal and Vertical Gene Transmission

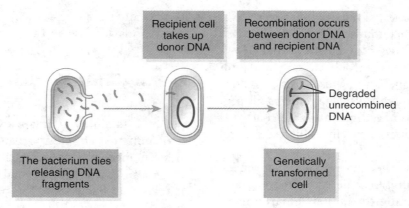

Recipient cell takes up donor DNA

Recombination occurs between donor DNA and recipient DNA

Degraded unrecombined DNA

The bacterium dies releasing DNA fragments

Genetically transformed cell

FIGURE 3-7 Transformation

a change in the genetic code that can range from having very little effect on a species to having drastic changes to the organism. Recombination, when referring to prokaryotes, includes three processes: transformation, transduction, and conjugation. Although distinct processes, they have several similarities[13]:

- All are unidirectional (genetic information goes from a source to a bacterial cell and not the other way around)
- Multiplication is *not* an outcome
- All are examples of horizontal gene transfer
- All occur naturally
- All involve integration of new "foreign" donor DNA into host DNA
- All result in new gene combinations, i.e., recombination

Transformation

Transformation, as shown in **FIGURE 3-7**, is the bacterial uptake of free, or "naked," fragments of DNA released by dead cells. In nature, bacterial cells capable of transformation take up DNA from a variety of sources, including bacteria in other genera. Once inside the cell, new transformed DNA must be integrated into the recipient DNA. If the DNA is a genetic match, integration will occur. If there is no "fit" between donor and recipient DNA, the donor DNA is disintegrated.[13]

Transduction

Transduction occurs when foreign DNA is introduced into the cell by a virus or viral vector. Viruses will be discussed in more depth in the next section. For now, know that certain viruses that infect

bacteria, called bacteriophages, can introduce viral DNA into a bacterium during the virus' replication cycle. This process can potentially lead to the release of both viral DNA and/or bacterial DNA to infect another bacterial cell. **FIGURE 3-8** illustrates this cycle.[13] In terms of bacterial genetics, this process can affect genetic diversity.

Conjugation

Bacterial conjugation is characterized by direct cell-to-cell contact between a mating pair (**FIGURE 3-9**). On the surface, it seems to be an underdeveloped form of sexual reproduction, but it lacks the characteristics. Though there is recombination of genetic material, neither donor nor recipient produce a new cell. Transmission is horizontal and unidirectional. Genetic transfer occurs through a specific kind of pili, known as sex pili, which act as a bridge between donor and recipient cells.[13] The actual process of conjugation is a little more complex, but the significance is clear: conjugation is a major recombination event leading to diversity.

The mechanism of genetic exchange in bacteria (i.e., transformation, transduction, conjugation), along with mutations, results in bacterial diversity. Diversity, in turn, leads to increased adaptability in new environments. This diversity in the form of new gene combinations is the foundation for Darwin's "survival of the fittest" at the genetic and molecular level. The "fittest" are the bacteria in a diverse population with genes that allow them to adapt, survive, and reproduce under hostile circumstances.[13] Public health specialists have to be constantly aware of the current state of bacterial and microbial genetics to combat infections and develop effective treatments.

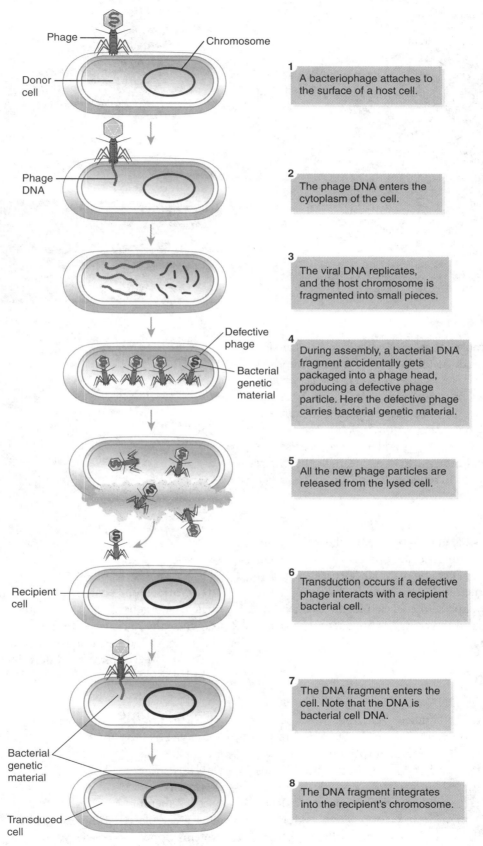

FIGURE 3-8 Generalized Transduction

1 A bacteriophage attaches to the surface of a host cell.

2 The phage DNA enters the cytoplasm of the cell.

3 The viral DNA replicates, and the host chromosome is fragmented into small pieces.

4 During assembly, a bacterial DNA fragment accidentally gets packaged into a phage head, producing a defective phage particle. Here the defective phage carries bacterial genetic material.

5 All the new phage particles are released from the lysed cell.

6 Transduction occurs if a defective phage interacts with a recipient bacterial cell.

7 The DNA fragment enters the cell. Note that the DNA is bacterial cell DNA.

8 The DNA fragment integrates into the recipient's chromosome.

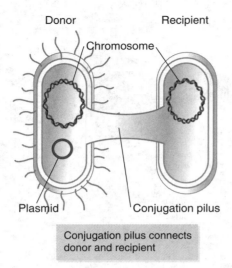

FIGURE 3-9 Bacterial Conjugation: Direct Transfer of DNA

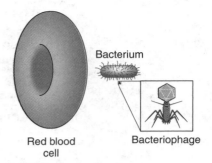

FIGURE 3-10 Viral Structure

▶ Viruses

Viruses are simpler than prokaryotic cells. Lacking the structural and metabolic components found in cells, these subcellular infectious agents consist of little more than genes packaged in a protein coat.[3] Viruses are responsible for a collection of diseases in humans, including smallpox, poliomyelitis, Ebola, severe acute respiratory syndrome (SARS), and influenza. Viruses are **obligate intracellular parasites**, meaning they must gain access into cells to replicate.[15]

Viral Structure

Viruses are a lot smaller than bacterial cells (**FIGURE 3-10**) Using an electron microscope, one can see viral structure and the type of genetic material. Viruses are generally simple in structure and may consist only of a nucleic acid wrapped in a protein coat, while others may have an envelope around the coat. A complete viral particle is called a **virion**.[15]

Nucleic Acids

Viruses can have DNA or RNA (ribonucleic acid), another molecule of nucleic acid, but never both. The presence of only RNA or only DNA is unique to viruses. *Cells*, whether prokaryotic or eukaryotic, contain both DNA and RNA. Further, some viruses are unique in that their genome is single-stranded DNA (ssDNA); others have double-stranded RNA (dsRNA). Other than these viruses, DNA is double-stranded and RNA is single-stranded. Thus, there are four categories of viruses in terms of nucleic acid content: dsDNA, ssDNA, dsRNA, and ssRNA (**TABLE 3-4**).[15]

TABLE 3-4 Virus Classification Based on Nucleic Acid Composition

Nucleic Acid	Virus(es)
dsDNA	Human papillomavirus, Epstein-Barr virus, adenovirus, herpes simplex virus, varicella-zoster virus (chickenpox and shingles), *Variola* virus (smallpox)
ssDNA	Parvovirus B19 (possibly slapped-cheek disease)
ssRNA	Hepatitis A virus, poliovirus, norovirus, rubella virus, Ebola virus, influenza virus, West Nile encephalitis virus
dsRNA	Rotavirus, Colorado tick fever virus, reovirus

Protein Coat

The viral protein coat is known as the **capsid**. The nucleic acid genome and the protein coat together are known as the *nucleocapsid*. The capsid consists of protein units called capsomeres. Three arrangements of these capsomeres have been described: helical, icosahedral, and complex.[15]

Viral Envelopes

Some viruses acquire a piece of the host cell's plasma membrane when emerging from the host cell. Viruses with this additional layer covering the capsid are called *enveloped viruses*. The envelopes are alterations of the host cell membrane where some of the membrane proteins are replaced with viral proteins. Some of these proteins appear as spikes as they protrude from the membrane. These "spikes" are important for subsequent attachment of viruses to host cells. The human immunodeficiency virus (HIV) for example, has spikes that attach

TABLE 3-5 Generalized Viral Replication Cycle[a]

Stage	Description
Adsorption (attachment)	Viruses attach to cell surface receptor molecules by spikes, capsids, or envelope.
Penetration	Entire viral particle or only nucleic acid enters via endocytosis or by fusion with cell membrane.
Replication	Process is complex, and details depend on particular viruses and their nucleic acid structure. Replication may occur in the nucleus or cytoplasm, viral nucleic acid replicates, and genes are expressed, leading to production of viral components.
Assembly	Components are assembled into mature viruses.
Release (exit)	Viruses are extruded from host cell by budding (HIV) or lysis of host cell membrane.

[a] Specific strategies vary with particular viruses.

to strategic white blood cells (T lymphocytes) of the immune system, leading to serious damage to the individual's ability to fight infection. Viruses lacking an envelope are referred to as naked or nonenveloped viruses.[15]

Viral Replication

Viruses are not the easiest thing to study because they are obligate intracellular parasites and need other cells to grow. Bacteriophages, a type of virus that infects bacteria, have been studied extensively because bacteria are easily grown. Much of our understanding of viral replication comes from the study of the T4 bacteriophage (a complex dsDNA phage) and *E. coli* as the bacterial host.

The replication of T4 in *E. coli* has provided a good model, though it should be noted that there is extensive variation in viral replication strategy.[15] The replication is divided into five stages shown in **TABLE 3-5**.

The first phase is *adsorption*, where the virus binds to the host cell. This process can occur though a number of different mechanisms depending on the virus and the type of host cell. Host cells have specific receptors that will match proteins on the virus. Consider a lock and key; the key can only fit into a certain lock. Specificity of the receptor is thereby required and establishes host range. Once the virus has bonded to the host cell, the virus must get inside. *Penetration* is the next step as the virus infiltrates the cell wall and/ or cell membrane and releases its nucleic acid contents into the host cell. Following penetration comes *replication* of the viral nucleic acid. Ultimately, viral components are synthesized within the host cell, again reflecting the obligate intracellular nature of viruses. Using the host cell's resources, viral genetic information is subsequently expressed into viral protein molecules specific for the particular virus. Think of the host cell as a factory for viral components analogous to an automobile factory. Instead of making fuel injectors, dashboards, air bags, and steering mechanisms, the products are tail fibers, capsids, nucleic acids, and envelopes. The blueprint is the nucleic acid of the virus that penetrated the cell. Following replication, *assembly* of all the parts must occur. Continuing with the analogy of the automobile plant, now that the parts have been made, the virus is assembled into a functional structure in a manner similar to that of a production line. The next and final stage for newly formed mature virions is *release*. The mechanism of release of virions varies depending on the virus, but they all end with new virions released to infect other host cells and start the cycle once again.[15]

Considering that each new virus produced is potentially infective, the overwhelming effects that occur when you acquire a viral infection are understandable. It should also now be evident why antibacterial drugs (antibiotics) are ineffective against viruses, because unlike bacteria, viruses lack a cell wall and other structures unique to bacteria that are targeted by antibiotics. There are some antiviral drugs, but they tend to be not as effective against viruses as antibiotics are against bacteria.[15]

▶ Microbial Disease

Public health microbiology focuses on infectious microbes that can cause human harm. From the research of Robert Koch, Louis Pasteur, and other early infectious disease scientists, the role of microbes as the causative

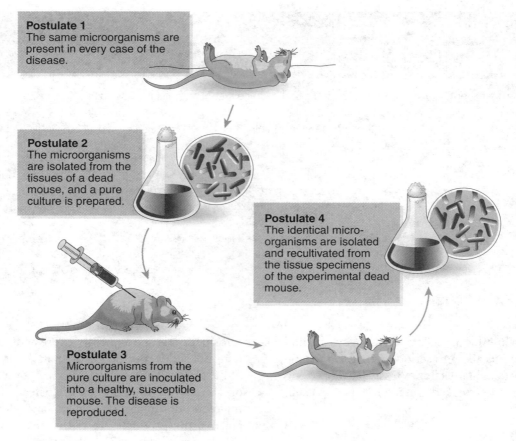

Postulate 1
The same microorganisms are present in every case of the disease.

Postulate 2
The microorganisms are isolated from the tissues of a dead mouse, and a pure culture is prepared.

Postulate 4
The identical micro-organisms are isolated and recultivated from the tissue specimens of the experimental dead mouse.

Postulate 3
Microorganisms from the pure culture are inoculated into a healthy, susceptible mouse. The disease is reproduced.

FIGURE 3-11 Koch's Postulates

agents of infection was uncovered. Specifically, Koch experimentally showed that specific microbes caused specific diseases. Koch's research on *Mycobacterium tuberculosis* (the causative agent of tuberculosis) led to the development of a series of four postulates, known as **Koch's postulates**, that are still used to establish if a particular organism is the cause of a particular disease (**FIGURE 3-11**).

1. *Association:* The causative agent must be present in every case of a specific disease.
2. *Isolation:* The causative agent must be isolated in every case of the disease and grown in pure culture.
3. *Causation:* The causative agent in the pure culture must cause the disease when inoculated into a healthy and susceptible laboratory animal.
4. *Reisolation:* Microbes identical to those identified in postulate 2 are isolated from the dead animal.

With advances in molecular biology, it is now possible to identify microbes through more complex genetic mechanisms without growth in culture, meaning that "classic" Koch's postulates may not always be fulfilled. However, these postulates have been critical

to public health microbiology and continue to play a significant role in infection identification.[16]

Epidemiology is the investigative methodology designed to determine the source and cause of diseases and disorders that produce illness, disability, and death in human populations. Epidemiologists focus on the frequency and distribution of diseases in populations and classify diseases into four categories listed in **TABLE 3-6**.[17]

The source and spread of epidemics can be described as **common-source epidemics** or **propagated epidemics**, illustrated in **FIGURE 3-12**. Common-source epidemics arise from contact with a single contaminated source, like a contaminated food or water source (**BOX 3-1**).[17] Storms and floods may also cause common source epidemics. In addition to the physical damage associated with storms and flooding (e.g., damaged buildings, power outages), there is also an increased risk of microbial outbreaks. Transmission of waterborne diseases like cholera and typhoid are frequently associated with serious storms and floods, especially in developing countries. The major risk factor during these events is the contamination of drinking-water facilities. Additionally, storms and flooding tend to increase human contact with contaminated drinking water sources. Individuals will commonly be unaware that the water

TABLE 3-6 Four Kinds of Disease Frequencies and Distributions

Sporadic	Occur only occasionally and at irregular intervals in a random and unpredictable fashion
Endemic	Continually present at a steady level in a population and pose little threat to the public health
Epidemic	Sudden increase in the *morbidity* (illness rate) and in the *mortality* (death rate) above the *usual,* causing a potential public health problem
Pandemic	Diseases that can spread across continents and may be worldwide

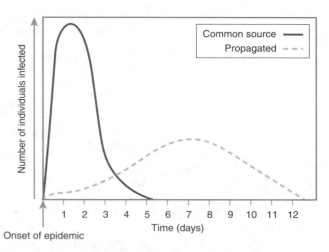

FIGURE 3-12 Comparison of the Courses of Common-Source and Propagated Epidemics

BOX 3-1 Jack-in-the-Box: An American Outbreak

In the early 1990s, children mysteriously started falling ill in the state of Washington. Though the cause of the illness was initially a mystery, the Washington state health department had a strong surveillance network in place and was able to carefully monitor health trends. After a number of children were being admitted to hospitals with symptoms of bloody diarrhea, it was clear that there was a serious outbreak taking place.

In mid-January 1993, a team of epidemiologists was called to action and alerted emergency departments to look for these characteristic symptoms. Further, patients were interviewed about where they had eaten recently. In less than a week, it became clear that the likely source was undercooked hamburgers served at Jack-in-the-Box restaurants.

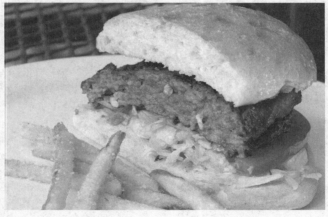

© Florence-Joseph McGinn/Shutterstock

This rapid outbreak investigation prevented 250,000 potentially contaminated hamburgers from being consumed, preventing an estimated 800 cases. The cause of the outbreak was a pathogenic strain of *E. coli*, *E. coli O157:H7*.[19] Ultimately, 623 people in the western United States became ill with *E. coli O157:H7*, and four children died. Many other individuals suffered long-term medical complications.

The Jack-in-the-Box incident was monumental in our appreciation of foodborne outbreaks. Lessons learned from the incident showed that outbreak surveillance and investigation are integral to preventing outbreaks from occurring and alleviating the effects of outbreaks that do occur.

Data from Bottemiller H. Outbreak Detection Since Jack in the Box: A Public Health Evolution. Food Safety News: Breaking news for everyone's consumption. http://www.foodsafetynews.com/2013/02/outbreak-detection-since-jack-in-the-box-a-public-health-evolution/#.WgI_c8anE2w. February 4, 2013. Accessed November 7, 2017.

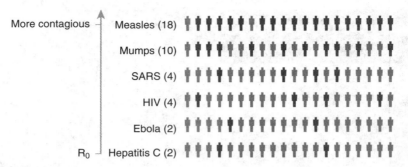

FIGURE 3-13 Basic Reproduction Rate (R_0)

is contaminated and assume it is *potable* (safe to drink). These instances can subsequently lead to outbreaks and epidemics.[18] Typically, in a common-source epidemic, many people become ill quite suddenly, and the disease peaks rapidly in the population.

A propagated epidemic, on the other hand, is the result of direct person-to-person contact; the microbe is spread from infected individuals to noninfected susceptible individuals. Relative to common-source epidemics, the number of infected individuals rises more slowly and decreases gradually. Chickenpox, measles, and mumps are examples of propagated epidemics.[17]

Epidemiology also measures the transmission of a disease. The basic reproduction rate, denoted as **R_0 (R-nought)**, is an important measure of transmission. Essentially, it is the mean number of secondary cases, occurring in a nonimmunized (susceptible) population in the wake of a particular infection. In other words, for every individual infected, "R_0" times as many noninfected people will become infected. See **FIGURE 3-13** and **TABLE 3-7**.

For an infection to spread, the R_0 value must be greater than 1; if less, the infection will die out.[17]

Microbial Mechanisms of Disease

The terms *infection* and *disease* are commonly used interchangeably, but they mean different things. **Infection** describes the multiplication of microbes on or in the body without producing definitive symptoms. **Disease** is a possible outcome of microbial invasion, whether by normal flora or exogenous (from the outside) microbes, resulting in impairment of health to some degree. Early symptoms of many infectious diseases include lethargy and a sense of ill health. Infectious diseases can range in severity from mild to moderate to severe to lethal. Some diseases are subclinical (asymptomatic) and some may result in death.[16]

Three major factors determine the chances of acquiring a particular infection and the severity of the accompanying symptoms[16]:

1. Dose (***n***): the number of microorganisms to which the potential host has been exposed

2. Virulence (***V***): a measure of pathogenicity, which encompasses those specific factors (for example, toxins) that enable pathogens to overcome host defense mechanisms and to multiply and cause damage

3. Resistance (***R***): The host's ability to defend itself in the form of the immune system

There is a continuous back-and-forth battle that occurs between a host's resistance and disease-producing microbes. The equation ***D = nV/R*** summarizes this struggle, with D representing the severity of the infectious disease.[16]

TABLE 3-7 Basic Reproduction Rate (R_0) Within Human Populations

Disease	Type of Causative Agent	R_0
Measles	Virus	12–18
Pertussis	Bacterium	12–17
Diphtheria	Bacterium	6–7
Smallpox	Virus	5–7
Poliomyelitis	Virus	5–7
Rubella	Virus	5–7
Mumps	Virus	4–7
HIV/AIDS	Virus	2–5
Influenza A	Virus	2–3
Ebola hemorrhagic fever	Virus	1
Rabies	Virus	< 1

Microbes that do wind up establishing disease have specific defensive strategies that allow them to escape destruction by the host immune system and offensive strategies (**TABLE 3-8**) that result in damage to the host. This can be compared to a football game—to win the game (analogous to establishing infection), the team (microbes) must have effective defensive strategies to counter the offensive strategies of its opponent (the host immune system). But that is not enough. The team must also have effective offensive strategies to move down the field and score points. Each group of pathogens has evolved unique defensive and offensive virulence factors, many of which are present in more than one group.[16] Infection that results in disease manifests in the general stages explained in Table 3-8.

Cycle of Microbial Disease

For infectious disease to exist at the population level, a chain of linked factors needs to be present. The cycle of microbial disease includes the infectious agent or pathogen, reservoirs, transmission, portals of entry, and portals of exit. To successfully break the chain and stop the spread of infectious diseases, we need to understand this cycle.[17] For example, if mosquitos are involved in transmission, as is the case in malaria, then controlling their population is a target[20]; for those microbes transmitted by drinking water, providing safe drinking water is the goal. In some instances, a combination of targets is preferable.[17]

Pathogen

For a particular disease to exist, there has to be a pathogen as the causative agent and a host in which the pathogen takes up residence. The potential for disease to occur and its outcome are a result of the complex interaction between the number of invading microbes and their virulence and the host immune system. *Communicable diseases* are infectious diseases in which the pathogen can be transmitted directly or indirectly from its reservoir to the host portal of entry.[17]

Reservoirs of Infection

A reservoir is a location in nature in which microbes survive (and possibly multiply) and from which they are transmitted. All pathogens have one or more reservoirs essential for their survival. Knowing what and where these reservoirs are is important, because they are prime targets for preventing and eliminating existing and potential epidemics. Reservoirs can be individual humans, but they can also be animals, plants, and even nonliving environments, such as water or soil.[17] **Zoonotic** diseases are diseases that can be transmitted from animals to humans and are cases where animals serve as the reservoir. The recent Ebola outbreak is a good example of this, as it is postulated that the outbreak may have originated from bats.[21]

Transmission

Transmission is the bridge between reservoir and portal of entry. Transmission explains how a disease spreads through the environment to another person, answering the question, "How do you get the disease?"

There are two major pathways of transmission, which can each be subdivided into three categories (**TABLE 3-9**). The first path is *direct* transmission, in which the infectious agent is directly and immediately transferred from a portal of exit to a portal of

TABLE 3-8 Stages of Microbial Disease

Stage	Description
Incubation	Period between initial infection and appearance of symptoms; considerable variation among diseases
Prodromal	Period in which early symptoms appear; usually short and not always well characterized
Illness	Period during which the disease is most acute and is accompanied by characteristic symptoms
Decline	Period during which the symptoms gradually subside
Convalescence	Period during which symptoms disappear and recovery ensues

TABLE 3-9 Modes of Transmission

Direct	Indirect
Contact (e.g., kissing, sneezing, coughing, singing, sexual contact)	Vehicles (fomites, e.g., doorknobs, eating utensils, toys, facial tissue)
Animal bites	Airborne (via aerosols created by, e.g., shaking bedsheets, sweeping, mopping)
Transplacental	
	Vectors (e.g., mosquitos, ticks, flies)

entry. Sexual contact, kissing, and touching are the most common examples. The second path is *indirect* transmission, which involves the passage of infectious material from a reservoir or source to an intermediate agent and then to a host. The intermediate agent can be living or nonliving. Living organisms, known as **vectors**, can transmit microbes from one host to another. Ticks, flies, mosquitos, lice, and fleas are the most common vectors.[17] In malaria, the mosquito is the vector and the malarial parasite is the pathogen.[20] Vehicle-borne transmission is accomplished by food, water, biologic products (organs, blood, blood products), and **fomites** (inanimate objects such as, for example, a doorknob).[17]

Portals of Entry

The portal of entry is the opening through which microbes get into body tissues. This can occur in a number of ways, but body orifices, including the mouth, nose, ears, eyes, anus, urethra, and vagina, as well as cuts or wounds in the skin, make it possible for microbes to gain access.[17]

Portals of Exit

To complete the cycle of infectious disease and allow the spread of disease into the community, pathogens need to find a way to leave the host and start the cycle anew.[17]

▶ Current Challenges to Public Health Microbiology

During the past century, public health has made many key advances and tackled a number of challenges. Vaccines, antibiotics, fortified foods, and access to clean water have all been ways to deal with these challenges throughout the 20th century. Advances in public health have greatly decreased the burden of microbial diseases both locally and globally, especially in industrialized nations like the United States. However, as the 20th century came to an end, the 21st century revealed a number of modern challenges of utmost importance to public health at the local and global scale.[22] These challenges include antibiotic resistance, biologic weapons, and some of the modern "plagues."

Antibiotic Resistance

The discovery of antibiotics has been one of the most important findings in the history of public health. These wonder drugs have allowed us to treat an array of microbial diseases. Antibiotics generally work by disrupting key structures and metabolic pathways in bacterial cells. Throughout the 20th century, we depended on antibiotics to fight the battle against pathogenic bacteria.[23] However, these drugs have been used so widely for so long that the targets of these antibiotics, bacteria, have had the chance to adapt. This adaptation manifests itself in the form of antibiotic resistance.

The U.S. Centers for Disease Control and Prevention (CDC) currently estimates that at least 2 million people become infected with antibiotic-resistant bacteria each year. Of those infected, it is estimated that 23,000 people die as a result.[24] This is truly a major public health problem contributing to the threat of emerging infections and demands attention.

Acquisition of Antibiotic Resistance

How does a bacterial cell become resistant to an antibiotic in the first place? If you recall from the section on bacterial genetics earlier in this chapter, antibiotic resistance is the product of Darwin's "survival of the fittest." To summarize, bacteria, like all cells, have genetic material in the form of DNA. This DNA can exist in their chromosome or it can exist in plasmids. As we just learned, plasmids can be transferred from one cell to another (horizontal gene transfer). Some of these plasmids have genes that confer resistance (R or resistance plasmids). These resistance factors are the result of gene mutation or gene recombination. In growing bacterial cells, mutations can occur spontaneously and *randomly*. Likewise, mutations are not caused by selective pressure. However, certain mutations will be selected if the mutation provides an advantage. If this is the case, only surviving cells will multiply and, in so doing, pass on their genes that confer survival advantages (vertical gene transmission), subsequently leading to the next generation possessing the new "survival gene."[23]

To apply these concepts to bacterial resistance, assume there is a colony of 100 bacterial cells. Say that they are all genetically identical cells, with the exception that 10 cells also possess a gene that confers resistance against an antibiotic. If the antibiotic is used on these 100 cells, all the cells without the resistant gene will die (90 cells). The 10 cells that had the resistant gene survived because they possess a gene that made them resistant to the antibiotic. Now, these surviving cells will multiply, and their offspring will all possess the resistant gene, creating a new population of cells that *all* confer resistance to this antibiotic. The original resistant 10 cells had a selective advantage compared to the other 90.

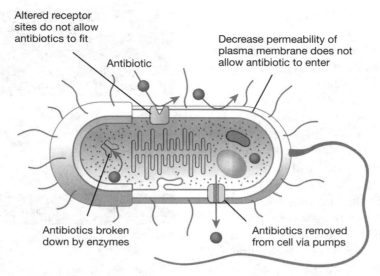

FIGURE 3-14 Mechanisms of Bacterial Resistance

Mechanisms of Antibiotic Resistance and Antibiotic Misuse

What does resistance really mean? Bacteria can counter the effects of antibiotics in a number of different ways as illustrated in **FIGURE 3-14**. Resistance has always been around; however, widespread antibiotic misuse among human populations has facilitated the emergence of antibiotic-resistant strains.

The concept of antibiotic misuse, though a problem everywhere, is defined as somewhat of a paradox when we look at developed and developing countries. In developing countries, misuse often occurs due to a *lack* of antibiotics. The drugs are either too expensive or simply unavailable, leading to unsafe practices such as taking part of the recommended dose and saving the rest for later. When an antibiotic is prescribed, it is essential to take the required dose as instructed to avoid evolutionary selection pressures.

Conversely, in developed countries, the problem is due to an *abundance* of antibiotics. In some countries, antibiotics can be purchased over the counter (absence of a prescription) in markets and pharmacies—and even where prescriptions *are* required, they are handed out far more frequently than is truly necessary. Frequently, patients request and receive antibiotics when they are not the appropriate treatment; for instance, antibiotic prescriptions are often written when the patient is sick with viral ailments like the flu and common cold (recall that antibiotics are *not* effective against viral illnesses).[23] If the disease is successfully running its course or if the disease is a virus, these are not times for antibiotics. Patients' misunderstanding of the medication adds to the problem. Even if antibiotics are needed, it is common for patients to stop taking them once they start

to feel better and dispose of the remaining dose. These practices favor selection of antibiotic resistance, as only the more susceptible strains will be wiped out by only a few doses, leaving the rest to survive and multiply. Misuse, many health professionals warn, could force us back to the pre-antibiotic era.[23] See **BOX 3-2**.

BOX 3-2   The Ultimate U.S. "Superbug"

In January 2017, the CDC released a report about a 70-year-old woman from Nevada who died from an infection resistant to all 26 antibiotics available in the United States.[25] Originally hospitalized in India, she had acquired an infection in her hip after fracturing her leg. Usually, in the United States, clinicians have last resorts in situations where certain treatments are ineffective. The antibiotic polymyxin E (Colistin) is an example of such a drug used as a last effort. In this instance, scientists tried whatever drugs they thought could be helpful, but none, not even polymyxin E, worked.

Due to the nature of her infection, the woman was isolated to contain this "superbug." Fortunately, no one in contact with the woman turned up positive for this pathogen, but its very existence is still cause for concern. It is still very likely other superbugs will emerge. Bacterial resistance factors are constantly swapped between bacteria. Your gut, for example, is full of bacteria that usually do not cause harm. However, they still have the ability to engage in horizontal transfer with other bacteria. These superbugs could be living inside us.

Data from Zhang S. A woman was killed by a superbug resistant to all 26 American antibiotics: She won't be the last. *The Atlantic*. Available at https://www.theatlantic.com/health/archive/2017/01/a-superbug-resistant-to-26-antibiotics-killed-a-woman-itll-happen-again/513050/. Published January 13, 2017.

The result of antibiotic overuse is also evident in healthcare settings. Due to the abundant use of antibiotics in these settings, healthcare environments are breeding grounds for antimicrobial-resistant pathogens, the result of which is the increasing risk of healthcare-associated infections (HCAIs) also known as **nosocomial infections**. This kind of infection occurs as a result of *being* in a healthcare setting, separate from the reason an individual went to that setting. HCAIs are usually associated with central lines, surgeries, and catheters. The common factor of each cause is a breach of individual barrier defenses, like the skin. This breach allows pathogens entry into the patient and can potentially cause infection. These pathogens are constantly adapting to their clinically based environment riddled with antibiotic use, posing a serious threat to public health.[26]

Another instance where antibiotics are frequently utilized is in food production, specifically with livestock. The U.S. Food and Drug Administration approves the use of antibiotics in food animals for disease treatment of sick animals, disease control for a group of animals when some animals are sick, and disease prevention for animals at risk of being sick. Again, widespread antibiotic use in this case poses a threat to public health. Though antibiotics will kill susceptible bacteria, resistant bacteria will survive and multiply. If this occurs, these bacteria can contaminate meat and other animal products when the animals are slaughtered and processed for consumption. Resistant bacteria can also get in the environment through animal stool and may spread to produce that has been irrigated with contaminated water. People can subsequently get infected with resistant bacteria from handling or eating raw or undercooked food from animals or contaminated produce, contacting animal stool, or caring for animals.[27]

In 2013, the CDC published a report highlighting the top 18 drug-resistant threats to the United States. The report breaks down the threats to varying levels of concern: urgent, serious, and concerning (**TABLE 3-10**). Urgent and serious threats tend to require increased monitoring and regular prevention activities. However, no matter the category, the CDC uses infectious disease epidemiology to address any gaps in its ability to detect for resistance and protect the public.[28]

The seriousness of antibiotic resistance is one of the biggest challenges faced in public health today. The critical point lies in the hands of physicians and patients, both of whom share the responsibility for the misuse and overuse of antibiotics resulting in the emergence of "superbugs." It is our job to ensure that the public and the clinical community are cognizant

TABLE 3-10 The CDC's List of Urgent, Serious, and Concerning Threats
Urgent
Clostridium difficile (CDIFF)
Carbapenem-resistant *Enterobacteriaceae* (CRE)
Neisseria gonorrhoeae
Serious
Multidrug-resistant *Acinetobacter*
Drug-resistant *Campylobacter*
Fluconazole-resistant *Candida*
Extended spectrum *Enterobacteriaceae* (ESBL)
Vancomycin-resistant *Enterococcus* (VRE)
Multidrug-resistant *Pseudomonas aeruginosa*
Drug-resistant non-typhoidal *Salmonella*
Drug-resistant *Salmonella* serotype *Typhi*
Drug-resistant *Shigella*
Methicillin-resistant *Staphylococcus aureus* (MRSA)
Drug-resistant *Streptococcus pneumoniae*
Drug-resistant tuberculosis
Concerning
Vancomycin-resistant *Staphylococcus aureus*
Erythromycin-resistant Group A *Streptococcus*
Clindamycin-resistant Group B *Streptococcus*

Reproduced from Centers for Disease Control and Prevention (CDC). Antibiotic/Antimicrobial Resistance: Biggest Threats. Available at https://www.cdc.gov/drugresistance/biggest_threats.html. Updated April 14, 2017. Accessed November 7, 2017.

and appreciative of this current challenge and the proper way to use antibiotics. The overuse of antibacterial products is everywhere. Moving forward we must be much more responsible and careful when using antibiotics if we plan to continue to reap their benefits.[23]

Biologic Weapons

For centuries, humans have attempted to harness the harmful effects of some microbial species and to weaponize them. Used in certain ways, these weapons can be highly detrimental. Biologic weapons are the tools of biologic warfare and bioterrorism. They are microbes deployed to grow in (or on) their target host or microbial products that are deliberately used to produce a state of clinical disease with the intent of incapacitating or killing individuals or producing mass casualties.[29]

Ironically, knowledge advancement about ways to combat and prevent disease has fostered improved ways to use these biologic agents as weapons. These weapons are deadly and can be deployed inside intercontinental missiles, in aerosol cans, by crop dusters, or even a mailed letter.[29]

Current Plagues

Throughout all of history, humans have been dealing with some widespread infectious disease or another. With the emergence and reemergence of a number of infectious diseases, this trend continues to this day and is of utmost concern. The occurrence of large-scale outbreaks of disease, commonly referred to as "plagues," is the result of the lack of adaptation between humans and microbes. Historically, the infamous examples of smallpox (a virus), and the Black Death (caused by the bacterium *Yersinia pestis*), decimated populations. As humans and microbes continue their battle, and new environments are explored, new diseases and new epidemics continue to emerge.[30]

Key Terms

Aerobes
Anaerobes
Autotrophs
Bacilli
Bacteria
Binary fission
Biogeochemical cycles
Biosphere
Capsid
Capsule
Cell wall
Chemosynthetic
Chemotaxis
Cocci
Common-source
   epidemics
Conjugation
Cultures
$D = nV/R$
Decomposers
Disease

Envelope
Epidemiology
Eukaryotes
Facultative anaerobes
Flagella
Fomites
Fungi
Gene
Generation time
Genus
Gram stain
Heterotrophs
Horizontal gene transfer
Infection
Infectious agents
Koch's postulates
Mutation
Nosocomial infections
Nucleoid
Obligate anaerobes
Obligate intracellular parasites

Organic
Organisms
Pathogens
Photosynthetic
Pili
Plasmids
Prokaryotes
Propagated epidemics
Protozoans
R_0 (R-nought)
Species
Spirilla
Transduction
Transformation
Unicellular algae
Vectors
Vertical gene transfer
Virion
Virulence
Viruses
Zoonotic

Discussion Questions

1. Compare eukaryotic and prokaryotic cells.
2. List the beneficial aspects of microbes. What is the goal of the public health microbiologist when it comes to microbes?
3. Explain what is meant by obligate intracellular parasite and explain how that relates to viral replication.
4. Compare bacteria and viruses.
5. The expression $D = nV/R$ expresses host–parasite relationships. Elaborate on this; identify each term (D, n, V, and R) in the equation. Create an example in real life of what each term could represent.
6. Distinguish between vertical and horizontal gene transfer and discuss the importance of genetic diversity within species.
7. List the cycle of microbial disease and discuss a preventative measure in each phase to try to break the cycle.

8. Explain how Darwin's concept of "survival of the fittest" relates to antibiotic resistance.

9. List three modern challenges in public health microbiology and potential ways to mitigate them.

References

1. Krasner RI, Shors T. Identifying the challenge. In: *The Microbial Challenge: A Public Health Perspective.* 3rd ed. Burlington, MA: Jones & Bartlett Learning; 2014:2-28.

2. Krasner RI, Shors T. The microbial world. In: *The Microbial Challenge: A Public Health Perspective.* 3rd ed. Burlington, MA: Jones & Bartlett Learning; 2014:29-47.

3. Reece JB, Urry LA, Cain ML, Wasserman SA, Minorsky PV, Jackson RB. *Campbell Biology.* 9th ed. French's Forest, N.S.W.: Pearson Australia; 2011.

4. Krasner RI, Shors T. Beneficial aspects of microbes: the other side of the coin. In: *The Microbial Challenge: A Public Health Perspective.* 3rd ed. Burlington, MA: Jones & Bartlett Learning; 2014:48-72.

5. Shaftel H. A blanket around Earth. Global Climate Change: Vital Signs of the Planet. Available at https://climate.nasa.gov /causes/. Updated October 30, 2017. Accessed October 31, 2017.

6. Krasner RI, Shors T. Bacteria. *The Microbial Challenge: A Public Health Perspective.* 3rd ed. Burlington, MA: Jones & Bartlett Learning; 2014:73-94.

7. Foster T. Staphylococcus. In: Baron S, ed. *Medical Microbiology.* 4th ed. Galveston, TX: University of Texas Medical Branch at Galveston; 1996. Chapter 12.

8. Patterson MJ. Streptococcus. In: Baron S, ed. *Medical Microbiology.* 4th ed. Galveston, TX: University of Texas Medical Branch at Galveston; 1996. Chapter 13.

9. Ng L-K, Martin IE. The laboratory diagnosis of *Neisseria gonorrhoeae. Can J Infect Dis Med Microbiol.* 2005;16(1):15-25.

10. Stepanović S, Ćirković I, Ranin L. Biofilm formation by *Salmonella* spp. and *Listeria monocytogenes* on plastic surface. *Lett Appl Microbiol.* 2004;38(5):428-432.

11. Donlan RM. Biofilms: microbial life on surfaces. *Emerging Infect Dis.* 2002;8(9):881-890. doi:10.3201/eid0809.020063.

12. Anderson JD, Eftekhar F, Aird MY, Hammond J. Role of bacterial growth rates in the epidemiology and pathogenesis of urinary infections in women. *J Clin Microbiol.* 1979;10(6):766-771.

13. Krasner RI, Shors T. Bacterial genetics. In: *The Microbial Challenge: A Public Health Perspective.* 3rd ed. Burlington, MA: Jones & Bartlett Learning; 2014:123-149.

14. Rogers K. Horizontal gene transfer. *Encyclopedia Britannica.* Available at https://www.britannica.com/science /horizontal-gene-transfer. Updated November 22, 2016. Accessed October 20, 2017.

15. Krasner RI, Shors T. Viruses and prions. *The Microbial Challenge: A Public Health Perspective.* 3rd ed. Burlington, MA: Jones & Bartlett Learning; 2014:95-122.

16. Krasner RI, Shors T. Concepts of microbial disease. In: *The Microbial Challenge: A Public Health Perspective.* 3rd ed. Burlington, MA: Jones & Bartlett Learning; 2014:152-172.

17. Krasner RI, Shors T. Epidemiology and cycle of microbial disease. In: *The Microbial Challenge: A Public Health Perspective.* 3rd ed. Burlington, MA: Jones & Bartlett Learning; 2014:173-200.

18. World Health Organization (WHO). Flooding and communicable disease fact sheet: Risk assessment and preventative measures. Available at http://www.who.int/hac /techguidance/ems/flood_cds/en/. Updated 2017. Accessed November 27, 2017.

19. Centers for Disease Control and Prevention (CDC). Update: multistate outbreak of *Escherichia coli* O157:H7 infections from hamburgers—western United States, 1992-1993. *MMWR Morb Mortal Wkly Rep.* 1993;42(14):258-263.

20. Nelson KE, Williams CM. Microbiology tools for the epidemiologist. In: *Infectious Disease Epidemiology.* 3rd ed. Burlington, MA: Jones & Bartlett Learning; 2014:187-218.

21. Marí Saéz A, Weiss S, Nowak K, et al. Investigating the zoonotic origin of the West African Ebola epidemic. *EMBO Mol Med.* 2015;7(1):17-23. doi: 10.15252/emmm.201404792.

22. Koplan JP, Fleming DW. Current and future public health challenges. *JAMA.* 2000;284(13):1696-1698. doi:10.1001 /jama.284.13.1696.

23. Krasner RI, Shors T. Control of microbial diseases. In: *The Microbial Challenge: A Public Health Perspective.* 3rd ed. Burlington, MA: Jones & Bartlett Learning; 2014: 379-410.

24. Centers for Disease Control and Prevention (CDC). Antibiotic/antimicrobial resistance. Available at https:// www.cdc.gov/drugresistance/index.html. Updated August 18, 2107. Accessed October 21, 2017.

25. Zhang S. A woman was killed by a superbug resistant to all 26 American antibiotics: She won't be the last. *The Atlantic.* Available at https://www.theatlantic.com /health/archive/2017/01/a-superbug-resistant-to-26 -antibiotics-killed-a-woman-itll-happen-again/513050/. Published January 13, 2017. Accessed January 17, 2018.

26. Centers for Disease Control and Prevention (CDC). CDC's Antibiotic Resistance Patient Safety Atlas. Available at https:// www.cdc.gov/hai/surveillance/ar-patient-safety-atlas.html. Updated March 3, 2016. Accessed November 7, 2017.

27. Centers for Disease Control and Prevention (CDC). National Antimicrobial Resistance Monitoring System for Enteric Bacteria (NARMS): Antibiotic Resistance. Available at https://www.cdc.gov/narms/faq.html. Updated December 16, 2016. Accessed November 7, 2017.

28. Centers for Disease Control and Prevention (CDC). Antibiotic/Antimicrobial Resistance: Biggest Threats. Available at https://www.cdc.gov/drugresistance/biggest _threats.html. Updated April 14, 2017. Accessed November 7, 2017.

29. Krasner RI, Shors T. Biological weapons. In: *The Microbial Challenge: A Public Health Perspective.* 3rd ed. Burlington, MA: Jones & Bartlett Learning; 2014:430-454.

30. Krasner RI, Shors T. Current plagues. In: *The Microbial Challenge: A Public Health Perspective.* 3rd ed. Burlington, MA: Jones & Bartlett Learning; 2014:455-495.

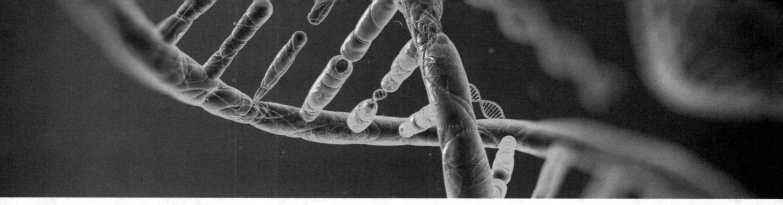

CHAPTER 4

Immunizations and Immunity

Carol A. Smith and Loretta DiPietro

LEARNING OBJECTIVES

By the end of this chapter, the student will be able to:

- Differentiate the two systems of immunity
- Identify elements of the innate immune system
- Compare humoral and cell-mediated immunity
- Explain B cell immunity as it relates to first antigenic exposure and subsequent exposure
- Differentiate active and passive immunity, giving examples of each
- Explain how a vaccine works to achieve resistance to an infectious organism
- List five types of vaccines, giving examples of each
- Define the term toxoid
- Identify the currently recommended childhood and adult immunizations in the United States
- Explain how herd immunity provides protection for the nonimmunized person

CHAPTER OUTLINE

▶ Introduction

Immunization is believed by many to be one of the most successful applications of immunologic principles. **Immunization** (which can occur via **vaccination**) is a procedure in which an infectious disease is prevented by prior exposure to a pathogen administered in a form that will not cause illness. The first widespread use of vaccination occurred during the late 18th century against smallpox, an infectious disease that was widespread in Europe. In 1796, Edward Jenner, an English physician, observed that individuals who had been infected by cowpox appeared to be resistant to smallpox, a similar disease in humans. Jenner introduced fluid from a pustule of a young dairymaid infected with cowpox into a wound of the 8-year-old son of his gardener. Six weeks later, he injected the young boy with fluid from a smallpox pustule. As Jenner anticipated, the boy did not develop smallpox. Jenner repeated his experiment with others during the following years and published his findings. Unbeknownst to Jenner, he had discovered a fundamental principle of immunization. By using a relatively harmless foreign agent, he had invoked an immune response that protected someone from an infectious disease.

Although immunization against smallpox spread rapidly, vaccination against other agents did not occur until the latter part of the 19th century when Louis Pasteur accidentally discovered a means for protecting against cholera. Pasteur had grown, in culture, the organism that caused fowl cholera. After returning from a summer vacation, he injected some chickens with an old culture of the organism and to his surprise, the chickens became ill with cholera but recovered. To save resources, he injected these recovered chickens with a fresh culture of the organism. The chickens that had been previously exposed to the organism did not develop cholera; however, chickens that had not previously been exposed did develop the disease. Pasteur hypothesized that the aging of the bacterial culture had altered the virulence of the organism, rendering it incapable of causing disease. In recognition of Jenner's earlier work, he named the aged culture a **vaccine**, which was derived from the Latin word *vaccinus* meaning "pertaining to cows." Pasteur subsequently experimented with other infectious organisms and developed more vaccines, including one for rabies. Although Jenner and Pasteur showed that immunization was effective in preventing disease, they did not understand how it worked. It was not until elucidation of the mechanisms of immunity in the 20th century that the "how" became known.

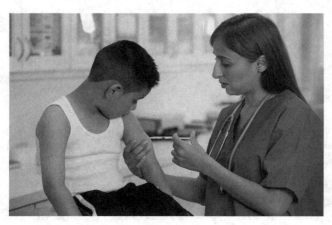

© Ariel Skelley/Blend Images/Getty Images

▶ Mechanisms of Immunity

The human body has a variety of mechanisms that provide protection against infectious agents. This protection is accomplished by complex processes that require detection of changes in an individual's cells or the presence of infectious organisms. There are two systems of **immunity** that work together to provide protection:

- Innate immune system
- Adaptive immune system

The innate system, which is present from birth, provides the first line of defense against infectious agents. The response of the innate system is *nonspecific* in that it does not differentiate between different challenges. It reacts in basically the same manner with all organisms. A wide range of anatomic and physiologic barriers creates an environment inhospitable to invading organisms (**BOX 4-1**). The physiologic processes of inflammation and phagocytosis facilitate movement of cells to infected sites where engulfment and clearance of microorganisms can occur (**FIGURE 4-1**).

BOX 4-1 Host Defenses of the Immune System

Innate Immunity
Anatomic barriers
Skin and mucosal membranes: provide mechanical barriers preventing entry of organisms

Physiologic barriers
Complement defense system
Acid environment of stomach: kills ingested organisms
Chemical mediators: lysozymes and other enzymes in secretions destroy organisms

Phagocytic cells
Neutrophils and macrophages with the aid of complement engulf and destroy ingested organisms

Inflammatory processes
Produce antibacterial activity and stimulate phagocytosis

Natural killer cells
Possess cytotoxic activity against tumor cells and some virus-infected cells

Adaptive Immunity
Humoral
B lymphocytes: production of antibodies and memory cells

Cell-mediated
T lymphocytes: cell-to-cell contacts, secretion of soluble products and memory cells

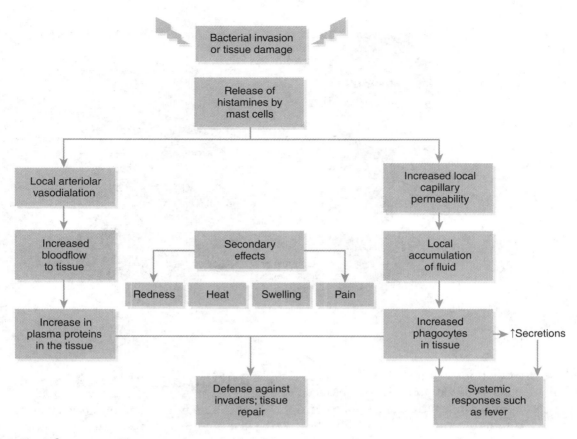

FIGURE 4-1 The Inflammatory Response

Modified from Sherwood L. *Human Physiology: From Cells to Systems*. 4th ed. Belmont, CA: Brooks/Cole; 2001.

When the innate immune response is insufficient to protect the individual from the invading organisms, the second form of immunity—**adaptive immunity**—is stimulated to respond to the challenge. Adaptive immunity, also known as *acquired* or *specific immunity*, involves the activation of immune cells and development of substances that will aid in the elimination of the organisms and facilitate the development of immunologic memory. It is this immunologic memory that is crucial to the success of a vaccine.

Unlike **innate immunity**, adaptive immunity demonstrates *specificity* for the foreign agent. Microorganisms possess surface molecules capable of stimulating an immune response. These molecules are known as **antigens**. Interactions between antigens and the cells of the adaptive system help clear the organism from the body.

Two Types of Adaptive Immunity: Humoral and Cell-Mediated

There are two major types of adaptive responses: cell-mediated (cellular) and humoral immunity. Each type involves different cells and molecules that help rid the body of extracellular and intracellular organisms. Although cell-mediated and humoral immunity are often discussed as separate entities, there is a great deal of cooperation between the two. The major cells involved in the adaptive response are T and B lymphocytes. **Cell-mediated immunity** primarily involves T lymphocytes (T cells), which are derived from bone marrow but undergo differentiation in the thymus. T lymphocytes develop into cells with specific functions. Three types of T cells are specialized to kill virus-infected host cells and to suppress other immune cells: (1) *cytotoxic T cells* (T_c or CD8 cells) are the "hit men" that destroy any infected host cells, cancer cells, and transplanted cells; (2) *helper T cells* (CD4 cells) enable Tc and B cells in their killing by secreting various cytokines; and (3) *suppressor T cells* suppress B-cell activity and T_c and helper T-cell activity. T lymphocytes are important in eliminating intracellular organisms such as viruses and certain types of bacteria. T cells also play an important role in presenting protein antigens to B cells in a form that the B cell can recognize. Activation of T cells leads to secretion of substances known as *cytokines*, soluble proteins

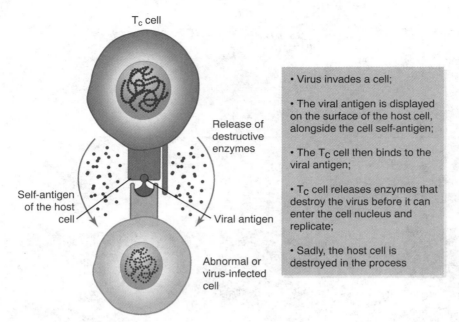

T_C cell

Release of destructive enzymes

Self-antigen of the host cell

Viral antigen

Abnormal or virus-infected cell

- Virus invades a cell;

- The viral antigen is displayed on the surface of the host cell, alongside the cell self-antigen;

- The T_C cell then binds to the viral antigen;

- T_C cell releases enzymes that destroy the virus before it can enter the cell nucleus and replicate;

- Sadly, the host cell is destroyed in the process

FIGURE 4-2 T-Cell Activity

that mediate the functions of the cells that secrete them and of other cells (**FIGURE 4-2**). Some cytokines play amplification roles while others are involved in regulation and communication of cells within the immune system. T-cell responses are very important with regard to defending the host from foreign invaders (for instance, see the chapter on HIV/ AIDS).

Humoral immunity (or antibody-mediated immunity) is a function of B lymphocytes (B cells) and is the primary defense against extracellular organisms. When B cells encounter an organism, they recognize parts of the antigens on the surface called antigenic determinants or **epitopes**.

These are smaller portions of the antigen that the cells recognize as foreign. Binding of the antigen to the B lymphocyte triggers the cell to transform into an antibody-producing cell known as a *plasma cell*. Plasma cells manufacture antibodies that are specific for the antigen that induced their production. **Antibodies**, which are proteins of the immunoglobulin class, are secreted by the plasma cell into plasma and function to help eliminate the foreign organisms. The five classes of antibodies produced by plasma cells are: IgM, IgG, IgA, IgD, and IgE. Each plays a role in supporting the immune system's functions, but their chief functions are to:

- Neutralize bacterial toxins
- Neutralize viruses
- Attach to bacteria promoting phagocytosis
- Activate components involved in the inflammatory response

▶ Antibodies at Work

When the body encounters a particular antigen for the first time, a primary immune response is initiated (**FIGURE 4-3**). The adaptive immune system becomes activated and antibody production occurs. A few days to a week after exposure to the antigen, IgM antibody specific for the antigen that stimulated its formation begins to appear in the blood. A short time later, IgG specific for the antigen appears. The antibody titer then rises in the blood, reflecting the antibody production. Levels will plateau and eventually decline over time after the organism is cleared from the body. Any excess antibody will be broken down into simpler molecules (catabolized). If the immune system encounters the same organism again in the future, memory cells that were formed during the first encounter will recognize

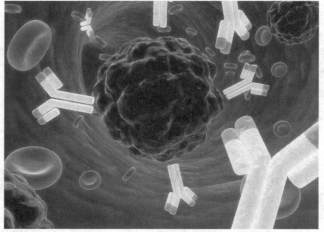

© Sebastian Kaulitzki/Shutterstock

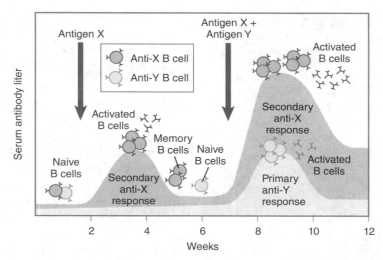

FIGURE 4-3 Specificity and Memory in Adaptive Immunity, Illustrated by Primary and Secondary Immune Responses

Reproduced from Abbas AB, Lichtman AH, Pillai S. *Cellular and Molecular Immunology*. 6th ed. Philadelphia, PA: Saunders Elsevier, 2010.

the organism, and the response of the immune system will be much quicker than during the first encounter (see Figure 4-3).

Antibodies will be made much faster and in greater amounts so they will be readily available to assist in clearing the organism quickly. Should an individual be exposed to the antigen a third time, the antibody response will be further amplified because of previously having encountered the antigen. These memory responses as well as the specificity of the antibodies produced are crucial to the effectiveness of vaccines.

Active and Passive Immunity

Immunity to microorganisms can be achieved through active or passive immunization (**TABLE 4-1**). In both cases, the immunity can be acquired or attained by natural means.

Active immunity occurs when an immunocompetent individual (i.e., someone who can produce a normal immune response) is exposed to a foreign organism and the person's immune cells respond by producing immune products such as antibodies and memory cells. Active immunity may be naturally developed if the person is naturally infected with the organism. It also may be acquired artificially by means of vaccination.

Passive immunity involves the transfer of preformed antibodies to an individual to protect against a challenge. The transfer of maternal antibodies to a fetus in utero is an example of natural passive immunity. Passive immunity also can be achieved by injecting an individual with preformed antibodies to an organism. This is used primarily when someone who was not previously immunized becomes exposed to an organism for which an immunoglobulin product is available. An example of this is the use of hepatitis

B immunoglobulin for someone who may have been exposed to the disease.

TABLE 4-1 Comparison of Active and Passive Immunity

Immunity	Type of Acquisition	Length of Protection
Active	Natural—infection Acquired—vaccination	Long term Long term
Passive	Natural—transfer in utero Acquired—injection of immunoglobulin	Short term Short term

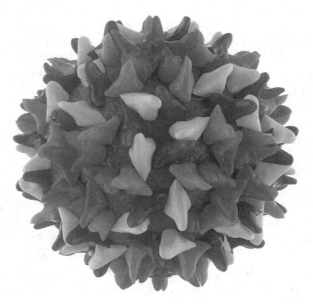

TABLE 4-2 FDA-Approved Monoclonal Antibodies for Cancer Treatment

Name of Drug	Type of Cancer It Treats
Alemtuzumab (Campath)	Chronic lymphocytic leukemia
Bevacizumab (Avastin)	Brain cancer Colon cancer Kidney cancer Lung cancer
Cetuximab (Erbitux)	Colon cancer Head and neck cancers
Ibritumomab (Zevalin)	Non-Hodgkin's lymphoma
Ofatumumab (Arzerra)	Chronic lymphocytic leukemia
Panitumumab (Vectibix)	Colon cancer
Rituximab (Rituxan)	Chronic lymphocytic leukemia Non-Hodgkin's lymphoma
Tositumomab (Bexxar)	Non-Hodgkin's lymphoma
Trastuzumab (Herceptin)	Breast cancer Stomach cancer

Data from Mayo Clinic. Monoclonal antibody drugs for cancer: how they work. 2017. Available at http://www.mayoclinic.org/diseases-conditions/cancer/in-depth /monoclonal-antibody/art-20047808?pg=2.

Development of active immunity to an organism generally provides long-term protection against future exposure to the organism. Because the individual's immune system is activated, memory cells are formed. Re-exposure to the organism will result in a rapid response of the immune system to clear the organism before illness can develop. The length of time from exposure to the waning of immunity varies by antigen, however. Passive immunity provides short-term protection. Memory cells are not formed and when the antibodies have been consumed or catabolized, there will be no remaining protection against future exposure.

Can the Immune System Help Protect Us from Cancer?

Cancer cells are recognized as "non-self" after cellular transformation and presentation of novel antigens on the surface. Some novel antigens on cancer cells include those from infecting viruses, such as the human papilloma virus (HPV), Ebola virus, and hepatitis B virus. Host gene products can also be expressed on transformed cells. For example, NY-ESO1 is produced by several tumors but is not expressed by normal cells. Some normal host proteins can also be altered and

therefore not recognized as "self." All of these mechanisms "mark" the cancer cell as foreign.

Recently transformed cells can initially be eliminated by an innate immune response, such as by natural killer cells. During tumor progression, however, even though an adaptive immune response can be provoked by antigen-specific T cells, immune selection produces variants in these cancer cells, and they may lose major histocompatibility with complex class I and II antigens. Furthermore, tumor-derived soluble factors can facilitate the escape of these tumor cells from immune attack, allowing progression and metastasis. Drug therapy for cancer can be based on the fact that tumor cells carry unique antigens on their surface. **TABLE 4-2** lists monoclonal antibodies (antibodies that derive from the same parent cell) that are used to treat certain types of cancers.

▶ Vaccines

Vaccines attempt to stimulate the immune system by mimicking a natural infection. The success of a vaccine depends on two key elements: immunological memory and specificity. These elements allow the immune system to mount a much stronger response on a second encounter with the organism.

The aim in vaccine development is to alter the organism in such a way that it does not cause disease but maintains its immunogenicity. The goal is to stimulate memory T and B cells in an individual to:

- Induce specific immunity
- Eliminate organisms that enter the host
- Neutralize bacterial toxins

A vaccine contains a killed or weakened form or derivative of the infectious organism. Use of such forms of the organism is possible because B and T cells recognize specific parts of the organism—the epitopes—and not the whole organism. There are several types of vaccines currently in use (**TABLE 4-3**).

Live, attenuated vaccines contain a weakened form of the microorganism. This weakening process, known as **attenuation**, occurs in the laboratory by growing the organism under abnormal culture conditions. An example of an attenuated vaccine is that which was developed by Pasteur for protecting against cholera. The resultant vaccine retains similar characteristics to the original organism but lacks its pathogenicity. Because a live, attenuated vaccine contains an altered organism similar to the causative organism, it is the closest thing to an actual infection and tends to produce strong cellular and humoral responses, resulting in long-term protection after just a few doses. Two disadvantages to using attenuated vaccines are the remote chance that

TABLE 4-3 Types of Vaccines

Vaccine Type	Examples of Vaccines
Live, attenuated vaccine	Measles, mumps, rubella, polio (Sabin) vaccine, varicella
Inactivated (killed) vaccine	Cholera, rabies, influenza, hepatitis A, polio (Salk) vaccine
Toxoid vaccine	Tetanus, diphtheria
Subunit vaccine	Hepatitis B, pertussis, pneumococcus (*Streptococcus pneumoniae*)
Conjugate vaccine	*Haemophilus influenzae* type B (HiB), pneumococcus (*Streptococcus pneumoniae*)

the organism could mutate back to a virulent form and the need for refrigeration of the vaccine.

Inactivated or killed vaccines are created by treating the microorganism with chemicals or heat. These types of vaccines are usually more stable and safer than live vaccines but tend to stimulate a weaker response. They do not require refrigeration and can often be shipped in freeze-dried form, which is an advantage in developing countries.

Some bacteria produce toxins that cause illness in an individual. These toxins can be made harmless by treating them with **toxoid** vaccines, created by treating bacterial toxins with formaldehyde. This treatment renders the toxin harmless but maintains its immunogenicity. Thus, the resultant toxoid can stimulate a strong antibody response that will help eliminate the harmful toxin.

Subunit vaccines are composed of selected epitopes or proteins from the organism rather than the entire antigen. This contributes to the specificity of the immune response that is mounted by T cells and antibodies. Because the vaccine is composed of only certain parts of the antigens, the chances of adverse reactions to the vaccine are minimized. The difficulty in creating subunit vaccines is identifying the epitopes from the organism that will best stimulate an immune response. Subunit vaccines and toxoids often contain **adjuvants**. Vaccine adjuvants, usually aluminum salts, increase the length of stay of the antigen in the body so that the immune system has more time to respond to the antigen. The choice of vaccine adjuvant is often as important to the vaccine as the antigen type.

Conjugate vaccines attempt to strengthen the immunogenicity of some organisms with polysaccharide capsules. Polysaccharide antigens associated with these organisms may be difficult for the immature immune system of infants and younger children to recognize. Conjugate vaccines couple these antigens

to a protein carrier. The antigen-protein complex becomes more readily recognizable by the immune system so that a strong response is made.

Mechanisms of protection stimulated by vaccines can be affected by many factors, including nutritional status, underlying diseases, and age. Immunization never confers absolute protection, so there will always be individuals who will not respond (poor responders). The size of the poor responder group will vary with the individual vaccine and the number of booster shots given.

▶ Future Vaccines

Several other types of vaccines are in experimental stages. Deoxyribonucleic acid (DNA) vaccines use the organism's own genetic material. When an organism's genes are introduced into the host, the DNA becomes incorporated in the host's cells, where it can instruct the cells to make antigens that are secreted and displayed on the cells. The displayed antigens can then stimulate the host's immune system. Somewhat similar to DNA vaccines are recombinant vector vaccines. These experimental vaccines use an attenuated virus or bacterium to introduce the microbe's DNA into the host's cells. These newer techniques are being tested for diverse diseases such as influenza, malaria, rabies, and measles.

One of the biggest hurdles faced by vaccine researchers is the ever-changing nature of many microorganisms. The organism responsible for human immunodeficiency virus (HIV) infection is a classic example of this problem. HIV often mutates, creating new forms of the virus and making it much more difficult to develop a single vaccine that is effective against all forms of the virus. Development of an effective malarial vaccine also has suffered from the fact that the malarial parasite is genetically complex and presents thousands of antigens. Determining which of these many antigens would be most effective in stimulating an immune response complicates the development of a vaccine. Despite these problems, many researchers believe it is only a matter of time before these challenges are conquered.

▶ Public Health Perspectives for the Health of the General Population and of High-Risk Groups

Immunization of Selected Groups

Immunization has proven to be a cost-effective means of preventing infectious diseases. Successful immunization programs have been responsible for the eradication of smallpox worldwide. The last reported case of a naturally acquired smallpox infection occurred in 1977. The success of this program led the World Health Organization (WHO) to call for a cessation of vaccination for smallpox in 1979 in all countries.[1] Immunization programs against polio also have been successful. Although childhood vaccination for polio is currently recommended, many believe that polio will be eradicated in the near future (see **BOX 4-2**).[2]

Immunizations play a central role in the U.S. Department of Health and Human Service's Healthy People 2020 framework.[3] In the project, immunization has been designated as 1 of the 10 leading health indicators, which is reflected by the fact that a significant number of the 2020 Health Objectives concern improving and expanding immunization coverage (see **TABLE 4-4**).

Childhood immunization programs have played an important role in reducing infection and deaths among children. In the United States, childhood immunizations are recommended starting at birth. The Centers for Disease Control and Prevention (CDC) publishes recommended immunization schedules on its website. These schedules are approved yearly by the

---

BOX 4-2 Vaccine-Preventable Diseases

The number of reported cases of vaccine-preventable diseases has generally decreased over the past several decades. In 2009, there were no reported cases of polio or smallpox in the entire United States, and no cases of tetanus or rubella among children under five years of age. In fact, the United States has been polio free since 1979. From 2006–2016, there were fewer than 5 reported cases of diphtheria (in total) and an average of 11 cases of rubella reported annually from 2005–2011.

Between 2008 and 2009, the number of reported cases of hepatitis A, measles, and meningococcal disease decreased among children under five years of age. The United States first saw a significant decline in childhood hepatitis A cases after the Centers for Disease Control and Prevention (CDC) recommended vaccination for children living in high-risk areas starting in 1996. In 2005, the CDC broadened that recommendation to include routine hepatitis A vaccination for all children, starting at 1 year of age. Rates of hepatitis B infection have steadily declined with the implementation of a national strategy to eliminate the disease. This strategy includes routine screening of pregnant women for the hepatitis B virus and routine vaccination of infants and children. It is important to note that because most hepatitis B infections among infants and young children are asymptomatic, the reported number of cases likely underestimates the **incidence** in these age groups.

There are still many cases of vaccine-preventable diseases reported annually in the United States. In 2013, there were 26 reported cases of tetanus, more than 28,000 cases of pertussis, 187 cases of measles, 584 cases of mumps, 9 cases of rubella, 1,781 cases of hepatitis A, and over 11,000 reported cases of varicella (chicken pox).

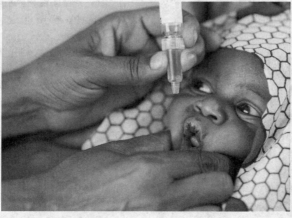

© ranplett/Vetta/Getty

TABLE 4-4 Selected Healthy People 2020 Objectives for Immunizations and Infectious Diseases

IID-1.6	Reduce cases of pertussis among children under 1 year of age to 2,500 cases from 2,777 cases reported in 2004–2008 (10% improvement goal).
IID-2.0	Reduce early-onset group B streptococcal disease from 0.30 newly reported cases among newborns aged 0 through 6 days per 1,000 live births to 0.25 new cases (10% improvement).
IID-5.0	Reduce outpatient visits for ear infections where antibiotics were prescribed to young children under 5 years to 70.0% from 77.8% in 2006–2007 (10% improvement).
IID-6.0	Reduce outpatient visits where antibiotics were prescribed for the sole diagnosis of the common cold to 21.0% from 28.6% in 2006–2007.
IID-7.1	Maintain an effective vaccination coverage level of 4 doses of the diphtheria-tetanus-acellular pertussis (DTaP) vaccine among children ages 19 to 35 months to 90% from 82.5% in 2012.
IID-8	Increase the percentage of children aged 19 to 35 months who receive the recommended doses of DTaP, polio, MMR, HiB, hepatitis B, varicella, and pneumococcal conjugate vaccine (PCV) to 80% from 68.4% in 2012.
IID-12.7	Increase the percentage of noninstitutionalized adults aged 65 years and older who are vaccinated annually against seasonal influenza to 90% from 66.6% in 2008 (maintain 2010 goal).

Reproduced from Office of Disease Prevention and Health Promotion, U.S. Department of Health and Human Services. *Healthy People 2020: 2020 Topics & Objectives: Immunization and Infectious Diseases*. Washington, DC: DHHS. Available at https://www.healthypeople.gov/2020/topics-objectives/topic/immunization-and-infectious-diseases/objectives. Accessed May 12, 2017.

CDC, the American Academy of Pediatrics, and the American Academy of Family Physicians. Vaccination too early following birth may be ineffective for some vaccines due to protective effects of passively transferred maternal antibodies. Efficacy depends on the vaccine and whether booster doses are administered. Most of these vaccines require multiple doses over a period of time. The heightened immune response that occurs with each exposure to the vaccine contributes to the development of effective immunity. Recommendations for adult immunizations are dependent on the risk group. For example, recommendations for older adults, those with underlying medical conditions, and those whose immune systems may be compromised include yearly influenza vaccine and immunization with pneumococcal vaccine.

Other vaccines may be recommended for travelers and those exposed to certain microorganisms through their work environment. The threat of bioterrorism has concerned many in recent years. Government and military agencies have ongoing research and development programs for vaccines against biologic threats. Anthrax and smallpox vaccines are currently licensed but recommended only for select groups such as military personnel, individuals working in research labs with these agents, and first responders. The vaccines are not available to the general public.

Vaccination is not always effective. A small group of individuals will respond poorly or not at all. Generally, these poor responders are not of concern when looking at the effectiveness of an immunization program. If most of the individuals who have been exposed to an infectious organism through vaccination have responded adequately, the chances of a poor responder encountering an infected person is small. "Herd" (community) immunity is the term often used to describe immunity to an infectious organism developed by a large group of vaccinated individuals; the goal of **herd immunity** is to stop transmission of the infectious disease. Impediments to the achievement of herd immunity are based on people who decline vaccination for themselves or their children due to concerns regarding adverse side effects and/or costs, especially costs of newer vaccines.

▶ Barriers to Achieving Widespread Coverage

In the Developed World

Expanding immunization coverage faces distinct barriers in the developed and developing world. In developed nations, immunizations are widely available, but access issues still occur among marginalized populations. Education materials may not exist for non-English-speaking populations, and immigrants are especially vulnerable to a lack of access to primary care. In general, new parents are very cautious about a newborn's health, so vaccine coverage for infants is not a large problem. However, as children age, they are less likely to come in for follow-up boosters and other immunizations.

Parents' fears and misunderstandings about immunizations also may prevent them from having their children vaccinated. Many people believe that a "bad batch" of a vaccine can actually cause the disease it is designed to prevent or will cause some other illness (e.g., autism). Indeed, this anti-vaccine movement has the potential to undermine a century of effective public health practice with regard to protecting the population from common communicable diseases that once were lethal (see the Case Report). Although certain vaccines are made from attenuated viruses that can mutate into a virulent form (e.g., Sabin OPV), none of the immunizations prescribed in the United States carries this risk. Parents may perceive that if a vaccine for HPV, a sexually transmitted infection, is provided to their adolescent child, it would encourage early initiation to intimate sexual behaviors. Finally, people may underestimate their risk for contracting a disease, which can prevent them from seeking immunizations.

In Developing Countries

Although many developing countries have achieved impressive child immunization rates, other countries fail to meet their vaccination goals. Although providing vaccine coverage costs relatively little, logistical issues can present a significant hurdle. Several types of vaccines must be refrigerated at all times, a feat that is difficult to accomplish in areas without electricity. In countries with large rural populations, poor infrastructure and a lack of roads pose problems to developing consistent supply chains. Many developing countries also suffer from a huge shortage of healthcare workers, which serves as a bottleneck to expanding vaccine coverage.

🔍 CASE REPORT

The Anti-Vaccine Movement

In 1998, many people in a region in southwest Wales refused to vaccinate their children for measles, fearing that the vaccine caused autism. Even after the autism link was disproven, resistance to the vaccine continued. Eventually, this refusal to vaccinate children caught up with the community; between November 2012 and July 2013, there were 1,219 cases of measles in this region. In the remainder of Wales, where vaccination had been accepted, there were a total of 105 cases of measles in all of 2011.

1. With regard to this scenario, explain what is meant by herd immunity.
2. Where was the reservoir for measles that fueled this re-emergence?
3. How robust is the measles vaccine?
4. From a public health perspective, what would you do to address this problem?

Key Terms

Active immunity	Cell-mediated immunity	Incidence
Adaptive immunity	Epitopes	Innate immunity
Adjuvants	Herd immunity	Passive immunity
Antibodies	Humoral immunity	Toxoid
Antigens	Immunity	Vaccination
Attenuation	Immunization	Vaccine

Discussion Questions

1. Why must individuals be inoculated against influenza every year?
2. How would you develop an immune globulin for passive protection of someone exposed to rabies?
3. What are the impediments to creating a vaccine for the common cold?
4. How are the Sabin and Salk polio vaccines different? Why does the U.S.-recommended immunization schedule no longer include the Sabin vaccine?

5. Develop a timeline showing changes in the U.S. immunization schedule over the last 30 years.

6. How does the U.S. immunization schedule differ from the schedules of other developed nations?

7. Despite evidence that immunizations are a cost-effective means of preventing specific infectious diseases, many people do not receive the recommended immunizations. Discuss possible reasons for the resistance to vaccination. Suggest means for overcoming these obstacles and for increasing the percentage of the immunized population.

References

1. World Health Organization. *Global Alliance for Vaccines and Immunization (GAVI): Fact Sheet No. 169*. Geneva, Switzerland: WHO; March 2005. Available at http://www.who.int/mediacentre/factsheets/fs169/en/. Accessed May 12, 2017.

2. United Nations Children's Fund (UNICEF). *Immunize Every Child: GAVI Strategy for Immunization Services*. New York, NY: UNICEF; February 2000. Available at https://www.unicef.org/chinese/immunization/files/immunize_every_child.pdf. Accessed May 12, 2017.

3. Office of Disease Prevention and Health Promotion, U.S. Department of Health and Human Services. *Healthy People 2020: 2020 Topics & Objectives: Immunization and Infectious Diseases*. Washington, DC: DHHS. Available at https://www.healthypeople.gov/2020/topics-objectives/topic/immunization-and-infectious-diseases/objectives. Accessed May 12, 2017.

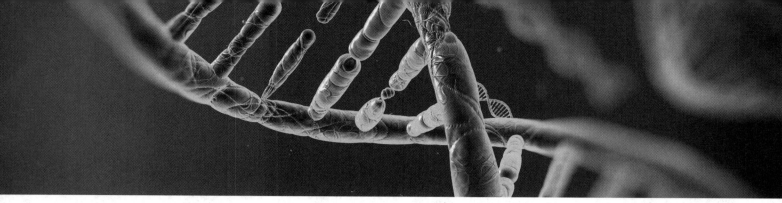

CHAPTER 5

Genetics in Public Health

Julie A. DeLoia

LEARNING OBJECTIVES

By the end of this chapter, the student will be able to:

- Describe the basic properties of DNA
- List the types of genetic mutations
- Explain the connection between genotype and phenotype
- Differentiate between mutation and normal variation
- Distinguish inheritance patterns of simple Mendelian genetics from multifactorial disorders
- List the goals of the Human Genome Project
- Apply the outcomes of the Human Genome Project to multifactorial disorders and public health

CHAPTER OUTLINE

▶ Introduction

The Human Genome Project (HGP), a global research effort to understand genetic factors in human disease, elevated the field of genetics from the domain of the subspecialist to the realm of public health. Molecular technology is now being used not only to identify specific deoxyribonucleic acid (DNA) sequence changes in single-gene disorders, but also to interrogate diseased tissues in the hope of developing specific and targeted therapy, and to provide patients with an individual prognosis. Current technologies, combined with an explosion in bioinformatics, have enabled research teams to begin the discovery process of identifying those genetic factors that put us at **risk** for developing complex diseases, helping clinicians to prescribe the most appropriate drug for any one person and to track outbreaks of infectious diseases. With these advances also come challenges, especially around issues of privacy, accessibility, and ownership of the information. Despite these challenges, most people now have at least some awareness that genetic information is more readily obtainable and being used in ever-increasing ways. This chapter will provide a high-level review of basic concepts of inheritance, as well as an introduction to the post-genomic era.

Basic Properties of DNA

DNA is the storage system in our cells that codes for all of the proteins that our bodies will ever use. The DNA molecule consists of a long strand of a 5-carbon deoxyribose alternating with a phosphate group. Four nitrogenous bases—thymine, adenine, guanine, and cytosine—provide the identity of the molecule. All of the information is stored in the sequence of these bases, a system that is both simple and elegant.

Within the cell, the DNA exists as a double strand, pairing with another DNA strand that has a complementary sequence, and bound by simple hydrogen bonds (**FIGURE 5-1**). The complete set of human DNA, known as the **genome**, contains approximately 3 billion base pairs.

Within these 3 billion-plus bases, the DNA is organized into discreet functional units, the **gene**. Genes can code for proteins or a variety of ribonucleic acid (RNA) molecules. The current estimate of the number of protein-coding genes in humans is around 20,000, which comprises less than 2% of all nuclear DNA. The remainder of the DNA codes for RNA molecules, regulatory sequences, repetitive sequences (used in DNA fingerprinting), and sequences of unknown function.

As mentioned, the gene-encoded proteins provide both form and function to the cell. The constellation of proteins produced in any given cell determines the identity and functions of that cell. Consequently, different cell types will have a unique set of genes expressed at any time. In order for the information contained within the nuclear DNA to be processed, or translated, into a protein, a portion of the genome is first transcribed to a messenger RNA molecule, processed, and then exported from the nucleus to the cytoplasm. Researchers interested in studying gene expression in cells isolate this exported RNA, the sum of which is known as the **exome**. Because exomes represent less than 1.5% of the genome and provide key insights into function, they can be sequenced much more readily than the entire genome. Exome sequencing is being used to identify genetic causes of both common diseases, such as Alzheimer's disease,[1] and rare genetic disorders, such as Miller syndrome.[2] Exome sequencing is also beginning to be used clinically for diagnosis, treatment choices, and sometimes, for prognosis.[3]

Inheritance

We owe much of our thinking about inheritance today to Gregor Mendel (1822–1884), an Augustinian monk and contemporary of Charles Darwin. Mendel spent several years breeding pea plants with different physical characteristics. Through detailed observation and meticulous note taking, he developed his ideas related to how physical traits are passed from one generation to the next—what we now know as inheritance. His work, which was first presented in 1865, went against the current thinking of the time and was largely ignored until the early 1900s, when it was rediscovered and began to be appreciated. His two most important conclusions, now known as Mendel's laws, were the Law of Segregation and the Law of Independent Assortment. The Law of

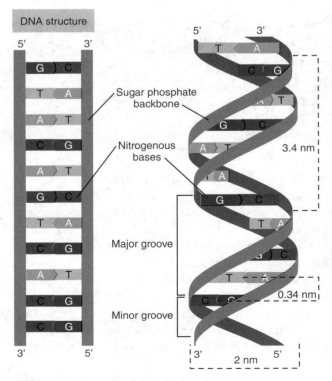

DNA structure

5'   3'

Sugar phosphate backbone

Nitrogenous bases

3.4 nm

Major groove

0.34 nm

Minor groove

2 nm

FIGURE 5-1 Diagram of DNA Molecule

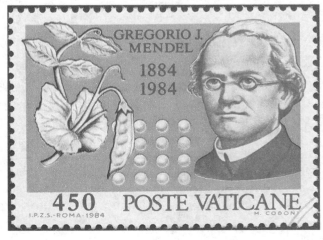

GREGORIO J. MENDEL
1884
1984

450   POSTE VATICANE

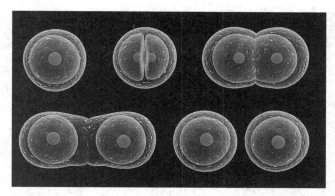

© Lukiyanova Natalia frenta/Shutterstock

Segregation states that every individual carries two copies (**alleles**) for any particular trait and that these alleles separate during cell division, with one copy going to one daughter cell and the other copy going to the other daughter cell. The implication was that within each offspring, one copy of a particular gene was (randomly) provided by the first parent and the other copy was (randomly) provided by the second. Mendel's second law (the Law of Independent Assortment) stated that two unrelated traits, such as peapod shape and flower color, segregate independently when passed from parent to offspring.

From Mendel, we also got the concepts of dominant, recessive, heterozygous, and homozygous. **Dominant** and **recessive** refer to the relationship of each allele to the other and zygosity refers to the identities of the two copies; if both alleles are the same, the individual is said to be **homozygous** at that locus, while if two different alleles are at a given locus, the individual is said to be **heterozygous**. **Hemizygous** refers to the unique situation of the sex chromosomes. The X chromosome is one of the largest chromosomes in the genome. Because females have two X chromosomes, they can be either heterozygous or homozygous for genes on the X. However, because males have only one X chromosome, they have only one copy of each gene on the X chromosome and are considered to be hemizygous for such alleles.

When Mendel performed his experiments, he chose only traits that had binary, or discontinuous, characteristics. He largely ignored the continuous (or quantitative) traits. We now recognize that most of these quantitative traits are impacted by more than one gene and oftentimes involve environmental factors. Such traits are known as **multifactorial** because many factors, both genetic and nongenetic, influence the final presentation of the trait.

▶ Human Genome Project

The Department of Energy and the National Institutes of Health began the HGP in 1990 (see **BOX 5-1** and **BOX 5-2**) with the goal of understanding all the genes that make

up humans. The project remains one of the largest and most collaborative scientific endeavors ever attempted. It could also be argued that the HGP was an extremely risky project for several reasons: (1) at the time, the technology for high-throughput sequencing was inadequate to support the scientific goals of the HGP; (2) the available **bioinformatics** was completely underdeveloped to store, organize, and analyze the data that were to be generated; and (3) perhaps most controversial, the data generated from the HGP had the potential to be misconstrued or misused in marginalized populations. Given these challenges and the enormity of the project, it should not be surprising that it took almost 5 years of discussion and argument before consensus was found on how to proceed.

The output of the HGP spawned numerous technologies, new fields of study, and even new industries. Because of the HGP, we can diagnose many diseases more accurately using molecular profiling (e.g., the Lymphoma/Leukemia Molecular Profiling Project [llmpp.nih.gov]); we are able to identify individuals at risk for specific diseases such as breast cancer (e.g., using new screening tests such as OncoVue®); and using a pharmacogenomics approach, we can prescribe treatment with better efficacy and fewer negative outcomes, though adoption of these new tests has been slow.[4] The use of companion diagnostic testing helps identify patients who are most likely to benefit or be harmed by a specific drug.[5] The U.S. Food and Drug Administration oversees this type of genetic testing and maintains a list of approved companion tests on its website.[6] Through the private sector, individuals can learn about their personal genetic history or potential

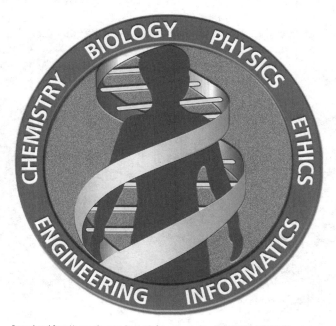

BOX 5-1   The Human Genome Project

Formally funded in 1990, the $3 billion undertaking was projected to be complete in 15 years. In addition to the United States, the consortium also included scientists from the United Kingdom, France, Australia, and China. The project was declared "complete" in April 2003, 2 years ahead of schedule. The stated goals of the HGP were to:

1. Sequence all 3 billion DNA base pairs of the human genome
2. Identify all of the genes in the human genome
3. Sequence model organisms important to medical research
4. Develop new bioinformatics tools
5. Make this information readily available to the public and private sectors
6. Address the ethical, legal, and social implications that may arise from the project

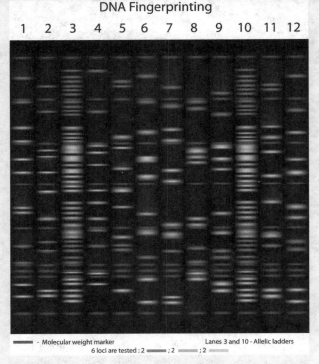

DNA Fingerprinting

1 2 3 4 5 6 7 8 9 10 11 12

━━━ - Molecular weight marker   Lanes 3 and 10 - Allelic ladders
6 loci are tested : 2 ━━━ ; 2 ━━━ ; 2 ━━━

© Alila Medical Media/Shutterstock

Data from National Institutes of Health. National Human Genome Research Institute (NHGRI). Available at https://www.genome.gov. Accessed October 30, 2017.

BOX 5-2   Ethical, Legal, and Social Implications Program

The Ethical, Legal, and Social Implications (ELSI) Program was launched in 1990 as an integral part of the HGP. Through the National Institutes of Health Revitalization Act of Congress in 1993, it was mandated that "not less than" 5% of the NIH Human Genome Project budget be set aside for research on the ethical, legal, and social implications of genomic science. It remains the only dedicated extramural bioethics research program at the NIH. The program's research priorities fall into four broad categories, as shown below.[7] The reason for committing significant long-term resources to ELSI stemmed from the fact that the planners of the HGP realized that the data generated from this project could have profound implications for individuals, families, and entire populations. Thus, ELSI was put in place to protect people from misuse of genomic information. The National Human Genome Research Institute commits more than $18 million annually to ELSI research.

Genomic Research

The issues that arise in the design and conduct of genomic research, particularly as it increasingly involves the production, analysis, and broad sharing of individual genomic information that is frequently coupled with detailed health information.

Genomic Health Care

How rapid advances in genomic technologies and the availability of increasing amounts of genomic information influence how health care is provided and how it affects the health of individuals, families, and communities.

Broader Societal Issues

The normative underpinnings of beliefs, practices, and policies regarding genomic information and technologies, as well as the implications of genomics for how we conceptualize and understand such issues as health, disease, and individual responsibility.

Legal, Regulatory, and Public Policy Issues

The effects of existing genomic research, health and public policies and regulations, and the development of new policies and regulatory approaches.

Data from McEwen JE, Boyer JT, Sun KY, Rothernberg KH, Lockhart NC, Guyer MS. The ethical, legal, and social implications program of the National Human Genome Research Institute: reflections on an ongoing experiment. *Ann Rev Genomics Hum Genet.* 2014;15:481-505. doi: 10.1146/annurev-genom-090413-025327.

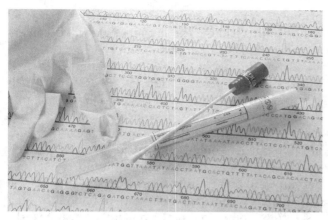

© Henrik Dolle/Shutterstock

risk factors via direct-to-consumer (DTC) genetic testing. Much of this progress has come as we have learned more about normal genetic variation.

▶ Genetic Variation

Unless you are an identical twin, there is no one in the world genetically just like you. With the completion of the HGP and the development of high throughput and rapid sequencing, it is now possible and affordable to sequence individuals. Whole genome analyses, or complete sequencing of an individual, are being conducted for diagnosis of individuals with both rare and common disorders such as autism spectrum disorder,[8] for risk assessment on patient populations,[9] and for prediction of patient outcomes following therapy.[10] These genome-wide association studies allow identification of genetic similarities between unrelated people who share similar **phenotypes** or clinical outcomes.

The fundamental unit of **genetic variation** in humans is the **single nucleotide polymorphism (SNP)**. One of the surprises from the HGP was the discovery that, as a species, we are quite similar. In fact, any two people on the planet selected at random are about 99.9% identical at the genetic level. These single nucleotide differences are what give any individual his or her unique genetic and biologic characteristics. The majority of these SNPs are found in the regions of DNA between genes and have little or nothing to do with functional differences. However, some SNPs are located within coding regions or in a regulatory region of a gene. These SNPs are proving useful to determine who might respond appropriately or poorly to a drug, who might be susceptible to a specific infectious agent, and who could be most impacted by an environmental toxin. Millions of these SNPs have now been catalogued and are available through open access sites, such as http://www.ncbi.nlm .nih.gov/projects/SNP/. Unlike Mendelian-type mutations, which have a strong correlation between the **genotype** of a person and the expression of the related trait (high **penetrance**) and are generally rare in the population, SNPs are much more common in the population, but have a much lower correlation to any one phenotype. SNPs may be included as a liability in the threshold model of disease, which posits that multifactorial diseases occur when an individual accumulates enough genetic and environmental factors to cause a disease. An example of a multifactorial disease is diabetes mellitus, a dichotomous trait. A person either has diabetes or does not. But the pathway to developing diabetes is influenced by genetic, environmental, and even economic factors. By cataloging genetic variation common among thousands of people who have type 2 diabetes, it has been possible to establish associations between genetic loci and type 2 diabetes.[11] With an estimated global burden of diabetes approaching 350 million,[12] being able to identify those at risk could support targeted behavioral modification to prevent disease onset. (See **BOX 5-3**.)

▶ Direct-to-Consumer Testing

As noted, one goal of the HGP was to make genetic information accessible to both private and public sectors. An offshoot of this goal was the significant growth of DTC genetic tests. Most of these tests are performed in laboratories that receive samples from home collections. The sample can be a blood sample, a swab from the inside of your cheek, or saliva. No physician's prescription is required. Currently there are about two dozen laboratories that will perform dozens of DTC tests. "Tests" can

---

BOX 5-3 The 1000 Genomes Project

The 1000 Genomes Project (www.internationalgenome.org) is an international collaborative project with the goal of finding the most common genetic variants in humans. There are over 2,500 samples that are being sequenced from East Asia, South Asia, Africa, Europe, and the Americas. Data from the 1000 Genomes Project will be made available through open-access databases. Projected uses of the data include:

1. Discovery of regions of the genome that are associated with a specific disease or trait
2. Cataloging all the genetic variants in these disease-associated regions
3. Investigating population structures and natural selection

Data from The International Genome Sample Resource. About IGSR and the 1000 Genomes Project. Available at http://www.1000genomes.org/about. Accessed October 30, 2017.

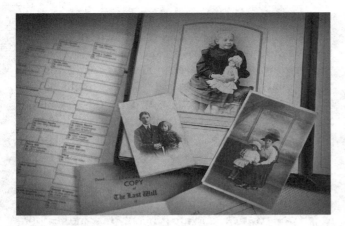

© Andrew Bret Wallis/DigialVision/Getty

include providing an assessment of risk for a particular disease, such as heart disease, cancer, or diabetes; ascertaining disease or carrier status; how a person's body will respond to prescribed drugs; or even how someone will withstand certain environmental exposures. These DTC tests are also available for nonmedical purposes, such as to establish paternity or ancestry.

Proponents of DTC genetic tests have cited privacy and personal empowerment as major reasons for supporting this option. Genetic information is highly charged and many people prefer to learn about their "genetic liability" without their doctor or insurer having that information. As well, knowing that you are at risk for certain diseases will hopefully inspire proactive behavioral changes. The relatively low cost and ease of access are also major drivers for this industry. In addition, some DTC companies provide significant patient education materials through the testing process, and commercial advertising for DTC tests has helped to raise public awareness. The current regulations regarding DTC testing are variable from state to state, and as such, it is difficult to ensure the same quality as a Clinical Laboratory Improvement Amendments-certified laboratory.

Opponents of DTC testing have raised concerns that patients can easily misinterpret the test results, especially when the test is about risk prediction and not actual diagnosis. It is also easy for patients to feel a false sense of "safety" if no genetic risk is found for a particular disease, with the potential to make poor health behavior choices. Finally, opponents believe that anyone who receives genetic test results would benefit from discussion with a physician or genetic counselor. Genetic counseling is the process of providing information to individuals and their relatives who may be at risk for an inherited disorder. Genetic counselors discuss genetic risks and advise clients on the nature and consequences of disorders for which they are at risk (for themselves or of passing to their children), the probability of developing or transmitting the disorder, and the options open to them with regard to disease management and family

planning. As genetic testing becomes even more widely available, the field of genetic counseling will become a mainstay of public health practice.

Given the public interest in obtaining personal genetic information and the relative ease with which people can obtain such tests, it is hard to imagine that DTC tests will go away. Consequently, instead of arguing whether or not DTC testing should exist, greater positive impact could be achieved by ensuring high standards of DNA testing, uniformity in regulations pertaining to DTC testing, and more education for the general public about the value and limitations of such test results. Some would call upon public health workers to provide the surveillance that is perhaps necessary with such technology available.

▶ Public Health Relevance

With the rapid genetic technology advances leading to significant insights into factors impacting human health, the intersection of genomics and public health continues to expand. The Centers for Disease Control and Prevention recognized this convergence early and formed the Office of Public Health Genomics (OPHG) in 1997.[13] OPHG has served the public by "identifying, evaluating, and implementing evidence-based genomics practices to prevent and control the country's leading chronic, infectious, environmental, and occupational diseases." Genomics is now playing a key role in many of the 10 essential public health services, especially in the domain of assessment, but also in policy development and quality assurance as well (**FIGURE 5-2**).

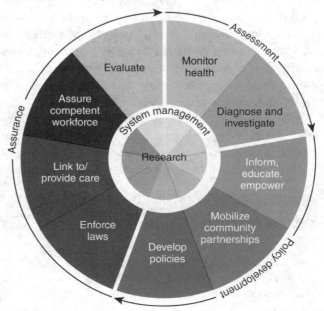

FIGURE 5-2 The Public Health Wheel

Reproduced from Centers for Disease Control and Prevention. State, Tribal, Local & Territorial Public Health Professionals Gateway: National Public Health Performance Standards. Updated September 19, 2017. Available at http://www.cdc.gov/nphpsp/essentialServices.html. Accessed October 30, 2017.

TABLE 5-1 Integration of Genetics and Public Health

Public Health Service	Genetics-Related Goal
Monitor health status of the community to identify community health problems	Identify opportunities to include genetic information in existing health programs
Diagnose health hazards and investigate health programs in the community	Identify genetic risk factors that will increase opportunities for early intervention, reduction of disease burden, and primary prevention
Inform, educate, and empower people about health issues	Inform the public and policy makers about genetics and its impact on health
Mobilize community partnerships at state and local levels to identify and solve health problems	Establish effective communication with community members regarding genetic issues
Develop and support policies and practices that encourage individual and community health efforts	Create a strategic plan to integrate genetics into public health practice and policies
Enforce regulations that protect health and ensure safety for community members	Provide guidance for public health genetic policies
Link people to health services, including genetic services, and assure the provision of health care when otherwise unavailable	Ensure the availability of high-quality, clinically valid genetic tests
Assure a public healthcare workforce competent in genetics	Create and maintain a competent genetics-aware public health workforce
Evaluate effectiveness, accessibility, and quality of personal and population-based health services, including genetics	Research, review, and evaluate the clinical utility and validity of genetic tests
Conduct research to obtain new insights and innovative solutions to health problems	Ensure that up-to-date genetic information is incorporated into the public health infrastructure

Data from Aswini YB, Varun S. Genetics in public health: Rarely explored. *Indian J Human Genet*. 2010;16(2):47-54. doi:10.4103/0971-6866.69326.

Genomics has enabled a deeper understanding of health risks and has provided methods and technology to monitor the public's health, and to investigate gene–environment interactions. Use of molecular technologies has enabled timely identification of health threats, such as the identification of the source of cholera during the 2013 Haiti outbreak,[14] and is now being evaluated for efficacy in monitoring the safety of our food supply.[15,16] The growth in diagnostic services and laboratory capacity also contributes to monitoring the health of populations and supports development of response plans to major health threats. We are learning more and more about susceptibility to infectious agents such as HIV[17] and, through whole-genome analyses, gaining crucial insights into pathological mechanisms that should provide more therapeutic targets.

Integrating genetics into public health policy and practice can be accomplished through areas identified by Aswini and Varun (2010)[18] with related goals, shown in **TABLE 5-1**.

Key Terms

Alleles	Genome	Penetrance
Bioinformatics	Genotype	Phenotype
Dominant	Hemizygous	Recessive
Exome	Heterozygous	Risk
Gene	Homozygous	Single nucleotide
Genetic variation	Multifactorial	polymorphism (SNP)

Discussion Questions

1. Explain the difference between normal variation and genetic mutation.
2. How would the environment impact a multifactorial trait like height in someone with normal genetic variation? How would environment impact someone with a mutation that results in dwarfism?
3. A normal genetic variation in the GST-1 gene has been found in 7% of a study population. People who carry two copies of this variant are 5 times more likely to develop lung cancer if they smoke a pack of cigarettes per day than people who have no copies of the variant. How could this information be used to talk about risk to this person?
4. The GST-1 variant can best be described as _____ prevalence and _____ penetrance.
5. The National Collegiate Athletic Association (NCAA) now screens all Division I and II athletes for sickle cell trait. How do you feel about testing for sickle cell anemia at birth vs. testing for the trait as a young adult?
6. Does the NCAA testing policy discriminate against athletes with the sickle cell trait? Does it discriminate based on race or ethnicity?

References

1. Reitz C. Genetic diagnosis and prognosis of Alzheimer's disease: challenges and opportunities. *Expert Rev Mol Diagn.* 2015;15(3):339-348. doi: 10.1586/14737159.2015.1002469.
2. Ng SB, Buckingham KJ, Lee C, et al. Exome sequencing identifies the cause of a Mendelian disorder. *Nat Genet.* 2010;42(1):30-35. doi: 10.1038/ng.499.
3. Stranneheim H, Wedell A. Exome and genome sequencing: a revolution for the discovery and diagnosis of monogenic disorders. *J Intern Med.* 2016;279:3-15. doi: 10.1111/joim.12399.
4. Cox SL, Zlot AI, Silvey K, et al. Patterns of cancer genetic testing: a randomized survey of Oregon clinicians. *J Cancer Epidemiol.* 2012;2012:294730. doi: 10.1155/2012/294730.
5. Canestaro WJ, Pritchard DE, Garrison LP, Dubois R, Veenstra DL. Improving the efficiency and quality of the value assessment process for companion diagnostic tests: The Companion Test Assessment Tool (CAT). *J Manag Care Spec Pharm.* 2015;21(8):700-712.
6. Food and Drug Administration. List of cleared or approved companion diagnostic devices (in vitro and imaging tools). Available at https://www.fda.gov/medicaldevices /productsandmedicalprocedures/invitrodiagnostics /ucm301431.htm. Accessed October 17, 2017.
7. McEwen JE, Boyer JT, Sun KY, Rothernberg KH, Lockhart NC, Guyer MS. The ethical, legal, and social implications program of the National Human Genome Research Institute: reflections on an ongoing experiment. *Ann Rev Genomics Hum Genet.* 2014;15:481-505. doi: 10.1146/annurev-genom-090413-025327.
8. Tammimies K, Marshall CR, Walker S, et al. Molecular diagnostic yield of chromosomal microarray analysis and whole-exome sequencing in children with autism spectrum disorder. *JAMA.* 2015;314(9):895-903. doi: 10.1001/jama.2015.10078.
9. Danforth DN, Warner AC, Wangsa D, et al. An improved breast epithelial sampling method for molecular profiling and biomarker analysis in women at risk for breast cancer. *Breast Cancer (Auckl).* 2015;9:31-40. doi: 10.4137/BCBCR. S23577.
10. Klco JM, Miller CA, Griffith M, et al. Association between mutation clearance after induction therapy and outcomes in acute myeloid leukemia. *JAMA.* 2015;314(8):811-822. doi: 10.1001/jama.2015.9643.
11. Mohlke KL, Boehnke M. Recent advances in understanding the genetic architecture of type 2 diabetes. *Hum Mol Genet.* 2015;pii: ddv264.
12. Danaei G, Finucane MM, Lin JK, et al.; Global Burden of Metabolic Risk Factors of Chronic Diseases Collaborating Group (Blood Glucose). National, regional, and global trends in fasting plasma glucose and diabetes prevalence since 1980: systematic analysis of health examination surveys and epidemiological studies with 370 country-years and 2.7 million participants. *Lancet.* 2011;378(9785):31-40. doi: 10.1016/S0140-6736(11)60679-X.
13. Centers for Disease Control and Prevention. Public Health Genomics: About Us. Available at http://www.cdc.gov /genomics/about/index.htm. Accessed October 17, 2017.
14. Eppinger M, Pearson T, Koenig SS, et al. Genomic epidemiology of the Haitian cholera outbreak: a single introduction followed by rapid, extensive, and continued spread characterized the onset of the epidemic. *MBio.* 2014;5(6):e01721. doi: 10.1128/mBio.01721-14.
15. Pielaat A, Boer MP, Wijnands LM, et al. First step in using molecular data for microbial food safety risk assessment; hazard identification of Escherichia coli O157:H7 by coupling genomic data with in vitro adherence to human epithelial cells. *Int J Food Microbiol.* 2015;pii: S0168–1605(15)00201-9. doi: 10.1016/j.ijfoodmicro.2015.04.009.
16. Lambert D, Carrillo CD, Koziol AG, Manninger P, Blais BW. GeneSippr: a rapid whole-genome approach for the identification and characterization of foodborne pathogens such as priority Shiga toxigenic Escherichia coli. *PLoS One.* 2015;10(4):e0122928. doi: 10.1371/journal.pone.0122928.
17. McLaren PJ, Carrington M. The impact of host genetic variation on infection with HIV-1. *Nat Immunol.* 2015;16(6):577-583. doi: 10.1038/ni.3147.
18. Aswini YB, Varun S. Genetics in public health: rarely explored. *Indian J Human Genet.* 2010;16(2):47-54. doi: 10.4103/0971-6866.69326.

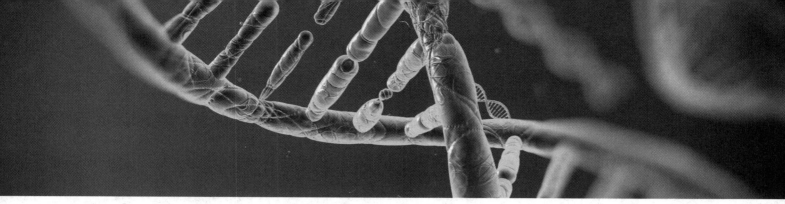

CHAPTER 6

Epigenetics in Human Health and Disease

Julie A. DeLoia

LEARNING OBJECTIVES

By the end of this chapter, the student will be able to:

- Describe the molecular mechanisms of epigenetic modification in humans
- Explain dosage compensation as it relates to the X chromosome
- Provide evidence for the influence of the environment upon the epigenome
- Explain how environmental stress can impact gene expression through generations
- Describe how we use epigenomic changes to monitor the impact of the environment

CHAPTER OUTLINE

▶ Introduction

The human body has multiple mechanisms to respond and adapt to external conditions and needs. The most obvious of these are the basic biochemical mechanisms of homeostasis—the body's immediate response to environmental stressors or challenges. This type of adaptation occurs within an individual and can last minutes to years. At the other end of the spectrum are evolutionary changes that occur over generations as a result of persistent selective pressure on populations. This type of natural selection of traits helps species adapt and survive over time. These changes transcend an individual's lifetime.

This chapter will focus on yet another mechanism of adaptation to the environment called **epigenetic modification**. Epigenetic modification occurs through covalent (molecular) modifications of either deoxyribonucleic acid (DNA) itself or the proteins that form the scaffolding for DNA packaging. Both of these types of molecular adaptations impact gene expression within an individual, *without changing the actual sequence of the DNA*. As a consequence, there can be a change in phenotype (e.g., a person's actual height) without a change in genotype (e.g., the genes for height). Of note, these epigenetic modifications can be passed on to future generations. They are both common and important in human health and thus have public health significance.

Mechanisms of Epigenetic Modification

Epigenetic modification has been shown in numerous taxa, including bacteria, protists, fungi, plants, and animals and via multiple mechanisms.[1] However, this chapter will focus primarily on humans. During formation of the egg and sperm (gametogenesis), regions of the DNA are tagged in accordance with the sex of the parent. These tags, or imprints, result in parent-specific gene expression and are maintained through mitotic divisions. The two most prominent mechanisms for tagging regions of the genome are DNA methylation and histone modification. DNA methylation occurs through transfer of methyl groups directly onto the DNA molecule by a group of highly conserved enzymes called methyltransferases. The sites in the genome that are methylated are not random but rather occur at imprinting control regions. Because the addition of a methyl group does not change the DNA sequence itself, the process can be reversed through demethylation, which can reverse repression of gene expression. It is estimated that approximately 1.5% of human DNA is methylated.[2]

Histones are positively charged proteins that help organize genetic material into higher order structure. DNA, which is negatively charged, wraps around histone proteins much like thread would be wound around a spool. There are several possible post-translational modifications that occur on histone proteins that can impact how tightly the DNA wraps around the histone core and, subsequently, whether or not the transcriptional machinery can access gene promoters. Histone acetylation, the addition of an acetyl group (COCH3), and deacetylation (the removal of the same group) are controlled by the enzyme families known as histone acetyltransferases (HATs) and histone deacetylases (HDACs). Acetylation creates accessible chromatin and allows gene expression, while deacetylation compresses chromatin in such a way that it becomes difficult for the transcription machinery to access promoter regions, with a consequent silencing of genes. In addition to DNA, histones can also be methylated, which mediates chromatin structure. Histone methylation can suppress gene expression, as occurs when lysine residues are methylated on histone H3, or promote gene expression, as occurs when arginine residues are methylated on H3 and H4 proteins.[3]

Most of these post-translational modifications occur on the extended tail of the histone proteins (see **FIGURE 6-1**). Methylation of DNA occurs near promoter regions and interferes with the transcriptional apparatus, thus silencing gene expression. Methylation can also occur on histone proteins and results in chromatin that is difficult to access, with consequent gene silencing. Acetylation of histones has the same impact, while deacetylation opens the chromatin and promotes gene expression.

Epigenetics and Development

There are two drivers of epigenetic modifications; some are established predictably as cells differentiate during development, while other changes occur as adaptations throughout an organism's life in response to both internal and external signals. In the first scenario, epigenetic modifications play a key role in how cells develop their identity. The DNA in every cell in the body, except germ cells, is identical—yet the function and form of different cell types varies dramatically. For example, an epithelial cell is very easy to distinguish from a nerve cell under the microscope. During normal development, cells acquire unique characteristics based on their location within the body and their local environment. By sensing the environment, cells turn on or turn off specific genes—the final result of which is the cell type. As an analogy, the keyboards on any piano are the same; however, the song that you hear will depend on the combination of keys that are pressed. The same is true for cell identity: the genes in each cell are the same, but the cell that emerges will depend on the combination of genes that are expressed. Once a cell is fully developed, it is important that this identity gets "locked in," because the cell has a specific job to do in the body. Epigenetic modification is one method a cell uses to maintain its specific identity and function—by expressing some genes and keeping other genes turned off. Consequently, much of the epigenetic changes that occur during development persist throughout an individual's life.

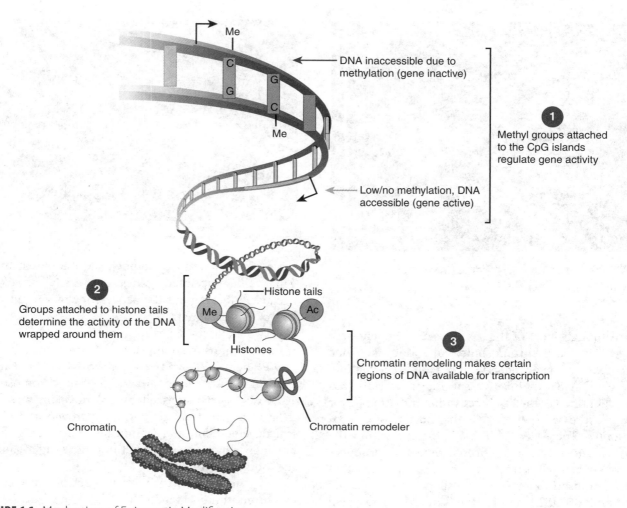

Me

C
G

G
C

Me

DNA inaccessible due to methylation (gene inactive)

Low/no methylation, DNA accessible (gene active)

1 Methyl groups attached to the CpG islands regulate gene activity

2 Groups attached to histone tails determine the activity of the DNA wrapped around them

Histone tails

Me

Ac

Histones

3 Chromatin remodeling makes certain regions of DNA available for transcription

Chromatin remodeler

Chromatin

FIGURE 6-1 Mechanism of Epigenetic Modification

Reproduced from Rajender S, Avery K, Agarwal A. Epigenetics, spermatogenesis and male infertility. *Mutat Res*. 2011;727(3):62-71.

One of the early examples of developmentally important epigenetic modification is inactivation of the X chromosome. In mammals, the two genders are distinguished by the sex chromosomes; males have one X and one Y chromosome, while females have two X chromosomes. The Y chromosome is much smaller in size than the X chromosome and holds only about 70 protein-encoding genes, 95% of which are male-specific.[4] These genes are critical for sex determination; without a Y chromosome, an organism will be female. In contrast, the X chromosome is much larger than the Y chromosome and represents approximately 800 protein-coding genes, of a total of 20,000–25,000 genes in the human genome. The majority of the genes on the X chromosome have little to do with sex determination but rather are important for a variety of cell functions.

To compensate for the difference in the number of X chromosomes between males and females, one of the X chromosomes is randomly and permanently inactivated early in embryonic development. This process is known as **X chromosome inactivation** or Lyonization (for Mary Lyon, who first discovered X inactivation in 1961). As a consequence of Lyonization, all female mammals are **mosaics**. An example of X inactivation can be seen readily in calico cats, which have white fur with patches of orange and black fur. The gene for fur pigmentation is located on the X chromosome. Variants of the gene produce either black or orange color fur. Early in development, one of the X chromosomes gets shut off, leaving only one coat-color gene active. Depending on which chromosome is left active, either an orange or black color results. Once chromosome inactivation occurs, all the cells that result down the lineage from mitosis will have the same X chromosome inactive. We see the end result as a cat that has patches of orange and black fur; the patches are the lineage of the original cell that had an X inactivated (**FIGURE 6-2**).

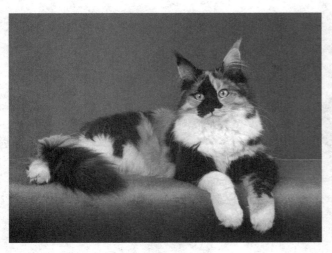

FIGURE 6-2 X-Inactivation Produces Characteristic Calico Pattern in Cats
© Linn Currie/Shutterstock

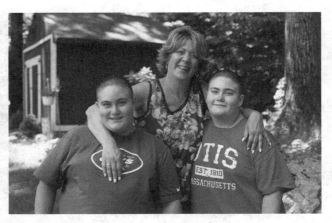

© Ruaridh Connellan/BarcroftImages/Barcroft Media via Getty Images

Although most of the sex-determining genes are located on the Y chromosome, the X does have one very important gene that is required for X inactivation. The gene, *XIST* (X-inactive specific transcript), has been identified as the key inactivation initiation factor and is expressed only in cells that have two X chromosomes. The RNA from *XIST* remains within the nucleus and "coats" the chromosome that produces it, which in turn attracts a variety of proteins that silence transcription. The gene silencing that occurs as a result of *XIST* transcription is quickly propagated along the entire X chromosome at sites known as X inactivation centers. To "lock in" gene silencing, chromosomes marked by *XIST* RNA are methylated. Thus, the transcriptional repression is maintained through cellular divisions.[5] See **BOX 6-1**.

▶ Genomic Imprinting

For reasons that remain unknown, there are some genes in the genome that are expressed on only one copy, even though two copies of that gene are present. Which copy of the gene is active depends on which parent passed on that gene. For example, some genes are expressed only when they are inherited from the father (paternally expressed), while others are expressed only from the maternally inherited copy. This phenomenon of specific gene silencing dependent on the parent of origin of that locus is known as **genomic imprinting** and results in **monoallelic expression** (expression of a singular allele). There are approximately 100 imprinted genes in the human genome (www.geneimprint.com/site/home). Most of these genes are in functional networks related to

growth and neural development. Mutations in these genetically imprinted genes are easily observed, because knocking out the active copy will result in a lack of gene product.

Two well-characterized syndromes that result from mutations in an imprinted region of the genome are Prader-Willi syndrome (PWS) and Angelman syndrome (AS). Both are located on chromosome 15. PWS is characterized by cognitive impairment, delayed motor development, poor growth and physical development, and significant and unusual food cravings, which usually result in rapid weight gain in the toddler period.

The mutation for PWS involves deletion of a region on chromosome 15 that includes the gene *SNRPN*, but the phenotype is apparent only when the mutation is inherited from the father. In the same region of the chromosome lies the root cause for AS, a phenotype seen only when the mutation comes from the mother. Children with AS can be misdiagnosed with cerebral palsy or autism due to lack of speech, seizures, significant developmental delay, and balance disorders. The gene for AS is *UBE31A*, which is expressed only on the maternal allele. Noteworthy is the observation that both of these syndromes involve neurologic impairment.

▶ The Dynamic Epigenome

For a long time, the study of imprinting was primarily in the domain of developmental biologists who were attempting to decipher the mechanism of cell determination. It remained unknown whether epigenetic patterns were static or continued to change over time. An early demonstration that the epigenome changed over time was through the study of **monozygotic** twins. Although monozygotic twins share identical genotypes, most have obvious phenotypic differences, including physical appearance and susceptibility to various diseases. In their landmark

BOX 6-1 Sex Chromosome Disorders and the Pseudoautosomal Region

About 1 in 400 infants will be born with an abnormal number of chromosomes, known as sex chromosome **aneuploidy** (SCA).[6] Unlike aneuploidies of non-sex chromosomes, or autosomes, SCA is generally compatible with life, and many individuals with SCA go undiagnosed. The most commonly occurring SCAs are Turner syndrome (45X), XXX females, Klinefelter syndrome (47 XXY), and XYY males. Turner syndrome has the most pronounced phenotype, characterized by short stature, a lack of female secondary sexual characteristics, and infertility. Some females with Turner syndrome also have mild mental retardation. Women with three X chromosomes are normal in appearance and are fertile. They may experience slight learning difficulties and are often taller than average.[7] Klinefelter syndrome is the most common SCA, affecting approximately 1 in 600 males.[8] Males with Klinefelter syndrome are tall, have low levels of testosterone related to hypogonadism, are infertile, and have incompletely developed secondary male sex characteristics. Males carrying an extra Y chromosome (XYY) are phenotypically normal males, though many are taller than average and have acne due to a higher level of testosterone. Most are unaware that they have an extra Y chromosome and fertility is normal. While individuals with SCA have far less severe phenotypes than other autosomal aneuploidies, there is a correlation with extra X chromosomes and learning. In fact, in individuals with additional X chromosomes, IQ is lowered by about 15 points with each additional X chromosome (48, XXXY; 49, XXXXY).[9]

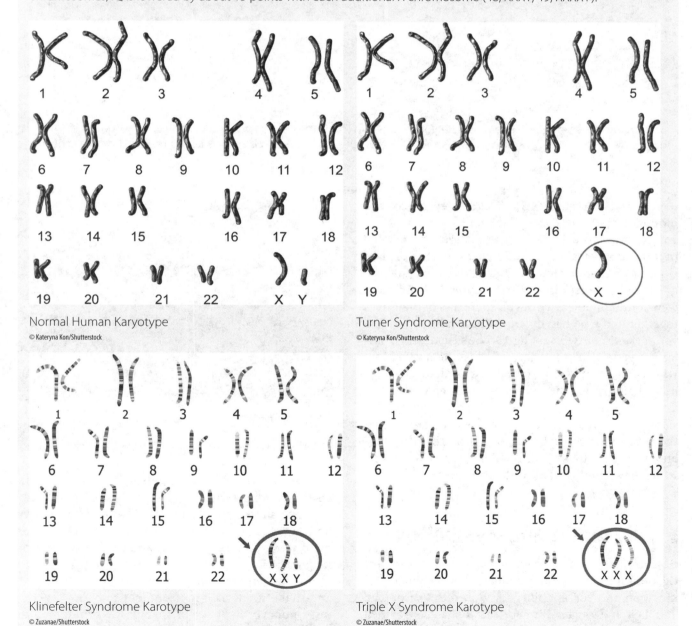

Normal Human Karyotype
© Kateryna Kon/Shutterstock

Turner Syndrome Karyotype
© Kateryna Kon/Shutterstock

Klinefelter Syndrome Karotype
© Zuzanae/Shutterstock

Triple X Syndrome Karotype
© Zuzanae/Shutterstock

(continues)

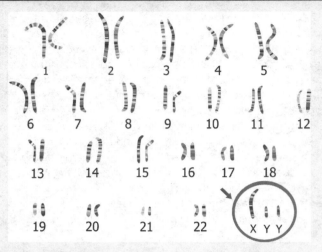

XYY Syndrome Karotype
© Zuzanae/Shutterstock

These observations raise the question of why there is any phenotype associated with extra X chromosomes if all extra X chromosomes are inactivated. The reason for the phenotype lies in the finding that even on the inactive X, not all of the genes are silenced. This is particularly true at the ends of the chromosome, in an area called the pseudoautosomal regions. Genes in this region of the X chromosome are also present on the Y chromosome, so that both males and females have two active copies of these genes, many of which are needed for normal development.

paper, Fraga et al. (2005) provided evidence that monozygotic twins can differ significantly in their epigenome—both in DNA methylation and histone modification—leading to differences in gene expression.[10] Most interesting was the observation that the greatest differences in the epigenomes of twin pairs were found in older twins who spent less of their lives together and who had divergent health histories. The youngest set of twins, at age 3 years, had very similar patterns of methylation and histone acetylation, while older twins who shared less of their environment had greater differences in their epigenomes.[10] These results supported the idea that gene expression is impacted by changes in the epigenome, that the epigenome changes over time, and that the epigenome seems to be impacted by external factors, which have implications for health and disease.

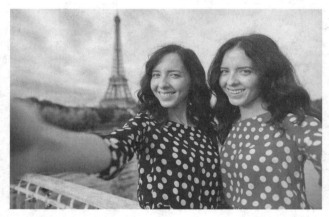

© Ekaterina Pokrovsky/Shutterstock

▶ Epigenetics and Metabolism

Both animal studies and human epidemiologic investigations have shown strong linkage between maternal nutrition and susceptibility to adult-onset disorders. The Dutch Hunger Winter (see **BOX 6-2**) provided a rare opportunity to evaluate the impact of severe calorie restriction on a population in an industrialized, modern country.

Overnutrition during fetal development can also have long-term, negative consequences. Studies have shown that mammals exposed to obesity and overnutrition (diabetes) *in utero* have greater birth weight, more fat tissue, and greater weight for height during childhood than offspring of healthy mothers,[13] and the long-term effects of the obese and diabetic uterine environment may not emerge until puberty in these offspring. Maternal glucose freely crosses the placenta; however, maternal

BOX 6-2 The Dutch Hunger Winter

Near the end of World War II, during the winter of 1944–1945, a convergence of events left the northern part of the Netherlands cut off from food sources. By the summer of 1944, allied troops had finally broken through German lines and advanced quickly through France, Luxembourg, and Belgium and the southern part of the Netherlands. However, retaking control of the northern part of the Netherlands, which held major population centers, proved to be more difficult, as the Germans retained control of the bridge across the Rhine River at Arnhem, thus slowing the move north.

At the same time, the Dutch government-in-exile called for a strike of the railways in support of the allies. In retaliation, the Germans stopped all food transport into the region. When the embargo was lifted in November of 1944, it was too late to transport food, as the canals and waterways, critical for water transport of food from the east, had frozen due to an exceptionally harsh and early winter. As a consequence, a population area of approximately 4.5 million suffered extreme food shortage over a period of several months.

In October of 1944, adult rations were about 1,400 calories; by late November, this fell to below 1,000 calories per day. During the worst of the famine, from December 1944 to April 1945, the official daily allotment for adults was between 400–800 calories. The liberation of the Netherlands finally arrived in early May of 1945, and by June 1945, rations were once again to 2,000 calories per day. Thousands of people died from malnutrition during this time, yet affected women continued to conceive and give birth. The children conceived during this period of extreme calorie restriction provided a unique opportunity to study the effects of maternal malnutrition during different stages of gestation.

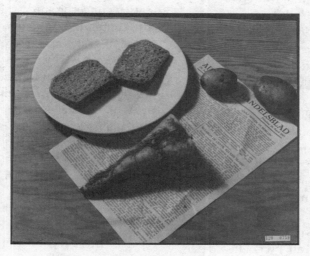

Lemaire, Frits / Anefo, Dutch National Archives / Rijksvoorringingsdienst Eigen, CC0

Children who were conceived during this defined time period were small for gestational age, and as adults experienced up to twice the risk of cardiovascular disease, suffered from higher rates of obesity and high blood pressure, and had overall higher rates of illness, as evidenced by hospitalization rates.[11] These observations provided evidence that conditions during gestation can impact health later in life. Children born to the adults who were nutritionally deprived *in utero* were also found to be small for gestational age, indicating that gestational effects can be transmitted to at least two generations.[12]

insulin does not, thus requiring the fetus to produce additional insulin to clear the high levels of glucose. As a consequence, the increased insulin produced serves as a fetal growth hormone promoting growth and adiposity. Babies are born heavy and are on their way to metabolic imbalance from a very early age. It is for these reasons that it is very important to monitor and control weight gain during pregnancy. A woman who enters pregnancy underweight should gain more weight during pregnancy (28–40 pounds) than a woman who enters pregnancy significantly overweight (11–20 pounds).

▶ Early Chemical Exposures and Long-Term Consequences

Nutrition in the fetal and early postnatal periods is not the only environmental stressor that has been linked to adult diseases through epigenetic modification. A growing body of literature provides compelling data on the link between chemical exposures during early development and later disease. An early example of this link was found in women with high-risk pregnancies who were treated with diethylstilbestrol (DES) to prevent miscarriages. DES, an **endocrine disruptor**, was used between 1938 and 1971 to treat between 5 and 10 million pregnant women. In 1971, the U.S. Food and Drug Administration (FDA) advised physicians to stop prescribing DES because it was observed that a small number of female children born of mothers treated with DES developed a rare form of vaginal cancer. Approximately one in every 1,000 women exposed to DES *in utero* later developed clear cell adenocarcinoma. In addition, women exposed *in utero* also had a greater risk of developing breast cancer after age 40.[14] Additional studies demonstrated an even stronger link between DES exposure *in utero* and the development of more benign problems, including reduced fertility, reproductive organ dysfunction, and some immune function problems.[15] Males exposed i*n utero* were not immune to developmental abnormalities, with a two-fold higher prevalence of both undescended testicles and epididymal cysts.[16] Data also showed consequences of children of females exposed to DES *in utero*, suggesting that the DNA in the eggs of the developing females could be affected by exposure.[17] In other words, the grandchildren of the woman who experienced the original exposure were susceptible to consequences. The key point in these studies is that the impact of gestational exposure was not witnessed for years after exposure and could be transmitted to the next generation.

A common prenatal exposure worldwide is cigarette smoke, which contains an estimated 5,000 chemicals, including over 70 known carcinogens.[18] Despite concerted efforts to educate pregnant women about the hazards of smoking, exposure remains a significant public health challenge. According to the Centers for Disease Control and Prevention, health hazards caused by intrauterine cigarette smoke exposure include prematurity, miscarriage, and some birth defects, such as cleft palate. Sudden infant death syndrome has also been associated with smoking during pregnancy. Smokers, in general, have less DNA methylation, suggesting that *in utero* exposure could alter methylation patterns important for cell lineage differentiation. In a study profiling genomic methylation of human fetuses, Chatterton et al. (2017) demonstrated reduced methylation in the brains of cigarette-smoke-exposed fetuses, which could potentially impact cellular differentiation.[19] They were also able to show a delay in expression of genes important in neuronal function, concluding that intrauterine smoke exposure can alter developmentally appropriate DNA methylation patterns in the developing human brain, leading to neurologic damage.

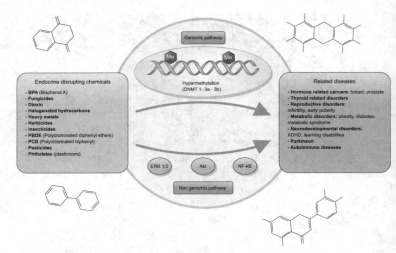

© ellepigrafica/Shutterstock

The pervasive use of plastics in our culture has raised concerns about the safety of phthalates, one of the compounds added to plastics to increase flexibility, durability, and longevity. Phthalates are of concern because they fall into the category of endocrine disruptors, similar to DES. It is estimated that almost 100% of the U.S. population has some detectable level of phthalates in their urine. Not surprising then, phthalate exposure in expecting mothers has been associated with both the risk of miscarriage and gestational diabetes.[20] Phthalate exposure also impacts males, with associated DNA damage to sperm and consequent reduction in male fertility.[21] Males exposed to phthalates during the preconception period had changes in the methylated regions of their sperm. These regions were enriched in genes important for growth and development, cell movement, and cytoskeleton structure and provide a possible mechanism for impact on offspring of this pre-exposure.[22]

▶ Epigenetic Changes as Biomarkers of Exposure

Throughout the world, environmental pollution is thought to cause more than 13 million deaths, many of which could be averted through prevention.[23] From the public health perspective, it is important to understand cause and effect in order to advocate for policy changes. However, it is often difficult to prove causation of an environmental insult that may have preceded overt disease by many years. It can be difficult, if not impossible, to measure the amount, type, and duration of an exposure from prior years. One way to potentially circumvent these limitations is to have a biomarker that would persist over time and be a good indication of the dose of exposure. A growing body of evidence supports the idea that pollutants such as metals, pesticides, chemicals such as benzene, synthetic hormones, and water pollution all can cause epigenomic changes that can persist for years. Further, many of these epigenomic changes could be mechanistically involved in disease initiation and progression.

Analyzing the epigenomes of people is a potentially powerful approach to gain insights into past exposures because epigenetic patterns are maintained through cell divisions, long after the hazardous exposure is gone. Measuring the epigenome could have a profound impact on epidemiologic studies if data could support its validity as a biomarker. To do so will require experimentation on potentially thousands of samples stored in repositories that have solid exposure data. Fortunately, the technology now exists to conduct such studies.

▶ Epigenetics and Cancer

Cancer is primarily a genetic disease; however, it is clear that carcinogenesis cannot be accounted for by genetic alterations alone. Over the past several years, mounting evidence has shown that changes in DNA methylation, histone modifications, and microRNAs are also consistently present in a variety of cancers. Detailed epigenetic analyses of multiple tumor types revealed consistent patterns of changes in DNA methylation. First, there is a global decrease in methylation that occurs at **retrotransposons**, repeat sequence, and other sites around the genome. The consequences of the reduced methylation include overexpression of proto-oncogenes and other growth factors, as well as an increase in overall genomic instability, which is a hallmark of cancer. Conversely, there is also hypermethylation of promoter regions in multiple genes involved in the DNA repair pathway and cell cycle control, which results in propagation of genetic mutations and an accumulation of DNA damage. The International Cancer Genome Consortium (icgc.org) serves as a continually updated resource for tracking these data.

Given the complexity of carcinogenesis and the fact that chromatin structure is critically important for DNA regulation, it is not surprising that there are also many modifications of histone proteins in cancers. In particular, global levels of lysine methylation change in cancers, as do the regulation of lysine methyltransferases and demethylases. These histone modifications then lead to long-term patterns of gene expression impacting cell growth and invasiveness. Furthermore, some of the genetic mutations have been shown to affect regulators of histone modification. Given the complexity of cancer-related histone modifications, a complete discussion is beyond the scope of this chapter. A good review on this topic is offered by Dawson and Kouzarides (2012).[24]

With recent advancements in high-throughput technologies such as next-generation sequencing platforms, chromatin immunoprecipitation techniques, and mass spectrometry, the cancer epigenome is now being interrogated at a rapid pace and opening up the possibility of using these data as therapeutic targets. There are currently several drugs in preclinical and clinical trials that are focused on modifying DNA methyltransferase, HAT and HDAC, and a few have received FDA approval such as panobinostat (Farydak) for multiple myeloma and vorinostat (Zolinza) for T-cell lymphoma.

However, encouraging, many hurdles still remain before this type of therapy becomes commonplace. The biggest hurdle is undoubtedly specificity of tissue targeting. More specific inhibitors will have to be created to limit side effects related to therapy because epigenetic modifications, as previously shown, are an important marker for normal cellular differentiation and gene function.

▶ Conclusion

In conclusion, the field of epigenomics shows great promise in helping to discern basic mechanisms of cellular differentiation, disease processes, and carcinogenesis. Accumulating data suggest that epigenomic modifications may provide historical information about a person's lifetime exposure to multiple environmental challenges. And finally, the epigenome may ultimately provide novel targets for therapeutic interventions for a variety of human diseases, especially cancers.

Key Terms

Aneuploidy	Genomic imprinting	Mosaics
Endocrine disruptor	Monoallelic expression	Retrotransposons
Epigenetic modification	Monozygotic	X chromosome inactivation

Discussion Questions

1. Explain how an inherited mutation can have different impacts on future offspring depending on which parent passed on the mutation.
2. What is the evidence that epigenetic "marks" can be passed on to future generations?
3. Why do individuals with an excessive number of sex chromosomes often show minimum phenotypes?
4. Why would a doctor encourage a woman with a body mass index (BMI) of 18 to gain significant weight during pregnancy, while admonishing someone with a BMI of 30 to limit weight gain? What are the impacts on the fetus of undernutrition versus overnutrition? How will this impact the offspring long term?
5. Explain ways in which knowledge of epigenetics can be used in public health.

References

1. Jablonka E, Raz G. Transgenerational epigenetic inheritance: prevalence, mechanisms, and implications for the study of heredity and evolution. *Q Rev Biol.* 2009;84:131-176.
2. Lister R, Pelizzola M, Dowen RH, et al. Human DNA methylomes at base resolution show widespread epigenomic differences. *Nature.* 2009;462:315-322.
3. Greer EL, Shi Y. Histone methylation: a dynamic mark in health, disease and inheritance. *Nat Rev Genet.* 2012;13:343-357.
4. Willard HF. Tales of the Y chromosome [Comment]. *Nature.* 2003;423(6942):810-811, 813.
5. Plath K, Mlynarczyk-Evans S, Nusinow DA, Panning B. Xist RNA and the mechanism of X chromosome inactivation. *Annu Rev Genet.* 2002;36:233-278.
6. Passarge E. *Colour Atlas of Genetics.* New York, NY: Thieme Medical Publishers; 1995:344.
7. Lauritsen JG. The cytogenetics of spontaneous abortion. *Res Reprod.* 1982;14:3-4.
8. Nielsen J, Wohlert M. Sex chromosome abnormalities found among 34,910 newborn children: results from a 13-year incidence study in Arhus, Denmark. *Birth Defects.* 1990;26:209-223.
9. Visootsak J, Graham JM Jr. Klinefelter syndrome and other sex chromosomal aneuploidies. *Orphanet J Rare Dis.* 2006;1:42.
10. Fraga MF, Ballestar E, Paz MF, et al. Epigenetic differences arise during the lifetime of monozygotic twins. *Proc Natl Acad Sci USA.* 2005;102:10604-10609.
11. Roseboom TJ, van der Meulen JH, Ravelli AC, Osmond C, Barker DJ, Bleker OP. Effects of prenatal exposure to the Dutch famine on adult disease in later life: an overview. *Mol Cell Endocrinol.* 2001;185(1–2):93-98.
12. Painter RC, Roseboom TJ, Bleker OP. Prenatal exposure to the Dutch famine and disease in later life: an overview. *Reprod Toxicol.* 2005;20(3):345-352.
13. McMillen IC, Edwards LJ, Duffield J, Muhlhausler BS. Regulation of leptin synthesis and secretion before birth: implications for early programming of adult obesity. *Reproduction.* 2006;131:415-427.
14. Camp EA, Coker AL, Robboy SJ, et al. Breast cancer screening in women exposed in utero to diethylstilbestrol. *J Womens Health (Larchmt).* 2009;18:547-552.
15. Giusti RM, Iwamoto K, Hatch EE. Diethylstilbestrol revisited: a review of the long-term health effects. *Ann Intern Med.* 1995;122:778-788.
16. Palmer JR, Herbst AL, Noller KL, et al. Urogenital abnormalities in men exposed to diethylstilbestrol in utero. *Environ Health.* 2009;8:37.
17. Tomatis L. Transgeneration carcinogenesis: a review of the experimental and epidemiological evidence. *Jpn J Cancer Res.* 1994;85:443-454.
18. Talhout R, Schulz T, Florek E, Van Benthem J, Wester P, Opperhuizen A. Hazardous compounds in tobacco smoke. *Int J Envir Res Public Health.* 2011;8(12):613-628.
19. Chatterton Z, Hartley BJ, Seok MH, et al. In utero exposure to maternal smoking is associated with DNA methylation alterations and reduced neuronal content in the developing fetal brain. *Epigenet Chromatin.* 2017;10:4.
20. Messerlian C, Wylie BJ, Mínguez-Alarcón L, et al. Urinary concentrations of phthalate metabolites and pregnancy loss among women conceiving with medically assisted reproduction. *Epidemiology.* 2016;27(6):879-888.
21. Hauser R, Meeker JD, Singh NP, et al. DNA damage in human sperm is related to urinary levels of phthalate monoester and oxidative metabolites. *Hum Reprod.* 2007;22(3):688-695.
22. Wu H, Ashcraft L, Whitcomb BW, et al. Parental contributions to early embryo development: influences of urinary phthalate and phthalate alternatives among couples undergoing IVF treatment. *Hum Reprod.* 2017;32(1):65-75.
23. Prüss-Üstün A, Corvalán C. Preventing disease through healthy environments: Towards an estimate of the environmental burden of disease. Geneva, Switzerland: World Health Organization; 2006. Available at http://apps.who.int/iris/bitstream/10665/43375/1/9241594209_eng.pdf. Accessed November 24, 2017.
24. Dawson MA, Kouzarides T. Cancer epigenetics: from mechanism to therapy. *Cell.* 2012;150:12-27.

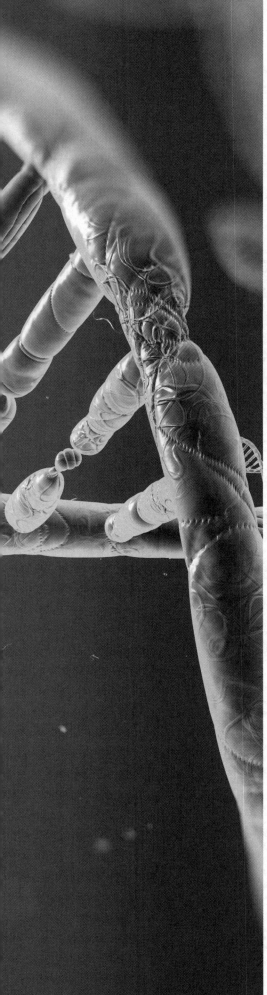

SECTION 2

Applications to Current Public Health Issues

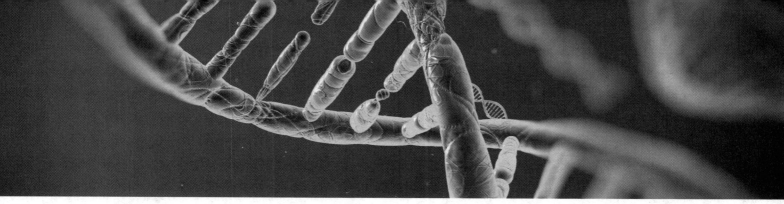

CHAPTER 7

A Public Health View of Cancer

Julie A. DeLoia

LEARNING OBJECTIVES

By the end of this chapter, the student will be able to:

- Explain why initiation of cancer is considered both a genetic and progressive disorder
- Describe how cancer cells differ from normal cells
- Name the two categories of cancer-related genes and provide examples of each category
- Distinguish hereditary and sporadic cancer traits and causes
- Design cancer prevention strategies based on knowledge of cancer biology

CHAPTER OUTLINE

▶ Introduction

Cancer is not a single entity. In fact, cancer includes more than 100 different diseases. Cancer can develop in virtually any of the body's tissues, and both hereditary and environmental factors contribute to its development. In this regard, cancer is a classic example of a multifactorial disorder. No single event or mutation can turn a normal cell into a cancerous cell.

Cancer is an old disease; dinosaur bones showed evidence of bone tumors, as did human mummies from ancient Egypt. Cancer is also quite common;

about one in two people in the United States will have cancer at some point in their lifetime, and one in four will die from cancer. An estimated 1,688,780 new cancer cases were diagnosed in 2017, with 600,920 cancer deaths in the United States alone.[1] The four major sites of cancer include colon and rectum, lung and bronchus, breast (women), and prostate (men).

Not too long ago, a diagnosis of cancer often meant inevitable death. However, with increasing understanding of cancer biology, more cancers are either being cured or becoming chronic conditions. However, that is not to say that cancer is under control. Cancer remains today a major challenge to both developed

---

BOX 7-1 Highlights of Progress in Cancer Research

1937: President Franklin D. Roosevelt establishes the National Cancer Institute to support research targeted at discovering the causes and treatment of cancer.

1943: Dr. George Papanicolaou introduces the Pap test, enabling doctors to detect and treat cervical cancers. Over the years, as a result of the Pap test, cervical cancer deaths dropped by nearly 70%.

1955: The National Cancer Institute establishes the Clinical Trials Cooperative Group Program to support large cancer treatment trials.

1950s–1960s: Studies show that cigarette smoking is a major cause of lung cancer. Secondhand smoke is identified as a threat to the health of nonsmokers.

1967: The fecal occult blood test is introduced as a means to screen for colorectal cancer, a common form of cancer. Sigmoidoscopy and colonoscopy follow within a few years. As a result, there is a decline of more than 40% in mortality.

1971: President Richard Nixon signs the National Cancer Act of 1971, resulting in a significant increase in funding for cancer research and granting broad authority to the Director of the National Cancer Institute to develop a National Cancer Program.

1970s: As a result of greater funding and collaboration, advances in cancer treatment accelerate. Some examples include introduction of computed tomography to detect cancers, first use of adjuvant chemotherapy (chemotherapy following surgery), breast-conserving surgery for breast cancer, and combination chemotherapy to cure testicular cancer.

1981: The first vaccine to prevent cancer is approved by the Food and Drug Administration (FDA). The vaccine was against hepatitis B virus, a major cause of liver cancer.

Late 1980s: Scientists prove a link between benzene, an occupational hazardous chemical, and lymphoma and leukemia.

1970s–1990s: Sun exposure is linked to melanoma.

1990: Deaths from cancer begin to decline.

1997: The first monoclonal antibody, rituximab, is approved by the FDA to treat B-cell non-Hodgkin lymphoma.

Late 1990s: Prophylactic surgery is shown to decrease risk of breast and ovarian cancers in women carrying genetic mutations (BRCA1 and BRCA2).

1998: Tamoxifen is approved as preventative therapy for BRCA mutation carriers.

1998: Obesity is linked to risk of common cancers.

2000: Radon in households is linked to lung cancer.

2003: Scientists announce completion of the Human Genome Project.

2005: The Cancer Genome Atlas project is launched to map the genetic and biochemical pathways in lung, ovarian, and glioblastoma cancers.

2006: The FDA approves vaccines against two strains of human papillomavirus to prevent cervical cancer.

2012: An all-time high of 13.7 million people in the United States are cancer survivors. This number is expected to reach 18 million by 2022.

Data from CancerProgress.Net. Cancer Progress Timeline. Available at https://www.asco.org/research-progress/cancer-progress-timeline. Accessed October 30, 2017.

---

and developing nations. The National Cancer Institute tracks cancer statistics in the United States and publishes these data regularly on their website as part of the Surveillance, Epidemiology, and End Results (SEER) program.[1] Statistics of global cancer rates can be found at the Centers for Disease Control and Prevention (CDC)[2] and World Health Organization (WHO)[3] websites.

History of Cancer Research in the United States

The history of changes in cancer incidence and mortality is a testament to the power of sustained and focused research. **BOX 7-1** highlights some of the progress that has been made in understanding cancer biology and implementing both prevention and cure.

The Biology of Cancer

A simple definition of cancer is uncontrolled cell growth. Recall from cell biology that cells are constantly surveying the environment to detect signals and to acquire nutrients. When conditions are appropriate, cells will initiate the cell cycle, in which they synthesize a copy of their deoxyribonucleic acid (DNA), grow and eventually divide. Cancer cells have unique properties that allow them to continue to divide regardless of conditions. Essential features of cancer cells include: (1) the ability to divide in the absence of growth signals; (2) the capacity to ignore anti-growth signals; (3) the ability to avoid **apoptosis**, even when carrying genetic mutations; (4) the ability to divide indefinitely without senescence; (5) production of signals to promote blood vessel growth (**angiogenesis**); (6) and finally, when metastasis occurs, the ability to break away from the tissue of origin and travel to other parts of the body to set up secondary tumors.

Cancer is a multi-step, multi-mutation process, and in that regard, can be considered a genetic disease. This idea was first proposed by Carl O. Nordling[4] in 1953 and later refined by Alfred Knudson.[5] Mutations occur in key genes that result in affected cells being able to outgrow and outcompete normal cells. Not surprising, it was later discerned that these cancer-promoting mutations included activation of genes that normally stimulate cell proliferation (**proto-oncogenes**) and deactivation of genes that guard against too much cell proliferation (**tumor suppressor genes**). Activation of proto-oncogenes (to become **oncogenes**) requires only a single mutation, and as such these mutations are considered **gain-of-function mutations**, while deactivation of tumor suppressors requires both alleles to be mutated and to be considered **loss-of-function mutations**.

Oncogenes include genes involved in growth promotion such as growth factors (fibroblast growth factor 3 in Kaposi's sarcoma), growth factor receptors

(human epidermal growth factor receptor type 2 [HER-2/neu] overexpression in up to 30% of breast cancers), signal transduction (ABL tyrosine kinase in chronic myelogenous leukemia), and nuclear transcription factors (Myc mutations in hematopoietic neoplasias).

Tumor suppressor genes can be further divided into "**gatekeepers**" and "**caretakers**." Gatekeeper genes are important in cell cycle progression; they normally function to prevent mutated cells from passing through cell cycle checkpoints, by either pushing a cell toward apoptosis or halting the cell cycle until the DNA can be repaired. Mutations in gatekeeper genes can lead to unrestricted cell proliferation and propagation of somatic mutations. Examples of gatekeeper genes include RB1 (mutated in retinoblastoma) and APC (mutated in familial adenomatous polyposis). Caretaker genes are primarily involved with DNA repair mechanisms and help ensure that DNA mutations do not accumulate. When DNA repair genes are mutated, genomic instability ensues and mutations accumulate quickly. Some examples of caretaker genes include BRCA1 (breast cancer) and MSH2 (hereditary nonpolyposis colorectal cancer). The p53 gene, which codes for a transcription factor, is unique in that it has functions of both gatekeeper and caretaker. It should not be surprising, then, that deregulation of p53 can be identified in about half of all cancers. **FIGURE 7-1** summarizes where in the cell cycle oncogenes and tumor suppressors function.

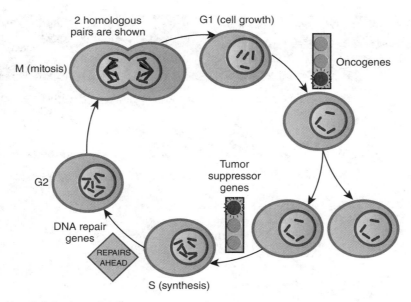

FIGURE 7-1 Mutations in the Cell Cycle and Cancer

Data from National Cancer Institute. Available at http://www.cancer.gov.

▶ Causes of Cancer

As noted, cancer initiation is a multi-step process and a multifactorial disease; no single event can cause cancer. It follows then, that there are many possible causes of cancer, both genetic and environmental. People can inherit a mutation in one of their "cancer genes." While it is possible to inherit a mutation in a proto-onco-gene, these types of mutations are rare. Much more common are mutations in one of the alleles of a tumor suppressor gene, which puts individuals at a much higher risk of developing cancer at some point in their lives. Recall that it takes two mutations or "hits" of a tumor suppressor gene to initiate cancer. People who inherit the first mutation carry that "hit" in every cell of their body, which is now more susceptible to cellular transformation with additional genetic insults.

Germline mutations in the tumor suppressor genes result in hereditary cancer syndromes, where many members of a family through multiple generations will develop specific types of cancers. A common example of a hereditary cancer syndrome is hereditary breast and ovarian cancer (HBOC), which occurs when either the BRCA1 or BRCA2 gene is mutated. Factors that should raise a concern of HBOC include:

- One or more women in a family with premenopausal breast cancer
- Cancer in both breasts
- Diagnosis of males with breast cancer
- Multiple generations with related cancers

- History of linked cancers such as prostate cancer, melanoma, and pancreatic cancer
- A higher-than-expected prevalence of ovarian cancer in the family
- Ashkenazi Jewish ancestry

In addition to inheriting a germline mutation, there is a myriad of environmental factors that can cause **somatic mutations** in cancer genes; namely, chemicals, radiation, and infectious agents. Somatic mutations are much more common in a population than germline mutations and, in general, result in cancers later in life. They are not associated with any identifiable pattern of inheritance and are known as sporadic cancers. **TABLE 7-1** lists the known environmental exposures and associated cancers.

These associations illuminate some very important concepts. For example, while most people recognize that chemicals and radiation are **carcinogenic**, many might not appreciate that lifestyle factors, such as obesity, tobacco use, and alcohol consumption remain major causes of cancer. The WHO estimates that about one-third of cancer deaths can be attributed to five major behavioral factors: low fruit and vegetable consumption, high body mass index, lack of physical activity, alcohol consumption, and tobacco use.[3] Even though lifestyle factors offer opportunities for prevention, behavior change remains challenging. For example, despite overwhelming data proving the link between tobacco and cancer and significant, sustained education campaigns, lung cancer remains the most preventable form of cancer death worldwide.[6]

TABLE 7-1 Known Environmental/Behavioral Risk Factors for Human Cancers	
Agent	**Associated Cancer**
Combustible tobacco	Lung, larynx, pharynx, esophagus, kidney, cervix, liver, bladder, pancreas, stomach, colon/rectum, myeloid leukemia
Smokeless tobacco	Mouth, tongue, cheek, gum, esophagus, pancreas
Ultraviolet radiation	Skin cancer, including basal cell, squamous cell, and melanoma
X-rays and gamma rays	Leukemia, multiple myeloma, lymphoma, cancers of the thyroid, bladder, breast, lung, ovary, colon, esophagus, stomach, liver, and skin
Radon	Lung cancer
Excess body weight	Breast, colon/rectum, endometrium, esophagus, kidney, pancreas
Alcohol	Cancers of the mouth, pharynx, larynx, esophagus, liver, colon/rectum, breast
Steroid hormones	Breast and endometrial cancers

Agent	Associated Cancer
Viral Infectious Agents	
Human papilloma virus	Cervical cancer
Hepatitis B and C viruses	Liver cancer
Human immunodeficiency virus	Anal cancer, Hodgkin disease, lung cancer, liver cancer, cancers of the mouth and throat
Human herpes virus 8	Kaposi sarcoma
Bacterial Infectious Agents	
Helicobacter pylori	Stomach cancer
Chlamydia trachomatis	Cervical cancer
Parasitic Infectious Agents	
Opisthorchis viverrini	Cancer of the bile duct
Clonorchis sinensis	Cancer of the bile duct
Schistosoma haematobium	Bladder cancer

Data from National Cancer Institute. Risk factors for cancer. Available at https://www.cancer.gov/about-cancer/causes-prevention/risk.

Infectious diseases are also a significant cause of many forms of cancer. Annually, of the over 12 million new cancer cases globally, it is estimated that approximately 16%, or around 2 million, had an infectious etiology.[7] Of particular importance to public health, prevention of the causative infections can result in significant reduction in cancer cases. A significant percentage of these infectious agents include pathogens such as human papillomaviruses (HPV), *Helicobacter pylori*, and hepatitis B and C viruses (HBV and HCV), all of which are either preventable through vaccines or treatable. Infection-attributable cancer cases are significantly higher in developing nations compared to developed countries, which highlights the importance of robust vaccine programs and reliable access to health care.

▶ Health Disparities and Cancer

The Office of Minority Health & Health Equity (OMHHE) of the CDC monitors the health of Americans and identifies differences in incidence and outcomes of major causes of death by geography, age, education, social class, disability, sexual orientation, ethnicity, and race (**FIGURE 7-2**). The OMHHE website publishes health trends in various groups over time.[8] While advances in prevention and treatment have increased life expectancy in recent years, there are still significant differences in incidence and mortality of some cancers.

The incidence rate of cancers in women has remained fairly constant for the past four decades, while it has fluctuated more in males. However, the death rate due to cancers has dropped in all populations studied. The persistently higher rates of death in African Americans, both men and women, in the United States are disturbing. Even though white women get more cancers, black women die at a greater rate. Reasons for these persistent differences for health outcomes vary

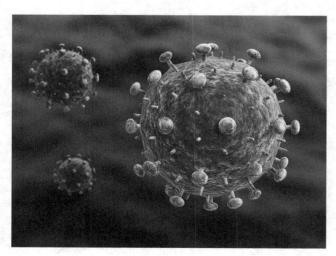

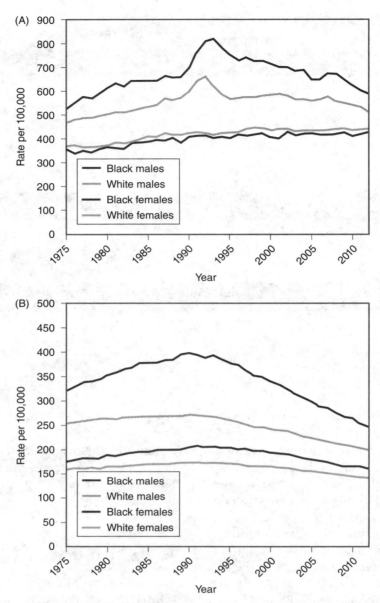

FIGURE 7-2 Trends in Cancer Incidence Rates* by Sex and Race, U.S. (A) 1975–2011 (B) 1975–2012

* Not included in these graphs are incidence rates and cancer deaths in Hispanic, Asian/Pacific Islander, and American Indian/Alaska Native populations, which are all lower than either Caucasian or African American populations.

(A) Data from Surveillance, Epidemiology, and End Results (SEER) Program, National Cancer Institute. Fast stats. Available at https://seer.cancer.gov/faststats/index.php. 2014.
(B) Data from Surveillance, Epidemiology, and End Results (SEER) Program, National Cancer Institute. Fast stats. Available at https://seer.cancer.gov/faststats/index.php. 2015.

depending on the cancer site. Obviously, lack of access to regular screening remains a major cause of health disparities.

▶ Reducing Cancer Disease Burden

Despite all we have learned about the etiology, biology, and treatment of cancers, it remains a major health burden in both developing and developed countries. Three major strategies to defeat cancer include prevention, early detection, and targeted therapy.

Cancer prevention relies on knowing risk factors and avoiding them or ameliorating their impact. Some successful strategies have included ultraviolet (UV) protection through use of sunscreen and UV-protective clothing; immunization against carcinogenic viruses such as HPV and HBV; condom use to prevent transmission of sexually transmitted infections; radon detection and reduction in the home;

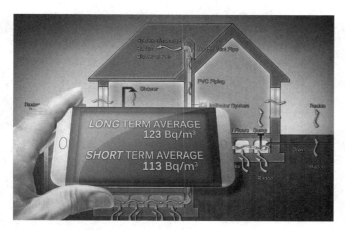

© Francesco Scatena/Shutterstock

reduction of medically used ionizing radiation; having a minimum age for purchase and consumption of tobacco products; regulating limits of carcinogenic chemicals in our environment; and promoting weight loss through physical activity and a healthy diet. For some people at a significantly higher risk of cancers, such as those with a germline mutation in a tumor suppressor gene, chemoprevention has been used to reduce the risk or delay the onset of cancer initiation. The National Institutes of Health conducts clinical trials to determine the efficacy of potential cancer prevention strategies.

Early detection of cancer is directly correlated with outcomes in most cases. For that reason, screening for various cancers is now part of routine medical care. The "Pap smear" for detection of early lesions in the cervix was introduced in the early 1940s. Since that time, there has been an estimated

70% decrease in cervical cancer deaths.[9] The CDC estimates that about 4,000 women in the United States still die from cervical cancer each year. Most of these women have not had recommended routine gynecologic care, including a Pap smear. The American Cancer Society recommends regular screening tests for cervical cancer, breast cancer, colon and rectal cancer, and prostate cancer (see **BOX 7-2**).[10]

The final strategy for lowering the disease burden of cancer is through highly effective and targeted therapy that would both kill the cancer cells and spare the healthy cells of the body. Many cancer treatment strategies have targeted rapidly dividing cells nonspecifically. Given the nature of cancer cells, this approach is rational. However, not all rapidly dividing cells are cancerous, and consequently there is often significant comorbidity associated with chemotherapy and radiation therapy. Two promising approaches to highly targeted therapy are immunotherapy and therapy targeting specific genetic mutations. Immunotherapy targets unique antigens on cancer cells and marks them for destruction by the host immune system. Molecular medicine, which is based on identifying and targeting specific gene mutations in an individual patient, has grown steadily with the successes of the Human Genome Project. The current standard of care at many hospitals is now to isolate tumor tissue and perform molecular testing at both the DNA and ribonucleic acid levels to try to pinpoint which of the cellular pathways discussed have been altered in an individual cancer. The National Cancer Institute

BOX 7-2 Colorectal Cancers: Can They Be Prevented?

Colorectal cancer (CRC) is a type of cancer that starts in either the colon or rectum, most often in the endothelial lining. Prior to overt **carcinoma**, most CRC begins with **neoplastic** or **dysplastic** cell growth in the form of polyps. CRC is the third most common cancer for both men and women in the United States, with an estimated 134,500 new cases in 2016.[11] CRC is also the third-leading cause of cancer-related deaths in this country with just under 50,000 deaths per year. Established lifestyle risk factors for CRC include overweight or obesity, physical inactivity, diets high in red meats or processed meats, smoking, and heavy alcohol use. Other risk factors include age, family history of CRC, and personal history of inflammatory bowel disease or polyps. About 5–10% of patients with CRC have an inherited family cancer syndrome, either familial adenomatous polyposis or hereditary non-polyposis colorectal cancer. Being African American is also a risk factor.

Screening and early detection have proven very effective in prevention of CRC. Tests used to screen for early lesions include testing stool samples for occult blood or DNA mutations in sloughed-off cells, colonoscopies, and double-contrast barium enema. The American Cancer Society recommends at least one of these screening tests by age 50. The 5-year survival rate of CRC is tightly linked with **stage** at diagnosis: stage I colon cancer has a 92% survival rate; stage II and III cancers have survival rates between 53–89%; and stage IV survival rate is about 11%. The CDC estimates that one in three adults between 50–75 years of age has not been screened for CRC, which represents about 20 million adults.[12]

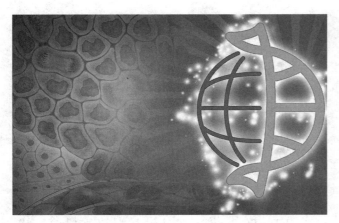

Courtesy of Ernesto del Aguila III, NHGRI

coordinates these types of data through The Cancer Genome Atlas project.

▶ Remaining Challenges

Despite significant progress in fighting cancer,[13] it remains one of the country's and world's most important health challenges (see **BOX 7-3**). Some of the remaining challenges include elucidating the cause(s) of many cancers, which will then inform early detection strategies, better treatment options, identifying people at risk, and creating behavior change. Many forms of cancer are still very difficult to detect at early stages, such as cancers of the ovary, lung, pancreas, and stomach. It is not surprising that these cancers also have higher mortality than those that are more readily detected.

Being able to identify people at risk for specific cancers would provide a significant advantage for monitoring and potentially using chemoprevention, as is done with women who carry BRCA mutations. With the completion of the Human Genome Project and the application of knowledge of genetic variation, it is hoped that sometime soon we will be able to genotype individuals and provide specific cancer risk estimates.

Advances in cancer treatment have had a profound impact on both morbidity and mortality, especially for some cancers such as breast and prostate, but other cancers are still difficult to treat. Cancer of the gallbladder, pancreas, liver, lung, esophagus, stomach, brain, and ovary all have a 5-year survival rate less than 50%.[1]

Lastly, even when solid scientific evidence identifies cancer risks and effective prevention strategies, effecting change can still be challenging. The WHO estimates that tobacco use is responsible for about 20% of cancer deaths globally, making it the most important and modifiable risk factor. The persistence of tobacco products and use demonstrates the challenges of both changing behaviors and sometimes fighting large multinational corporations, such as tobacco companies. Evidence suggests that the available HPV vaccines are effective at reducing cervical cancer incidence. Yet administering a vaccine against a sexually transmitted virus has met with considerable parental resistance.

Key Terms

Angiogenesis
Apoptosis
Carcinogenic
Carcinoma
Caretakers
Dysplastic

Gain-of-function mutations
Gatekeepers
Germline mutations
Loss-of-function mutations
Neoplastic
Oncogenes

Proto-oncogenes
Somatic mutations
Stage
Tumor suppressor genes

Discussion Questions

1. What category of cancer-related mutation would you expect to be inherited and why?
2. When would you suspect that a family was passing on a mutation in the Rb gene?
3. Explain the mechanistic link between HBV and liver cancer. How can this information be used to decrease liver cancer burden worldwide?

4. In the United States, why do African Americans die at a greater frequency than Caucasians from cancer, even today?

5. About 70% of all cancer deaths occur in low- and middle-income countries. Deaths from cancer worldwide are projected to continue to rise to over 13.1 million in 2030. What are some possible reasons for this projected trend?

References

1. Howlader N, Noone AM, Krapcho M, et al., eds. SEER Cancer Statistics Review, 1975-2014. National Cancer Institute: Bethesda, MD. Available at https://seer.cancer .gov/csr/1975_2014/, based on November 2016 SEER data submission posted to the SEER website, April 2017. Accessed October 20, 2017.

2. Centers for Disease Control and Prevention. Cancer data and statistics. Available at https://www.cdc.gov/cancer /dcpc/data/index.htm. Updated August 15, 2017. Accessed October 20, 2017.

3. World Health Organization. Cancer. Available at http://www .who.int/cancer/en/. Updated 2017. Accessed October 20, 2017.

4. Nordling C. A new theory on cancer-inducing mechanism. *Br J Cancer.* 1953;7:68-72.

5. Knudson AG Jr. Mutation and cancer: statistical study of retinoblastoma. *Proc Natl Acad Sci USA.* 1971;68:820-823.

6. Malhotra J, Malvezzi M, Negri E, La Vecchia C, Boffetta P. Risk factors for lung cancer worldwide. *Eur Respir J.* 2016;48:889-902.

7. de Martel C, Ferlay J, Franceschi S, et al. Global burden of cancers attributable to infections in 2008: a review and synthetic analysis. *Lancet Oncol.* 2012;6:607-615.

8. Centers for Disease Control and Prevention, Office of Minority Health & Health Equity. Health equity. Available at https://www.cdc.gov/minorityhealth/index.html. Updated June 28, 2017. Accessed October 20, 2017.

9. Cramer DW. The role of cervical cytology in the declining morbidity and mortality of cervical cancer. *Cancer.* 1974; 34:2018-2027.

10. American Cancer Society. American Cancer Society guidelines for the early detection of cancer. Available at https://www.cancer.org/healthy/find-cancer-early/cancer -screening-guidelines/american-cancer-society-guidelines -for-the-early-detection-of-cancer.html. Updated April 6, 2017. Accessed October 20, 2017.

11. American Cancer Society. Key statistics for colorectal cancer. Available at http://www.cancer.org/cancer /colonandrectumcancer/detailedguide/colorectal-cancer -key-statistics. Accessed October 20, 2017.

12. Centers for Disease Control and Prevention. Press Release: colorectal cancer screening rates remain low. Available at https://www.cdc.gov/media/releases/2013/p1105-colorectal -cancer-screening.html. Posted November 5, 2013. Accessed October 20, 2017.

13. Miller KD, Siegel RL, Lin CC, et al. Cancer treatment and survivorship statistics, 2016. *CA Cancer J Clin.* 2016;66:271-289.

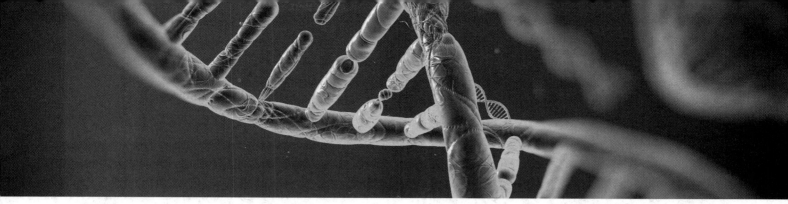

CHAPTER 8

Nutrition and Public Health

Kim Robien

▸ Introduction

The field of public health nutrition is a specialty practice area bridging the fields of nutritional science and public health. Nutritional science is the study of how food components, especially individual nutrients, affect health and risk of disease. The goals of those working in public health nutrition are to improve the health of communities and populations through nutrition-related education, community interventions, policy, administration, and research efforts. Public health nutritionists work toward ensuring that all people, at all times, have access to sufficient, safe, and nutritious food in order to meet their dietary needs for an active and healthy life.[1]

▸ The Science of Nutrition

Calories

Calories are units of energy provided by the foods we eat. The specific definition of a **calorie** is the amount of energy required to increase the temperature of one gram of water by one degree Celsius. Daily human caloric requirements are actually in the hundreds of thousands of calorie range, so kilocalories (1,000 calories) are more relevant to human nutrition. Although inaccurate, the terms "calories" and "kilocalories" are often used interchangeably. Adults typically require 1,800–3,000 kilocalories (kcal)/day to maintain body weight, depending on gender, body composition, and

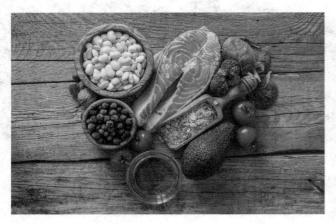

activity level. Energy balance is a term that is widely used to refer to the balance between calories consumed from diet and calories expended through physical activity and metabolic processes. When individuals are in positive energy balance, they will gain weight, typically as adipose tissue. When individuals are in negative energy balance, they will lose weight.

Macronutrients

The **macronutrients**—carbohydrates, proteins, and fats—are the nutrients we consume in the largest quantities and the source of calories in our food. On average, carbohydrates and proteins provide approximately 4 kcal per gram, and fats provide 9 kcal per gram. Most foods contain at least some amount of all three macronutrients, although the ratios of macronutrients may vary. For example, grains, fruits, and vegetables are predominantly carbohydrates, although they also provide a small amount of proteins and fat, whereas meat and fish are predominantly protein, although they also provide fats. Alcohol, while not traditionally considered a nutrient, is also a source of calories and provides 7 kcal per gram.

Humans must consume at least some of all three macronutrient categories in order to obtain the essential micronutrients. **Essential nutrients** are defined as nutrients that are required for human health, but cannot be synthesized *in vivo*, and thus must be obtained through diet. Typically, diets in which approximately 10–35% of calories come from protein, 20–35% from fat (especially unsaturated fats), and 45–65% from carbohydrates (especially complex carbohydrates such as those found in whole grains, fruits, and vegetables) will meet essential nutrient requirements and have been associated with the lowest rates of chronic diseases such as cardiovascular disease, diabetes, and cancers.[2]

Carbohydrates

The term carbohydrate refers to a broad class of sugars and starches. The most basic unit of carbohydrates is the monosaccharide, which is an aldehyde (R-(C=O)-H) or a ketone (R-(C=O)-R) with varying numbers of hydroxyl (C-H$_2$O) groups in the R position. Mono- and disaccharides (which include glucose, sucrose, and fructose) are referred to as "sugars." Complex carbohydrates, such as oligosaccharides and polysaccharides, are longer, more complex chains of monosaccharides that include starches and glycogen. These larger molecules typically require enzymatic cleavage in the intestinal tract in order to be absorbed; thus they tend not to increase blood sugars as rapidly as free mono- and disaccharides.

Metabolically, sugars serve as sources of energy in the body. Polysaccharides in the form of glycogen can be stored in the body and broken down into smaller saccharide units for energy as needed. Monosaccharides are also important components of deoxyribonucleic acid (DNA) and ribonucleic acid, as well as many biochemical cofactors and cell signaling molecules. Polysaccharides play an important role in maintaining bowel health by adding bulk to stools and in serving as a substrate for intestinal microflora.

Although sugars occur naturally in many fruits and dairy products, public health practitioners are concerned about the health effects of excessive calorie intake as a result of sugars added to processed foods, candy, and desserts. The 2015–2020 U.S. Dietary Guidelines for Americans recommended that Americans limit their intake of "added sugars" to less than 10% of daily caloric intake. Added sugars were defined as "sugars added to foods during processing, preparation, or at the table."[2] In 2015, the World Health Organization introduced a guideline for sugar intake among adults and children based on the amount of "free sugars," an even more inclusive term that was defined

Chemical structures of main saccharides

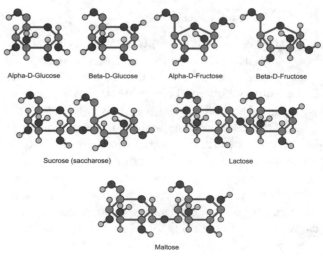

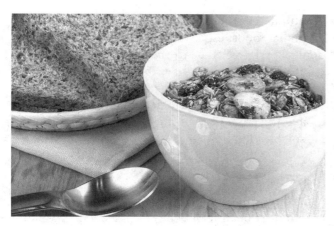

as the "monosaccharides and disaccharides added to foods and beverages by the manufacturer, cook, or consumer, and sugars naturally present in honey, syrups, fruit juices, and fruit juice concentrates."[3]

The term *dietary fiber* refers to the indigestible polysaccharides in plant foods. While humans may lack the ability to digest dietary fibers, they still serve important biologic functions and are part of a healthy diet. Dietary fibers are typically categorized into two categories: soluble fibers, which dissolve in water, and insoluble fibers, which do not dissolve in water. Both forms of dietary fiber add bulk to the stool and help to maintain regularity. Both forms of fiber are also fermented by intestinal bacteria. Dietary fibers help to regulate blood sugars by slowing the absorption of simple sugars. Fibers also help to lower total and low-density lipoprotein cholesterol levels by binding bile acids and preventing their reabsorption. Dietary fibers may also provide a sense of satiety and fullness without providing calories, thus decreasing overall caloric intake.

Protein

Proteins are molecules made up of one or more chains of amino acids. Amino acids, the key building block of proteins, are characterized by an amino group (R-NH) at the head (α end) of the molecule and a carboxyl group (R-(C=O)-OH) at the terminal end, with varying side chains in between. Proteins are synthesized according to the templates encoded in our genes and play a wide range of roles within the body. Perhaps the best-known role of proteins is their structural role as the primary components of muscle fibers, connective tissue, hair, nails, and cell walls. However, proteins also function as enzymes, hormones, receptors, antibodies, and in a wide variety of other cell signaling and ligand-binding functions. Humans can synthesize most amino acids from other compounds. However, there are nine essential amino acids (histidine, isoleucine, leucine, lysine, methionine, phenylalanine, threonine, tryptophan, and valine) that cannot be synthesized in the body and therefore must be obtained from dietary sources.

Fat

The main building block of fats includes fatty acids, which are organic compounds with a carboxyl group (R-(C=O)-OH) at the α end of the molecule followed by varying lengths of methyl (CH_2) groups. Fatty acids are typically described as being short (less than 6 carbons), medium (6–12 carbons), or long (13 or more carbons), and being either saturated (no double bonds between the carbon atoms) or unsaturated (one or more double bonds). Because fatty acids are similar to amino acids, humans are able to synthesize most of them from other compounds, with the exception of two essential unsaturated fatty acids, linoleic and alpha-linolenic acids, which must be obtained from dietary sources (such as flaxseed, walnuts, canola oil, and pumpkin seeds).

Unsaturated fatty acids are described by the location of the first double bond from the terminal methyl ("omega") end of the chain; thus omega-3 fatty acids have the first double bond at the third carbon from the final methyl group, and omega-6 fatty acids have the first double bond at the sixth carbon from the final methyl group.

Trans-fatty acids (trans fats) are a form of fatty acids where the hydrogen atoms of the carbon molecules around a double bond are on opposite sides of the molecule, rather than the usual formation where the hydrogen atoms are on the same side of the molecule (cis-fatty acids). This conformational change makes the trans-fatty acids more rigid, and foods containing these trans-fatty acids tend to be solids at room temperature. Dietary trans-fatty acids are primarily found in processed foods, in which manufacturers have purposely added hydrogen groups (hydrogenated) to polyunsaturated fatty acids to create a more stable, solid fat, which in turn tends to increase the

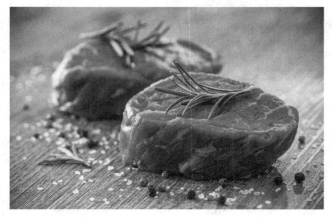

shelf life of the food product. However, trans-fatty acids have consistently been found to be associated with higher risk of cardiovascular diseases, and many health organizations have called for their elimination from the food supply.[4] In 2015, the U.S. Food and Drug Administration (FDA) ruled that trans-fats are no longer considered "Generally Recognized As Safe" food ingredients, and starting in 2018, manufacturers will be required to receive prior FDA approval to use trans-fats in foods sold in the United States.[5]

Fats serve as a concentrated source of energy, with adipose tissue as the storage form of excess calories. Fats are also important components of cell membranes and cell signaling molecules.[6] Dietary lipids and lipids synthesized in the liver are distributed to peripheral tissues in the form of triglycerides (three individual fatty acids joined to a glycerol molecule) and cholesterol (a lipid sterol molecule). Because lipids are hydrophobic, these lipid molecules must be surrounded by proteins (lipoproteins) in order to mix with the aqueous circulatory system. Elevated circulating levels of both cholesterol and triglycerides, especially when part of low-density lipoprotein molecules, have been associated with higher risk of coronary heart disease and stroke.

Fats and oils used in food preparation tend to be a mixture of different types of fatty acids, although one type of fatty acid may be present in greater quantities than others. For example, butter and other animal-derived fats tend to be comprised predominantly of saturated fatty acids, whereas plant-derived dietary fats such as olive and corn oils tend to be predominantly

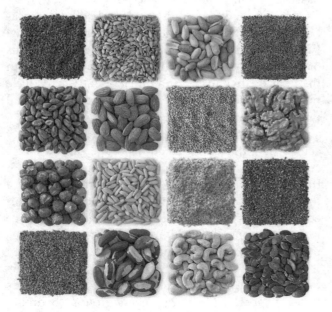

© Elena Schweitzer/Shutterstock

unsaturated fatty acids. Dietary cholesterols are found in animal foods, especially egg yolks, beef, pork, and poultry. Triglycerides are found in all dietary fats. While "low-fat" diets have been popular over the past 30 years, some dietary fat intake is necessary to provide the essential fatty acids that our bodies are unable to synthesize, and to allow for absorption of fat-soluble vitamins.

Micronutrients

Micronutrients are the other group of nutrients that are vital to health, but they are needed in smaller quantities than macronutrients and do not provide calories. Vitamins and minerals are the primary categories of micronutrients. **TABLE 8-1** lists the individual vitamins and minerals, as well as their role in human health and good food sources of each nutrient.

Vitamins

The term "vitamin" was originally coined by Casimir Funk in 1912 and comes from combining the words "vital" and "amine."[7] In this early period of vitamin discovery, it was erroneously thought that these essential compounds were made up of amino acids, similar to proteins. We now know that vitamins are not proteins, but the term remains. Vitamins are generally classified according to their solubility in either water or fat. The fat-soluble vitamins are vitamins A, D, E, and K, whereas the others are water-soluble. Fat-soluble vitamins require dietary fat as a vehicle for absorption from the aqueous environment of the intestinal tract.

Minerals

Minerals are inorganic elements required by the body in small amounts for health as outlined in Table 8-1. Minerals are typically divided into two categories—major minerals that are required in larger quantities, and trace minerals that are required in very small amounts (typically with some toxicity at higher amounts). Some minerals serve structural roles in the body, such as calcium in bone, while others are components or cofactors for enzymes involved in a wide variety of physiologic processes. Electrolytes (such as sodium, potassium, calcium, magnesium, and chloride) in circulation contribute to osmotic gradients that are important for fluid balance within the body. Mineral content of foods of plant origin may vary significantly, as mineral content will be determined by the mineral content of the soil in which the plants were grown.

TABLE 8-1 Recommended Daily Intake of Vitamins and Minerals

Nutrient	Recommended Daily Intake (Adults)	Role in the Body	Deficiency Syndrome	Good Food Sources
Vitamins				
A	900 mcg	Vision, immune function, antioxidant	Night blindness	Vegetables (especially orange vegetables)
Thiamine (B$_1$)	1.2 mg	Coenzyme in energy metabolism	Anorexia, neurologic disorders (*beri beri*)	Enriched grain products, whole grain products
Riboflavin (B$_2$)	1.3 mg	Coenzyme in energy metabolism	Mouth sores, dermatitis, anemia	Enriched grain products
Niacin (B$_3$)	16 mg	Coenzyme in protein metabolism	Dermatitis (*pellagra*), mouth sores, diarrhea	Enriched grain products
Folic acid	400 mcg	Methyl group donor	Anemia	Enriched grain products, green leafy vegetables
Pyridoxine (B$_6$)	1.3 mg	Coenzyme in protein metabolism	Weakness, insomnia, mouth sores	
Cobalamin (B$_{12}$)	2.4 mcg	Coenzyme in protein metabolism	Anemia	Enriched grain products
C	90 mg	Antioxidant	Scurvy	Fruits, vegetables
D	15 mcg (600 IU)	Calcium absorption, acts as a hormone	Rickets	Fortified dairy products, fish
E	15 mg	Antioxidant	Neuromuscular, vascular, reproductive issues	Nuts, seeds, oils
K	120 mcg	Assists in blood clotting	Inability to form blood clots	Green leafy vegetables
Major Minerals				
Calcium	1,000 mg	Bone health	Rickets	Dairy
Phosphorus	700 mg	Bones/teeth, metabolism	Rickets, osteoporosis	Meats, milk
Potassium	4.7 g	Build muscle, nerve conduction	Muscle weakness, increased blood pressure	Many foods – meat, fish, vegetables, fruits

(continues)

TABLE 8-1 Recommended Daily Intake of Vitamins and Minerals *(continued)*

Nutrient	Recommended Daily Intake (Adults)	Role in the Body	Deficiency Syndrome	Good Food Sources
Major Minerals				
Sodium	< 2,300 mg	Blood pressure and volume	Nausea, lethargy, cramps, seizures, loss of consciousness	Salt, processed foods
Chloride	2.3 g	Fluid balance, digestive juices	Vomiting, diarrhea, excessive sweating	Salt, vegetables
Magnesium	400 mg (M) 310 mg (F)	Cofactor in many enzyme systems	Cramps, anorexia, fatigue, insomnia, irritability	Green leafy vegetables, whole grains
Trace Minerals				
Iron	8 mg (M) 18 mg (F)	Component of red blood cells, oxygen delivery	Anemia	Animal meats, breakfast cereals
Iodine	150 mcg	Component of thyroid hormones	Goiter (enlarged thyroid)	Iodized salt
Zinc	11 mg (M) 8 mg (F)	Cofactor for numerous enzyme systems	Impaired growth, susceptibility to infections, diarrhea	Seafood, red meat, poultry, beans, nuts, whole grains
Selenium	55 mcg	Component of selenoproteins involved in reproduction, thyroid hormone metabolism, DNA synthesis, and protection from oxidative stress	Cardiomyopathy, exacerbation of iodine deficiency	Seafoods, meats, cereals and grains, dairy products
Fluoride	4 mg (M) 3 mg (F)	Bones and teeth	Tooth decay, osteoporosis	Fluoridated water, seafood, tea, gelatin
Molybdenum	45 mcg	Cofactor for catabolism of amino acids, DNA	Deficiency rare	Legumes, grains, nuts
Copper	900 mcg	Component of enzymes and proteins involved in electron transport and oxygenation	Anemia-like symptoms, impaired growth, bone abnormalities	Shellfish, whole grains, beans, nuts, organ meats, dark leafy greens, cocoa, black pepper
Manganese	2.3 mg (M) 1.8 mg (F)	Cofactor for many enzyme systems	Impaired growth, wound healing, glucose tolerance, reproductive function	Nuts, legumes, tea, whole grains

Data from NIH Office of Dietary Supplements. Dietary Supplements Fact Sheets. Available at https://ods.od.nih.gov/factsheets. Accessed October 30, 2017; Oregon State University Linus Pauling Institute. Micronutrient Information Center. Available at http://lpi.oregonstate.edu/mic. Accessed October 30, 2017.

Bioactive Food Components

Despite the long list of macro- and micronutrients that have been identified and studied for their importance to human health, nutritional scientists now recognize that there are still many thousands of chemical components of the foods we eat that have yet to be isolated and identified. Over the past two decades, it has become increasingly clear to nutritional scientists that there is a need to recognize a new category of nutrients that may not be essential, but nevertheless contribute to human health. This category of nutrients has been given the name **bioactive food components**, which has been defined as "constituents in foods or dietary supplements, other than those needed to meet basic human nutritional needs, that are responsible for changes in health status."[8] Examples of bioactive food components include: lycopene, a red pigment found in tomatoes, papayas, and watermelons that has antioxidant activity[9]; epigallocatechin gallate, a compound found in tea that has been found to have anti-inflammatory properties[10]; and resveratrol, a compound found in the skins of grapes, blueberries, and raspberries that has been reported to have anti-inflammatory and antioxidant activity.[11] It is important to note that although these nutrients have been used in traditional medicine for thousands of years, research into activities and health effects of most bioactive food components is only in the early stages, and in most cases, the findings to date in humans have been inconsistent.

▶ Human Nutritional Requirements

In North America, the Food and Nutrition Board of the U.S. National Academy of Sciences' Institute of Medicine (now known as the Health and Medicine Division [HMD]) and Health Canada collaborate to develop and publish the **Dietary Reference Intake (DRI)** recommendations for macro- and micronutrients.[12] The DRI recommendations are developed by expert panels of nutritional scientists and are based on all of the scientific evidence for the given nutrient. The recommendations are updated whenever sufficient scientific evidence indicates a revision is indicated. Methodologic challenges in defining human requirements and the lack of consistent scientific evidence on the human health effects have prevented the HMD from making dietary recommendations for bioactive food components at this time.[13]

For each macro- and micronutrient, the DRI report provides four reference values that can be used in evaluating and planning to meet the nutrient needs for healthy individuals in a population: Estimated Average Requirement (EAR), the Recommended Dietary Allowance (RDA), the Adequate Intake (AI), and the Tolerable Upper Intake Level (UL). The EAR represents the daily intake level for the nutrient that would be expected to meet the nutritional requirements of half of the population. The RDA is the daily intake level that would be expected to meet the nutritional requirements of nearly the entire (97–98%) healthy population. The AI is used in situations where the RDA cannot be estimated and represents the daily intake levels that are assumed to be adequate for groups of healthy people based on observational or experimental data. The UL represents that highest intake level of a nutrient that is likely to pose no adverse health effects to most individuals in the general population.[14] DRI recommendations vary by age, gender, and for women, by pregnancy and lactation status. A full review of the DRI recommendations for each of the more than 40 nutrients that have been evaluated is beyond the scope of this chapter; however, the DRI reports and tables are available on the HMD website.[15] It is important to keep in mind that the DRIs for each nutrient are established for healthy individuals, and there may be individuals or groups within a population who need higher or lower levels of a given nutrient. For example, people with a documented deficiency in the nutrient or people taking medications that can deplete body stores of a certain nutrient may be encouraged to consume higher quantities of the nutrient, whereas people with health conditions that lead to accumulation of the nutrient (such as iron for a person with hemochromatosis) may be instructed to decrease or avoid a given nutrient. Health behaviors may also alter nutrient requirements. Smokers have been found to require higher vitamin C intake to avoid deficiency symptoms,[16] and athletes who routinely engage in vigorous exercise tend to require higher amounts of calories, protein, and many micronutrients.

When assessing and planning the nutritional requirements of individuals, the RDA is the most appropriate of the DRI values to use. However, when assessing and planning for the nutritional requirements of communities and populations, the goal is to meet the nutritional needs of the majority of individuals in the population without exceeding the nutritional needs of others. Thus, the EAR is the most appropriate of the DRI values to use in population-level nutrition assessment and planning.[17]

A number of online tools and applications have been developed to help individuals identify their own specific nutritional requirements. Two scientifically validated tools include the SuperTracker program (https://www.supertracker.usda.gov/) and the DRI Calculator app (available as a free download from iTunes or Google Play) from the U.S. Department of Agriculture (USDA). The SuperTracker program also offers the Body Weight Planner module, which can help identify appropriate caloric intake and physical activity goals to achieve a specified weight loss within a given time frame.

Dietary supplements were originally developed for the medical treatment of nutrient deficiencies, but we now know that it is also possible to have adverse health outcomes related to excessive vitamin intake, resulting in the need for a UL recommendation as part of the DRIs. Reaching UL level intake of specific nutrients is difficult to achieve through diet alone and typically happens in the setting of dietary supplement use (usually when taken in doses higher than the supplement label recommends). Dietary supplements have now become a significant industry in the United States with sales of $36.7 billion in 2014[18] and are often used by healthy individuals looking to further improve their health. Yet for people without a specific nutrient deficiency, whole foods (with a variety of different bioactive food components, many of which may not have even been discovered) are generally going to be better sources of nutrition compared to supplements. There are likely thousands of important chemical compounds in foods that we have yet to identify, and foods provide many different nutrients, usually in well-balanced quantities. There is also a growing appreciation of the fact that nutrients interact with each other in order to function optimally. Thus, most nutrition professionals and health organizations now specifically recommend that healthy individuals use foods rather than dietary supplements to meet their nutritional needs.[19-21]

At the population level, food fortification is a potential strategy for addressing common nutrient deficiencies. However, food fortification programs must be carefully evaluated for potential unfavorable unintended consequences prior to implementation. While food fortification in the United States is not mandatory, the FDA has established a Food Fortification Policy (21 CFR Sect 104) that is guided by the following principles: (1) a significant portion of the population must consume the nutrient in quantities below the estimated requirements, (2) the food to be fortified is consumed in sufficient quantities by the population to expect that fortification would have the desired effect, (3) the nutrient being fortified is stable under the conditions that it would be used to fortify the food item, (4) the nutrient would be physiologically available after consuming the food item, (5) the fortified nutrient would not create imbalances of other nutrients, and (6) the fortified nutrient would not reach potentially toxic intake levels when the food item is consumed in usual quantities.[22] Food fortification efforts in the United States are summarized in **TABLE 8-2**. These efforts have resulted in a number of public health successes—fortification of liquid milk with vitamin D has resulted in significant decreases in the incidence of rickets, fortification of salt with iodine has virtually eliminated the incidence of goiter, and fortification of enriched grain products with folic acid has substantially decreased the incidence of neural tube defects in the United States.[22]

TABLE 8-2 Food Fortification in the United States	
Date	**Nutrient for Fortification**
1924	Iodized salt introduced in Michigan
1930s	Iodized salt available throughout the United States, iodine deficiency virtually eliminated
1930s	Vitamin D added to milk to prevent childhood rickets (amount not standardized until the 1950s)
1940s	Vitamin A added to low-fat and skim milk
1942	FDA formally established a standard of identity for enriched white flour (which is enriched with iron, thiamine, and niacin)
1943	Riboflavin added to standard identity for enriched white flour
1998	Folic acid added to enriched flours and other grain products

▶ Nutrition Surveillance and Dietary Recommendations for Disease Prevention

The National Health and Nutrition Examination Survey,[23] an annual data collection effort conducted by the National Center for Health Statistics of the Centers for Disease Control and Prevention (CDC) among 5,000 U.S. residents from across the country, is the primary source of nutritional surveillance data on the adequacy of the American diet. The data have consistently shown that Americans tend to exceed daily recommendations for calories, added sugars, saturated fats, refined grain products, and salt, and do not meet recommendations for fruits and vegetables, whole grains, dietary fibers, calcium, and vitamin D.[2]

To address these issues, the U.S. Congress has directed the USDA and the Department of Health and Human Services to develop the **Dietary Guidelines for Americans (DGAs)** every 5 years. The DGAs are intended to provide science-based advice on food and nutrition choices to help all Americans aged 2 years or older meet nutritional needs, achieve and maintain a healthy weight, and minimize risk of chronic diseases. The DGAs also serve as the basis for all federal nutrition policy—including federal nutrition assistance programs, the National School Lunch Program, and military meal service and rations. In developing the DGAs, expert food and nutritional scientists from across the country are appointed to serve on the Dietary Guidelines Advisory Committee, where they review the latest nutrition science research and revise the previous set of guidelines as needed. Starting with the 2005 Dietary Guidelines development process, the scientific literature used to develop the DGAs is now compiled and made publicly available in the Nutrition Evidence Library.[24] Once the scientific updates have been completed, the USDA's Center for Nutrition Policy and Promotion develops nutrition education to educate the public on the DGAs, which recently has included the Choose My Plate (www.choosemyplate.gov) and SuperTracker (https://www.supertracker.usda.gov) websites and apps.

While the DGAs are intended for addressing the basic nutritional needs and chronic disease prevention in a generally healthy population, other health organizations undertake similar processes to address nutritional requirements and recommendations for prevention and management of specific disease states. For example, the World Cancer Research Fund/American Institute for Cancer Research regularly reviews the scientific literature and generates nutrition recommendations related to cancer prevention, treatment, and survivorship, and the American Heart Association and American Diabetes Association do the same for their specific chronic diseases. Despite a few disease-specific issues, the general nutrition recommendations from all of these groups are to: (1) achieve and maintain a healthy body weight throughout life, (2) eat at least five servings of fruits and vegetables each day, (3) choose whole-grain foods whenever possible, (4) limit alcohol intake to no more than 1 drink/day for women and 2 drinks/day for men, and (5) minimize salt intake by avoiding salting food during cooking or at the table, and (6) minimize the use of highly processed or preserved foods.

▶ Malnutrition and Food Insecurity

The word "malnutrition" is a broad term referring to the situation where an individual has not consumed calories (under-nutrition and over-nutrition) or nutrients in the appropriate quantities. We tend to think of malnutrition as a deficiency in a specific nutrient, but the term can also refer to excess intake of calories or nutrients. Kwashiorkor (severe protein-calorie malnutrition characterized by severe wasting, abdominal distention, swelling of the hands and feet, hair and tooth loss) and marasmus (severe energy deficiency characterized by extreme wasting) are disease states associated with severe and long-term malnutrition that are more commonly seen in

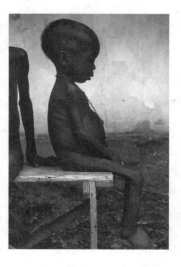

CDC/Dr. Lyle Conrad

developing countries, while in developed countries, malnourished individuals typically consume sufficient or excess calories overall but have micronutrient deficiencies and thus typically do not appear to have the characteristic wasting.

Alleviating hunger and malnutrition in populations is one of the primary missions of the field of public health nutrition. Most people understand the meaning of "hunger"; however, the word does not differentiate between the temporary experience we have if we go too long between meals and the more significant problem of chronic lack of sufficient food to eat. Thus, many public health practitioners prefer to use the term **food insecurity**, which has been defined as existing whenever the availability of nutritionally adequate and safe foods or the ability to acquire acceptable food in socially acceptable ways is limited or uncertain. "Hunger, in its meaning of the uneasy or painful sensation caused by a lack of food, is in this definition a potential, although not necessary, a consequence of food insecurity."[25] The Economic Research Service of the USDA further differentiates food insecurity into two categories: Low Food Security, which refers to "reports of reduced quality, variety, or desirability of diet but with little or no indication of reduced food intake"; and Very Low Food Security, which refers to "reports of multiple indications of disrupted eating patterns and reduced food intake."[26] In 2015, 12.7% of U.S. households experienced some degree of food insecurity.[27] The Healthy People 2020 goal related to food security (NWS-13) calls for reducing food insecurity to 6%.[28] (See **BOX 8-1**.)

In the United States, food insecurity is most often a result of poverty, but globally, food insecurity may also be the result of natural disasters, famine, and political unrest. A number of nutrition-assistance programs exist as a social safety net for food security in the United States, including the **Supplemental Nutrition Assistance Program**, formerly known as Food Stamps), the **Special Supplemental Nutrition Program for Women, Infants, and Children**, **The Emergency Food Assistance Program**, and the **Child and Adult Care Food Program**. While these and other nutrition assistance programs are vital to meeting the nutritional needs of food-insecure individuals, the programs are designed to supplement an individual's food supply, not to serve as the sole source of food. Thus, many people who participate in these programs must also rely on food from food banks, food pantries, soup kitchens, and other charitable organizations. The nutrition assistance programs are also intended to be temporary assistance until the individual can regain sufficient financial footing to provide for food needs. Many have argued that the best and most sustainable solution to food insecurity, especially in the United States and other developed countries, is to address the underlying issue of poverty through job-training programs and/or increasing minimum wage requirements. Similarly, at the global level, developed countries are moving away from the model of sending food surpluses to food-insecure areas of the world, and are instead helping local farmers in these regions to develop climate-adapted and culturally relevant crops and agricultural methods to become more self-sufficient.

BOX 8-1   Selected Health Objectives for Nutrition: Healthy People 2020

Objective: Increase the proportion of school districts that require schools to make fruits or vegetables available whenever other food is offered or sold.

Baseline: 6.6% in 2006
Target: 18.6% in 2020

Objective: Eliminate very low food security among children.

Baseline: 1.3% in 2008
Target: 0.2% in 2020

Objective: Reduce consumoption of calories from solid fats in people aged 2 years and older.

Baseline: 18.9% in 2004
Target: 16.7% in 2020

Objective: Reduce consumption of calories from added sugars in people aged 2 years and older.

Baseline: 15.7% in 2004
Target: 10.85% in 2020

In the United States and other developed countries, it is not uncommon for food-insecure individuals to be obese rather than emaciated. This situation has been described as the "hunger/obesity paradox"[29] and is likely the result of several different factors. First, the least expensive foods tend to be the highest in calories. For example, by taking advantage of volume purchasing and production efficiencies in all aspects of their food supply chain, large fast-food restaurants can offer full meals for a fraction of the cost of preparing a meal at home. These meals tend to be high in calories and sodium, but are missing many of the micronutrients needed for good health. Secondly, many food-insecure individuals live in areas where there is limited access to grocery stores, but there are a large number of fast-food outlets. Thus, fast foods are cheap, convenient, and readily available, whereas healthier food options are more difficult to locate. Third, there is some evidence to support the theory that inconsistent access to food (having plenty of food for a few weeks of each month, and then several weeks of little or no food intake) may lead to overeating, and that chronic, significant variations in caloric intake lead to increased fat storage over time.

▶ Food Systems in Public Health

Agriculture has always been a very labor-intensive process and subject to the forces of weather and nature (pests). Alternating periods of feasts and famines have been commonplace. However, since the industrial revolution in the late 1700s, food production has become increasing mechanized. Efficiencies of scale learned in other industries have been increasingly applied to food production. As a result, the modern food system in developed countries is often referred to as an **industrialized food system**, where large farming operations, food-processing facilities, and food retail establishments predominate. In many developed countries, the industrial food system is actually able to produce more food (and calories) than is necessary to feed the population, leading to what many have referred to as an **obesogenic environment**. In fact, the average number of calories available in the marketplace per U.S. resident on a daily basis has increased by 700 kcal between 1970 and 2010.[30] Public health nutrition professionals are working at many different levels (individual, social, physical, and macro-level environments) to develop and implement policy, systems, and environmental changes that create healthier food environments.[31]

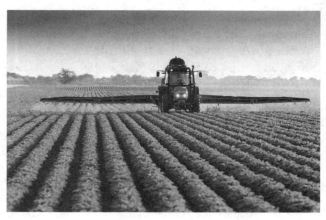
© Fotokostic/Shutterstock

Public health nutrition professionals also work to ensure the safety of the food supply. Food and water provide needed nutrients but are also vehicles of microbial and environmental toxicant exposure. (Microbiological contamination of food items is discussed in greater detail in other chapters in this book). The CDC maintains the Food Net Surveillance Program[32] to track trends in foodborne illnesses across the country. The USDA and the FDA are charged with ensuring the safety of the food supply, through inspections of food producers. The USDA's Food Safety and Inspection Service (FSIS) is responsible for ensuring the safety of the nation's commercial supplies of meat, poultry, and egg products, and that these products are correctly labeled and packaged. The FDA's Center for Food Safety and Applied Nutrition oversees the safety of dietary supplements, bottled water, food additives, infant formulas, and all other food items not under the purview of the USDA's FSIS program. The FDA also regulates all aspects of food labeling, except for meat, poultry, and egg products. The CDC, USDA, and FDA also jointly provide food safety education for the general public through the Foodsafety.gov website.

Concerns about health effects as a result of foodborne exposure to chemicals such as the agricultural chemicals used in the production of plant (e.g., pesticides, fertilizers) and animal foods (e.g., antibiotics, growth hormones), food additives, and chemicals used in food processing and packaging (e.g., bisphenols and phthalates) have led to increased interest among the general public in understanding where their food is coming from and how it is produced. As an example, the Organic Trade Association reports that sales of organic foods have experienced double-digit growth each year since the 1990s, and reached more than $39 billion in 2014.[33] Similarly, the number of farmers' markets in the United States has grown from 1,755 in 1994 to 8,669 in 2016,[34] indicating growing consumer interest in purchasing directly from local food producers, as well as having the opportunity to interact with the individuals producing their food.

The goals of Public Health Nutrition concern the improvement of community and population health through nutrition education, community interventions, research, and policy. A primary focus of this field is creating an environment in which all people have access to sufficient amounts of safe and nutritious food in order to meet the energy demands of a healthy, productive, and enjoyable life. It is important to remember that food policy is public health policy and that (similar to clean water) access to healthy food is a basic human right that must be protected for all.

Key Terms

Bioactive food components

Calorie

Child and Adult Care Food Program

Dietary Guidelines for Americans (DGAs)

Dietary Reference Intake (DRI)

Essential nutrients

Food insecurity

Industrialized food system

Macronutrients

Obesogenic environment

Special Supplemental Nutrition Program for Women, Infants, and Children

Supplemental Nutrition Assistance Program

The Emergency Food Assistance Program

Trans-fatty acids (trans fats)

Discussion Questions

1. Using the USDA's SuperTracker program, determine your individual nutritional requirements. Next, keep a record of your food intake for three days using the Food Tracker section of the program. How does your actual nutrient intake compare with your nutritional targets?

2. What is the hunger/obesity paradox? What are the factors that contribute to this situation?

3. What factors should be considered when planning a food fortification program?

4. How necessary and effective is the daily multivitamin for Americans?

5. How is food insecurity defined?

6. Why have some people referred to the food system in developed countries as an "industrial food system"?

References

1. Rome Declaration on World Food Security and World Food Summit Plan of Action. Rome: World Food Summit; 1996.

2. U.S. Department of Agriculture. Department of Health and Human Services. Dietary Guidelines for Americans 2015-2020. Alexandria, VA: USDA/DHHS; 2015.

3. World Health Organization. Guideline: sugars intake for adults and children. Geneva, Switzerland: World Health Organization; 2015.

4. Brownell KD, Pomeranz JL. The trans-fat ban—food regulation and long-term health. *N Engl J Med*. 2014;370(19):1773-1775.

5. U.S. Food and Drug Administration. FDA cuts *trans* fat in processed foods. Available at http://www.fda.gov /ForConsumers/ConsumerUpdates/ucm372915.htm. Accessed May 30, 2017.

6. Calder PC. Functional roles of fatty acids and their effects on human health. *J Parenter Enteral Nutr*. 2015;39(1 suppl):18S-32S.

7. Semba RD. The discovery of the vitamins. *Int J Vitam Nutr Res*. 2012;82(5):310-315.

8. Office of Public Health and Science, Office of the Secretary, U.S. Department of Health and Human Services. Solicitation of written comments on proposed definition of bioactive food components. *Fed Regist*. 2004;69(179):55821-55822.

9. Story EN, Kopec RE, Schwartz SJ, Harris GK. An update on the health effects of tomato lycopene. *Ann Rev Food Sci Technol*. 2010;1:189-210.

10. Legeay S, Rodier M, Fillon L, Faure S, Clere N. Epigallocatechin gallate: a review of its beneficial properties to prevent metabolic syndrome. *Nutrients*. 2015;7(7):5443-5468.

11. Bitterman JL, Chung JH. Metabolic effects of resveratrol: addressing the controversies. *Cell Mol Life Sci*. 2015;72(8): 1473-1488.

12. Institute of Medicine. *Dietary Reference Intakes: The Essential Guide to Nutrient Requirements*. Washington, DC: Institute of Medicine; 2006.

13. Ellwood K, Balentine DA, Dwyer JT, Erdman JW, Jr., Gaine PC, Kwik-Uribe CL. Considerations on an approach for establishing a framework for bioactive food components. *Adv Nutr (Bethesda)*. 2014;5(6):693-701.

14. Schectman G, Byrd JC, Gruchow HW. The influence of smoking on vitamin C status in adults. *Am J Public Health*. 1989;79(2):158-162.

15. Health and Medicine Division, The National Academies of Sciences, Engineering, and Medicine. Dietary Reference Intake Tables and Application. Available at http://www .nationalacademies.org/hmd/Activities/Nutrition/Summary DRIs/DRI-Tables.aspx. Accessed October 23, 2017.

16. Institute of Medicine. *Dietary reference intakes for calcium, phosphorus, magnesium, vitamin D, and fluoride*. Washington, DC: Institute of Medicine, Standing Committee on the Scientific Evaluation of Dietary Reference Intakes; 1997.

17. Nutrition Business Journal. *NBJ's Supplement Business Report 2015*. San Diego, CA: Penton Media, Inc.; 2015.

18. American Heart Association. Vitamin supplements: healthy or hoax? Available at http://www.heart.org/HEARTORG /Conditions/Vitamin-Supplements-Healthy-or-Hoax _UCM_432104_Article.jsp. Accessed June 2, 2017.

19. World Cancer Research Fund / American Institute for Cancer Research. *Food, Nutrition, Physical Activity, and the Prevention of Cancer: A Global Perspective.* Washington, DC: AICR; 2007.

20. Academy of Nutrition and Dietetics. Position of the American Dietetic Association: Nutrient Supplementation. *J Acad Nutr Dietet.* 2009;109(12):2073-2085.

21. Nutritional Quality Guidelines for Foods. *Code of Federal Regulations Title 21, Section 104.20.* Available at http://www .accessdata.fda.gov/scripts/cdrh/cfdocs/cfcfr/CFRSearch .cfm?fr=104.20. Accessed June 1, 2017.

22. Dwyer JT, Wiemer KL, Dary O, et al. Fortification and health: challenges and opportunities. *Adv Nutr (Bethesda).* 2015;6(1):124-131.

23. Centers for Disease Control and Prevention. National Health and Nutrition Examination Survey. Available at http://www .cdc.gov/nchs/nhanes.htm. Updated October 18, 2017. Accessed October 23, 2017.

24. U.S. Department of Agriculture. Nutrition Evidence Library (NEL). Available at http://www.cnpp.usda.gov /nutritionevidencelibrary. Accessed October 23, 2017.

25. Anderson SA. Core indicators of nutritional state for difficult-to-sample populations. *J Nutr.* 1990;120(suppl 11):1559-1600.

26. Economic Research Service, U.S. Department of Agriculture. Definitions of Food Security. Available at http://www.ers .usda.gov/topics/food-nutrition-assistance/food-security -in-the-us/definitions-of-food-security.aspx. Updated October 4, 2017. Accessed October 23, 2017.

27. Economic Research Service, U.S. Department of Agriculture. Household Food Security in the United States in 2015. Available at https://www.ers.usda.gov/publications /pub-details/?pubid=79760. Updated September 7, 2016. Accessed June 1, 2017.

28. Office of Disease Prevention and Health Promotion, U.S. Department of Health and Human Services. Nutrition and Weight Status. Available at http://www.healthypeople .gov/2020/topics-objectives/topic/nutrition-and-weight -status/objectives. Accessed June 1, 2017.

29. Dietz WH. Does hunger cause obesity? *Pediatrics.* 1995; 95(5):766-767.

30. Economic Research Service, U.S. Department of Agriculture. Food Availability (Per Capita) Data System. Available at https://www.ers.usda.gov/data-products/food-availability -per-capita-data-system/. Updated July 26, 2017. Accessed October 23, 2017.

31. Story M, Kaphingst KM, Robinson-O'Brien R, Glanz K. Creating healthy food and eating environments: policy and environmental approaches. *Annu Rev Public Health.* 2008;29:253-272.

32. Centers for Disease Control and Prevention. Foodborne Diseases Active Surveillance Network (FoodNet). Available at http://www.cdc.gov/foodnet. Updated March 3, 2017. Accessed October 23, 2017.

33. Organic Trade Association. State of the Industry: 2015. Available at https://ota.com/sites/default/files/indexed_files /OTA_StateofIndustry_2016.pdf. Accessed October 23, 2017.

34. Agricultural Marketing Service, U.S. Department of Agriculture. Farmers Markets and Direct-to-Consumer Marketing. 2016. Available at http://www.ams.usda.gov /services/local-regional/farmers-markets-and-direct -consumer-marketing. Accessed May 25, 2017.

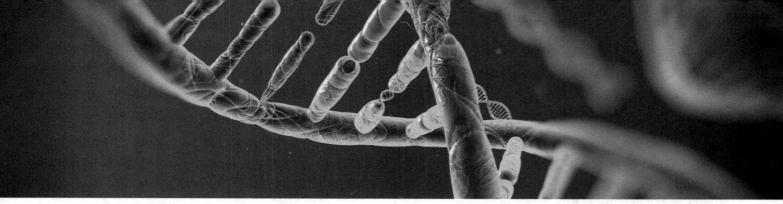

CHAPTER 9

Overfeeding, Disuse, and Cardiometabolic Outcomes

Loretta DiPietro

LEARNING OBJECTIVES

By the end of this chapter, the student will be able to:

- Describe the basic components of substrate metabolism
- Explain the ways in which the body maintains normal glucose levels
- Summarize the consequences of the modern lifestyle to the subsistence efficiency ratio and to cardiometabolic health
- Differentiate between type 1 and type 2 diabetes with regard to etiology and treatment
- Explain the mediating role of excess adiposity in the pathway between disuse and cardiometabolic disease
- Compare behavioral versus policy interventions with regard to mitigating cardiometabolic risk across the life span

CHAPTER OUTLINE

▸ Introduction

The modern-day lifestyle is characterized by a majority of time spent sitting and reclining throughout the day.[1] This prominence of sedentary living has been especially evident over the last several decades, as occupational-related energy expenditure has declined[2] and passive leisure-time activity (internet use, video games, television/movie viewing) has increased. Several studies have confirmed the deleterious association between prolonged (i.e., uninterrupted) periods of daily sitting and cardiometabolic risk,[3-6] as well as all-cause, cardiovascular, and cancer mortality,[7-10] even after adjustment for leisure-time

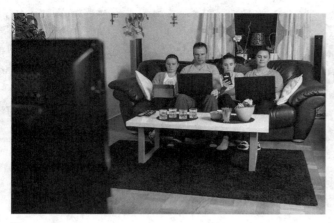

© Piotr Wawrzyniuk/Shutterstock

physical activity (which has not changed substantially over the past decades).[11] More recent evidence suggests that the deleterious relationship often reported between sedentary time and cardiometabolic risk may be attributable to the fact that sedentary time displaces time spent in health-accruing lower-intensity activity.[12]

Modern-day prosperity has also resulted in an abundant and omni-available food supply for the majority of the developed world. Indeed, "hunting and gathering" today is characterized by shopping at a supermarket and by opening a refrigerator (keep in mind that some supermarkets now will shop for you, deliver the food, and store the food for you). Although caloric intake has not increased appreciably since WWII, the composition of these calories has shifted considerably toward greater fat and refined carbohydrate density. Thus, an overabundance of food with no need for expending energy to obtain it results in overfeeding and overstorage of nutrients in the cell.[13] This chapter will discuss the implications of overfeeding and disuse (very low levels of daily physical activity) to the metabolic and cardiovascular disease currently observed globally.

▶ Substrate Metabolism

Substrate metabolism refers to the body's preference for fuel to support basal function, as well as all working activity. As discussed previously, energy is manufactured in the mitochondria of the cell, and the first law of fuel metabolism is that energy must first be stored before it can be released and utilized. The cell takes nutrients from food and, via the citric acid (Krebs) cycle and electron transport chain, converts the nutrients into ATP [Food + $O_2 \rightarrow CO_2 + H_2O$ + ATP = Energy]. The more oxygen that is combined with fuel sources, the more energy is produced.

Food is ingested in the forms of the common macronutrients: protein, carbohydrates, and fats. Once digested in the stomach, these nutrients transform into

absorbable units (substrates) before entering the bloodstream (**FIGURE 9-1**). Proteins circulate in the form of amino acids, carbohydrates circulate as glucose, and fats as free fatty acids and monoglycerides. Each of these substrates is then stored in a third form in different organs and tissue. Amino acids are stored as body protein, primarily in the muscle. Glucose is stored as glycogen, primarily in the liver and in the muscle, while fatty acids are stored as triglycerides in adipose (fat) tissue and in some cases in the muscle (**TABLE 9-1**).

The second law of fuel metabolism is that the brain must be continuously supplied with glucose, as it cannot metabolize proteins or fatty acids. Therefore, the body needs to ensure it has an adequate supply of glucose in the circulatory system to support brain function. The liver is a key organ in maintenance of an adequate blood glucose level. The liver first stores glucose in the form of glycogen through the process of **glycogenesis**. When circulating levels of glucose fall too low (due to fasting or to prolonged work activity), the liver will break down glycogen and release it back into the bloodstream in the form of glucose. This process of **glycogenolysis** is an example of negative feedback that results in a consequent rise in blood sugar. The liver can also convert amino acids to glucose through **gluconeogenesis**, although this is not desirable as it results in muscle wasting. Importantly, adipose tissue can help maintain blood glucose levels by breaking down stored fats for fuel via the process of **lipolysis**, thereby sparing precious glucose as well as muscle protein. **Metabolic flexibility** refers to the ability of the cellular machinery to switch rapidly from one substrate source to another in response to fuel availability, insulin, or to exercise. Blunted or delayed shifts in substrate utilization in response to various metabolic demands have been linked to insulin resistance and subsequent type 2 diabetes.

To maintain homeostasis, fuel metabolism is under tight hormonal control. There are hormones that promote the storage of fuel and hormones that promote the mobilization and release of fuel into the bloodstream. *Insulin* is a storage hormone secreted by the beta cells of the pancreas. The release of insulin is stimulated by a rise in blood sugar, and its role in metabolism is to lower blood sugar by increasing glucose uptake by the muscles. Insulin also increases glycogenesis (conversion of glucose into glycogen) and suppresses glycogenolysis and glyconeogenesis (conversion of glycogen or amino acids back to glucose), as well as lipolysis (fat mobility). In contrast, *glucagon* is secreted by the alpha cells of the pancreas in response to hypoglycemia (low blood sugar). Glucagon secretion causes a rise in blood glucose and free fatty acids by stimulating glycogenolysis in the liver.

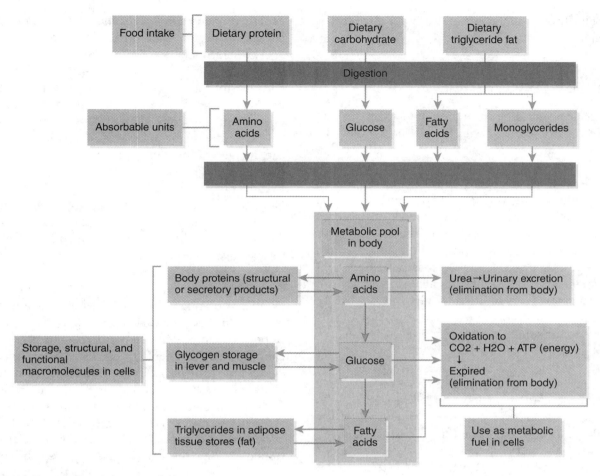

FIGURE 9-1 Nutrient Breakdown and Absorption

Reproduced from Sherwood L. *Human Physiology: From Cells to Systems*. 4th ed. Belmont, CA: Brooks/Cole; 2001.

TABLE 9-1 The Storage of Metabolic Fuel

Fuel	Circulating Form	Storage Form	Storage Site
Carbohydrate	Glucose	Glycogen	Liver, muscle
Fat	Free fatty acids	Triglycerides	Fat tissue
Protein	Amino acid	Body protein	Muscle

Remember that humans are designed to respond to environmental stressors, thereby requiring release of several stress hormones to ensure that there is adequate fuel in the bloodstream for *fight-or-flight*. *Epinephrine* is one such hormone that is stimulated both by immediate stress and by exercise. Its role is to suppress insulin secretion, promote glucagon secretion, and increase glycogenolysis, gluconeogenesis, and fat mobilization in order to increase circulating levels of glucose and fatty acids. *Cortisol* is stimulated by chronic stress and performs in a manner similar to epinephrine in that it increases circulating levels of substrates and ensures the mobilization of fuels necessary to adapt to long-term stress. One must remember that in Paleolithic times, these stress (or anti-insulin) hormones were a survival advantage for outrunning or fighting predators and for hunting. With modern-day stressors (traffic jams, work deadlines, poverty), however, the frequent secretion of these hormones becomes a survival disadvantage, as we no longer need to fight off predators or to hunt for food. Thus, the constant oversupply of fuel in the bloodstream, with few opportunities to "work it off," results in metabolic dysregulation, as there is a build-up of fuel at the cellular level.

▶ Subsistence Efficiency

Humans evolved to be in motion, and we are genetically programmed for cycles of feast or famine subsistence. Various fasting and satiety stimuli initiate different hormonal activations.[13] When there is a decrease in stored glycogen and fat, the body initiates a drive to hunt. The work activity of hunting initiates a cascade of hormones and proteins that bring glucose into cells to fuel the muscles. Aerobic fuel metabolism is more efficient over the long term than anaerobic because hunting takes time. A successful hunt and consequent large food intake initiates a sleep response for better storage of glucose and triglycerides. A thrifty (i.e., conservative) storage trait was a survival advantage due to the sometimes long intervals between successful hunts.

During Paleolithic times, energy intake and output were inextricably linked. *Subsistence efficiency* refers to the amount of food intake needed to support the work necessary to obtain that food. Over 100,000 years ago, our ancestors consumed approximately 3,000 calories per day and expended about 1,000 calories a day in work activity, for a **subsistence efficiency ratio (SER)** of 3:1.[14] Modern humans enjoy a relatively unlimited food supply; because we do not need to hunt or gather, we rarely exhaust our fuel storage. On average, modern humans ingest about 2,100 calories per day, but expend only about 300 in work activity. This results in a SER of 7:1, which—because we are nearly genetically identical to our Paleolithic ancestors—is not ideal for our metabolic functioning. As stated previously, the combination of overfeeding and disuse (inadequate levels of work activity) is the precursor of metabolic dysregulation at the cellular level. Modern-day humans need to add back approximately 400 kilocalories of daily energy expenditure to attain an SER of 3:1. This level of daily energy expenditure can be achieved by performing about 45 minutes of moderate-intensity activity (e.g., brisk walking, cycling, yard work).

▶ Weight Gain and Obesity

The body adapts to overfeeding and a chronic oversupply of fuel by getting bigger, as increased body mass will burn more energy at rest. An individual's rate of weight gain and risk of becoming obese, defined in public health as a body mass index (BMI) ≥ 30 kg body weight (kg)/height (m),^{2} has a strong genetic influence. Indeed, some people are quite susceptible to weight gain with a positive energy balance, whereas others are more resistant. For example, those carrying a common variant of the fat-mass and obesity-associated *FTO* gene (about 16% of the population) tend to be heavier than those without it. On average, one copy of the risky variant adds up to 3.5 extra pounds of weight, while having two copies can increase a person's risk of becoming obese by over 50%. More recent evidence, however, suggests that the obesity risk associated with this gene variant has been amplified substantially by environmental changes over the past several decades. Prior to WWII, daily work activity may have been sufficient protection against excessive weight gain, even among those most susceptible. In contrast, the drastic decline in both work and leisure-time energy expenditure since WWII, combined with a high-fat/high-sugar diet, has resulted in this gene variant having a greater relative importance to obesity risk. This effect of risk modification by environmental factors has been especially evident over the past 25 years and is corroborated by National Health and Nutrition Examination Survey (NHANES) data that demonstrate a rather marked spike in obesity prevalence after about 1985[15] (however, the validity of NHANES data has been questioned).[16] (See the Case Report at the end of the chapter.)

▶ Insulin Resistance and Type 2 Diabetes

As discussed previously, when the body consumes more energy than it expends, the result is a build-up of substrate within the cell. This build-up has several consequences to normal metabolic function. One such consequence is an increase in the production of reactive oxygen species. **Reactive oxygen species (ROS)** are the products of normal aerobic metabolism and include oxygen ions, free radicals (superoxide and hydroxyl radicals), and peroxides (hydrogen peroxide). These ROS are small and highly reactive molecules with important cell-signaling roles when maintained at proper cellular concentrations. Energy build-up in the cell will cause ROS levels to increase, resulting in increased oxidative stress. An excess production or decreased scavenging of ROS has been implicated in the metabolic dysregulation leading to type 2 diabetes, as it impairs mitochondrial biogenesis and insulin action within the cell (**FIGURE 9-2**).

Excess intracellular fuel accumulation can also lead to the build-up of adipose tissue in other parts of the body. Visceral (deep abdominal) fat accumulates

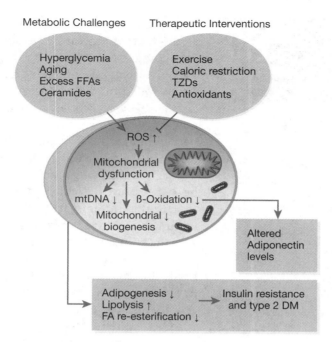

FIGURE 9-2 Substrate Build-Up Within the Cell

Reproduced from Kusminski CM, Scherer PE. Mitochondrial dysfunction in white adipose tissue. *Trends Endocrinol Metab*. 2012;23(9):435-443.

around the organs and comprises hypertrophied (enlarged) adipocytes that are highly metabolically active, relative to hyperplastic lower-body fat. The portal vein will deliver mobilized visceral fat directly to the liver, where again, insulin action is compromised. Remember that the liver protects against hypoglycemia by converting stored glycogen into glucose. If the liver becomes fatty, it will not read the insulin signals to shut down glucose production, thereby resulting in high blood sugar (hyperglycemia). Excess fuel accumulation can result in fatty tissue deposits in the muscle. Because the muscle is the primary site for insulin action, this has serious consequences for peripheral glucose disposal. Finally, the fat cells themselves can become impaired with regard to their ability to suppress fat mobilization and increase fat re-esterification in response to insulin. Impairment in insulin action

in the muscle, liver, and adipose tissue is termed multi-tissue **insulin resistance**, and it is a problem at the cell, tissue, and systems level. *With insulin resistance, there is no shortage of insulin produced by the pancreas.* Rather, insulin action in connection with glucose disposal (storage) is impaired—primarily through defects in insulin binding, insulin signaling, glycolysis, and glucose oxidation, or glucose transport into the cell.

Insulin resistance is the precursor to type 2 diabetes. Early-stage insulin resistance may go undetected because people are able to maintain relatively normal glucose levels (i.e., 100 mg/dL), albeit at a higher insulin cost. Without treatment, insulin resistance will progress to impairments in glycemic tolerance until eventually the person presents with clinical symptoms of chronic hyperglycemia. Type 2 diabetes is defined as a fasting glucose level ≥ 126 mg/dL and/or a 2-hour post-meal blood glucose level ≥ 200 mg/dL.

It is important to note that the etiology and progression of types 1 and 2 diabetes are very different (see **TABLE 9-2**). Type 1 diabetes is considered an autoimmune disease and is characterized by a deficiency in insulin production and secretion by the beta cells of the pancreas. In contrast, type 2 diabetes is considered a lifestyle disease and is defined by reduced insulin sensitivity in target tissue (primarily muscle, fat, and liver). Type 1 diabetes used to be termed "juvenile-onset" or "insulin-dependent" diabetes, and type 2 diabetes was referred to as "adult-onset" or "non-insulin-dependent" diabetes. However, these terms are no longer appropriate, as

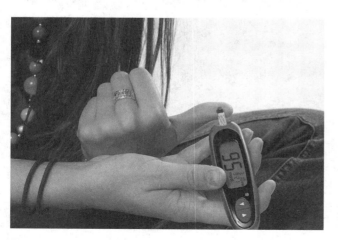

CDC/Amanda Mills

TABLE 9-2 Differences Between Type 1 and Type 2 Diabetes

Type 1	Type 2
β-cell deficiency	Reduced insulin sensitivity in target cells
Childhood or adolescent onset; occurs less commonly in infants or adults over age 19	Adolescent or adult onset
Approximately 10% of diabetes	Approximately 90% of diabetes
Requires insulin for treatment and diet/exercise for management	Weight loss, diet, and exercise for treatment
Rapid development	Slow development

type 1 diabetes is diagnosed in adults with increasing frequency, while type 2 diabetes can develop in children and its prevalence is growing steadily in pediatric populations.

▶ Factors for Cardiometabolic Risk

Three primary biologic factors that increase cardiometabolic risk are hypertension, hyperglycemia, and **dyslipidemia**. These three risk factors often appear as a cluster, especially in the presence of excess abdominal fat and low physical activity. The "*metabolic syndrome*" is defined by several biomarker cut-points related to blood pressure, waist circumference, fasting blood glucose, triglycerides, and cholesterol levels, and by resting systolic and diastolic blood pressure (see **TABLE 9-3** for criteria).

Another indicator of cardiometabolic risk is elevated level of glycated hemoglobin (HbA1c). Normal levels of glucose produce a small amount of HbA1c; however, as the average amount of blood glucose increases, the proportion (%) of HbA1c increases in a predictable way. Thus, HbA1c levels reflect total glycemic exposure over two to three months and are a good indication of chronic hyperglycemia. Normal HbA1c levels are approximately

5–6%, and every 1% increase above this predicts a 20% increase in cardiometabolic risk. For example, going from 6% to 7% can increase risk by 20%. The biggest contributor to high HbA1c levels is postprandial hyperglycemia (rather than fasting hyperglycemia), which makes controlling post-meal glucose excursions imperative among people at risk for cardiometabolic disease. A key factor in the mechanistic pathway between chronic hyperglycemia and cardiovascular disease may be **osteopontin**, which is a glycoprotein linked to chronic inflammation. Chronic inflammation within the micro- and macrovascular system damages the epithelial tissue, resulting in atherosclerotic plaque formation, hardening, and calcification. The final consequences of chronic inflammation are peripheral circulatory impairments and cardio- and cerebrovascular disease.

One often-cited strategy for cardiometabolic risk reduction is weight loss. It should be noted, however, that there are many people who are not overweight or obese, yet are "metabolically obese." Metabolic obesity can occur in those having a normal BMI (22–25 kg/m^2) but with a phenotype characterized by high ratio of body fat to lean mass, which is most likely attributable to low levels of physical activity. Conversely, there are many people who meet the BMI criterion for obesity, yet have a normal metabolic profile, more than likely due to regular physical activity and careful nutrition. If overfeeding at the cell level is a primary factor for metabolic dysregulation, then strategies to increase daily energy expenditure should become a priority in public health. Moreover,

TABLE 9-3 Criteria for Metabolic Syndrome[a]

Men	Women
Waist circumference > 102 cm	Waist circumference > 88 cm
TG ≥ 1.69 mmol·L^{-1}	TG ≥ 1.69 mmol·L^{-1}
HDL-C < 1.04 mmol·L^{-1}	HDL-C < 1.29 mmol·L^{-1}
SBP ≥ 130 or DBP ≥ 85 mmHg	SBP ≥ 130 or DBP ≥ 85 mmHg
Fasting glucose ≥ 6.1 mmol·L^{-1} (126 mg/dL)	Fasting glucose ≥ 6.1 mmol·L^{-1} (126 mg/dL)

[a] Metabolic syndrome defined as three or more of these factors.

BOX 9-1 Selected Health People 2020 Objectives for Cardiometabolic Diseases

Objective: Increase the proportion of the diabetic population aged 18 years and older with an HbA1c value < 7%.

Baseline: 53.5% in 2008.
Target: 58.9% in 2020.

Objective: Increase the proportion of persons at high risk for diabetes with prediabetes report increasing their levels of physical activity.

Baseline: 51.8% in 2008.
Target: 57.0% in 2020.

Objective: Increase the proportion of persons at high risk for diabetes with prediabetes who report increasing their levels of physical activity.

Baseline: 44.6% in 2008.
Target: 49.1% in 2020.

Objective: Increase the proportion of persons at high risk for diabetes with prediabetes who report trying to lose weight.

Baseline: 50.0% in 2008.
Target: 55.0% in 2020.

because skeletal muscle is the primary site for glucose disposal, any intervention that improves muscle quantity and quality (increased physical activity) will improve insulin sensitivity and lower cardiometabolic risk (see **BOX 9-1** for related Healthy People 2020 Objectives).

▶ Implications for Public Health Practice

As previously discussed, metabolic and cardiovascular diseases are becoming quite prevalent in both developed and developing countries. Fortunately for public health practice, most cardiometabolic risk factors are modifiable if addressed early on. Whereas the obesity epidemic (which is now endemic) is an important public health concern, there are factors that precede obesity that are more easily amenable to behavior and policy changes—namely, physical activity and nutrition. Current U.S. Public Health Service Recommendations for Physical Activity call for 150 minutes per week of moderate-intensity activity or 75 minutes per week of vigorous activity, with strength-training activity on 2 days per week.[17] The recommendation for children aged 5–17 is 60 minutes of moderate-to-vigorous intensity activity every day.[18] The World Health Organization recommends achieving 10,000 steps per day. In addition, Healthy People 2020 objectives target physical activity (see **BOX 9-2**). It is

important to note that these recommendations are for purposes of *prevention* and may not be sufficient for reversing established obesity or frank chronic disease—especially among people reporting more than 8–12 hours/day sitting. On the other hand, there is ample evidence that these recommendations can result in cardiometabolic risk reduction *independent* of weight loss. Unfortunately for public health practice, when obesity reduction is the primary endpoint of an intervention, the benefits of physical activity to risk reduction are often minimized.

Approximately 31% of adults and about 81% of adolescents across the world fail to meet these physical activity recommendations and are considered inactive.[19] The global estimate of the **population attributable fraction** for premature mortality

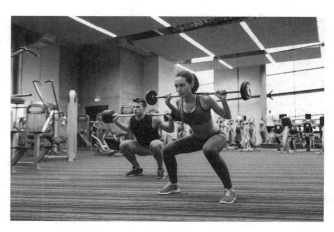

BOX 9-2 Selected Healthy People 2020 Objectives for Physical Activity

Objective: Increase the proportion of adults who engage in aerobic physical activity of at least moderate intensity for at least 150 minutes/week of vigorous intensity, or an equivalent combination.

Baseline: 43.5% in 2008.
Target: 47.9% in 2020.

Objective: Increase the proportion of adolescents who meet current Federal physical activity guidelines for aerobic physical activity.

Baseline: 28.7% in 2008.
Target: 31.6% in 2020.

Objective: Increase the proportion of the Nation's public and private elementary schools that require daily physical education for all students.

Baseline: 3.8% in 2008.
Target: 4.2% in 2020.

Objective: Increase the proportion of children and adolescents aged 6–14 years who view television, videos, or play video games for no more than 2 hours a day.

Baseline: 78.9% in 2008.
Target: 86.8% in 2020.

Reproduced from Office of Disease Prevention and Health Promotion, U.S. Department of Health and Human Services. Physical Activity. Available at https://www.healthypeople.gov/2020/topics-objectives/topic/physical-activity/objectives. Accessed June 1, 2017.

resulting from physical inactivity is 9%,[20] compared with 9% attributable to smoking and 5% attributable to obesity.[21] In this regard, public health has not been successful in counteracting the modern-day lifestyle. Indeed, considering the similar impact of inactivity and smoking to premature mortality, imagine the public outcry if 81% of adolescents reported smoking cigarettes rather than being inactive!

Public health practice is often a balance between behavioral strategies targeted to the individual versus collective strategies or policies that affect a community equally. Although there are effective behavioral and social strategies to help the individual achieve a more active lifestyle, these have been less effective at increasing population levels of physical activity. Most public health practitioners now agree that environmental approaches to increase physical activity at the community and population level are essential for success. These multisector (or systems) approaches involve several nontraditional public health partners (e.g., urban planners, transportation engineers, architects) working together to eliminate environmental hazards that affect the ability of the public to be physically active.

Traditionally, the most effective public health strategies have been *passive* in nature—that is, they have bypassed individual decision-making. Consider fluoridating drinking water, garbage pick-up, air bags in automobiles, lead removal, and improved highway design as examples of effective passive public health policies.[22] Following are five examples of multisector

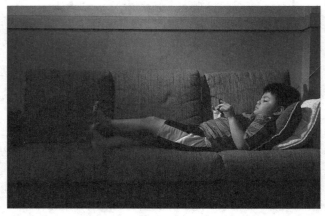

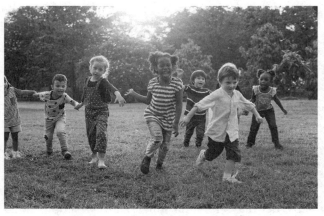

policy changes that could result in increased physical activity among the population, were they enacted.

- Reinstating physical education and recess as core requirements in the school curriculum
- Requiring that school drop-off points be a half mile from the school
- The promotion of stringent building design codes among communities, including Health Impact Statements
- The promotion of workplace policies that encourage movement throughout the building (incentives for stair use and standing desks)
- Requiring physician assessments of both physical activity and sitting behavior as part of standard care

Finally, similar to access to safe and nutritious food, access to safe and enjoyable ways to be physically active needs to also be considered a basic human right. Unfortunately, the application of research to policy efforts toward the promotion of an active lifestyle has yet to be fully realized. Indeed, even though physical inactivity has emerged as a significant public health threat, physical activity policy lags far behind policies directed at food, smoking, or obesity control. Physical activity policies are, in fact, prevention policies for obesity, diabetes, cardiovascular, and other noncommunicable diseases that have a far greater return on investment than policies directed toward treatment or curative actions. We cannot ignore the opportunity to leverage past public health successes in enacting such policies.

⌕ CASE REPORT

The Gene-Environment Interaction in Pima Indians

The Pima Indians of Arizona called themselves "river people" primarily because until the 1900s, they made their living via agriculture (subsistence farming) alongside the Gila River. Their lifestyle changed, however, with the European invasion and the building of several large dams (namely, the Hoover Dam) upriver. Over the years, their lifestyle transitioned from traditional to a more modern lifestyle.

The Pima Indians have among the highest prevalence of diabetes in any population group in the world.[23] They are one of the most studied groups due to the high heritability of type 2 diabetes in their population, which presents classically, with obesity and insulin resistance.

1. Why is the prevalence of obesity and type 2 diabetes so much higher in the Pima compared with their European counterparts, when both currently are living similar lifestyles?
2. How should public health respond to this? What key intervention strategies would you suggest?

Key Terms

Dyslipidemia
Gluconeogenesis
Glycogenesis
Glycogenolysis

Insulin resistance
Lipolysis
Metabolic flexibility
Osteopontin

Population attributable fraction
Reactive oxygen species (ROS)
Subsistence efficiency ratio (SER)

Discussion Questions

1. Explain why a child who goes to school without eating breakfast would have difficulty concentrating on schoolwork.
2. Explain why caloric restriction alone would not be a feasible way to attain a 3:1 SER. List several other strategies for achieving a 3:1 SER.
3. Describe three cellular impairments resulting from substrate build-up in the cell. How do these cellular impairments relate to whole-body metabolic function?
4. Rank the risk factors of obesity, smoking, hypertension, and physical inactivity according to their level of public health burden. Be ready to justify your ranking.
5. In addition to the multisector strategies for improving population levels of physical activity described at the end of the chapter, list five of your own. How feasible would your strategies be to enact?
6. Does a ban on the sale of large sugary drinks (think Big Gulp or Double Gulp at 7-Eleven) make sense for public health practice? Why or why not?

References

1. Matthews CE, Chen KY, Freedson PS, et al. Amount of time spent in sedentary behaviors in the United States, 2003–2004. *Am J Epidemiol.* 2008;167:875-881. doi: 10.1093/aje/kwm390.

2. Church TS, Thomas DM, Tudor-Locke C, et al. Trends over 5 decades in U.S. occupation-related physical activity and their associations with obesity. *PLoS ONE.* 2011;6:e19657. doi: 10.1371/journal.pone.0019657.

3. Proper KI, Singh AS, van Mechelen W, Chinapaw MJM. Sedentary behaviors and health outcomes among adults: A systematic review of prospective studies. *Am J Prev Med.* 2011;40:174-182. doi: 10.1016/j.amepre.2010.10.015.

4. Bey L, Hamilton MT. Suppression of skeletal muscle lipoprotein lipase during physical inactivity: a molecular reason to maintain daily low-intensity activity. *J Physiol.* 2003;551:673-682. doi: 10.1113/jphysiol.2003.045591.

5. Healy GN, Dunstan DW, Salmon J, Shaw JE, Zimmet PZ, Owen N. Television time and continuous metabolic risk in physically active adults. *Med Sci Sports Exerc.* 2008;40:639-645.

6. Gennuso KP, Gangnon RE, Matthews CE, Thraen-Borowski KM, Colbert LH. Sedentary behavior, physical activity, and markers of health in older adults. *Med Sci Sports Exerc.* 2013;45:1493-1500.

7. Katzmarzyk PT, Church TS, Craig CL, Bouchard C. Sitting time and mortality from all causes, cardiovascular disease and cancer. *Med Sci Sports Exerc.* 2009;41:998-1005.

8. Thorp AA, Owen N, Neuhaus M, Dunstan DW. Sedentary behaviors and subsequent health outcomes in adults: a systematic review of longitudinal studies, 1996–2011. *Am J Prev Med.* 2011;41:207-215.

9. Van der Ploeg HP, Chey T, Korda RJ, Banks E, Bauman A. Sitting time and all-cause mortality risk in 222,497 Australian adults. *Arch Intern Med.* 2012;172:494-500.

10. Patel AV, Bernstein L, Deka L, et al. Leisure time spent sitting in relation to total mortality in a prospective cohort of US adults. *Am J Epidemiol.* 2010;172:419-429. doi: 10.1093/aje/kwq155.

11. Centers for Disease Control and Prevention. Trends in leisure-time physical activity in the United States: BRFSS, 2001–2007. Available at http://www.cdc.gov/physicalactivity/data/surveillance.html. 2013.

12. Maher C, Olds T, Mire E, Katzmarzyk PT. Reconsidering the sedentary behavior paradigm. *PLoS ONE.* 2014;9:e86403. doi: 10.1371/journal.pone.0086403.

13. Chakravarthy MV, Booth FW. Eating, exercise, and "thrifty" genotypes: connecting the dots toward an evolutionary understanding of modern chronic diseases. *J Appl Physiol.* 2004;96:3-10.

14. Cordain L, Gotshall RW, Eaton SB. Physical activity, energy expenditure and fitness: an evolutionary perspective. *Int J Sports Med.* 1998;19:328-335.

15. Centers for Disease Control and Prevention. National Health and Nutrition Examination Survey. Available at https://www.cdc.gov/nchs/nhanes/index.htm. Updated October 18, 2017. Accessed October 24, 2017.

16. Archer E, Hand GA, Blair SN. Validity of U.S. Nutritional Surveillance: National Health and Nutrition Examination Survey Caloric Energy Intake Data, 1971–2010. Johannsen D, ed. *PLoS ONE.* 2013;8(10):e76632. doi:10.1371/journal.pone.0076632.

17. Centers for Disease Control and Prevention. How much physical activity do adults need? Available at https://www.cdc.gov/physicalactivity/basics/adults/. Updated June 4, 2015. Accessed June 11, 2017.

18. World Health Organization. Global Strategy on Diet, Physical Activity, and Health: Physical activity and young people. Available at http://www.who.int/dietphysicalactivity/factsheet_young_people/en/. Accessed June 11, 2017.

19. Hallal PC, Andersen LB, Bull FC, Guthold R, Haskell W, Ekelund U; Lancet Physical Activity Series Working Group. Global physical activity levels: surveillance progress, pitfalls, and prospects. *Lancet.* 2012;380(9838):247-257. doi: 10.1016/S0140-6736(12)60646-1.

20. Lee I-M, Shiroma EJ, Lobelo F, Puska P, Blair SN, Katzmarzyk PT. Effect of physical inactivity on major non-communicable diseases worldwide: an analysis of burden of disease and life expectancy. *Lancet.* 2012;380(9838):219-229. doi: 10.1016/S0140-6736(12)61031-9.

21. World Health Organization. Global health risks: Mortality and burden of disease attributable to selected major risks. Geneva, Switzerland: WHO; 2009. Available at http://www.who.int/healthinfo/global_burden_disease/GlobalHealthRisks_report_full.pdf. Accessed October 24, 2017.

22. Kohl HW 3rd, Craig CL, Lambert EV, et al. The pandemic of physical inactivity: global action for public health. *Lancet.* 2012;380(9838):294-305. doi: 10.1016/S0140-6736(12)60898-8.

23. Pearson ER. Dissecting the etiology of type 2 diabetes in the Pima Indian population. *Diabetes.* 2015;64(12):3993–3995. doi: 10.2337/dbi15-0016.

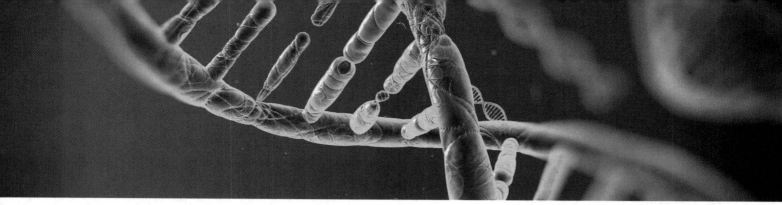

CHAPTER 10

Maternal Biology

Madeline Bundy

LEARNING OBJECTIVES

By the end of this chapter, the student will be able to:

- Apply a life-course perspective to maternal and infant health outcomes
- Describe the major functions of the menstrual cycle
- Compare methods of contraception by efficacy and major mechanism of action
- Differentiate embryonic and fetal development
- Summarize major maternal adaptations in pregnancy
- Explain the major mechanisms involved in labor and parturition
- Discuss the evolution and significance of drug safety assessment in pregnancy
- Identify the major infectious causes of adverse perinatal outcomes
- Describe the primary elements and goals of prenatal and postpartum care
- List the leading causes of maternal mortality globally
- Describe the current status of maternal health in the United States

CHAPTER OUTLINE

▶ Introduction

The life-course perspective is a popular conceptual framework for understanding the development of disease and health-related outcomes in women and children across generations. The life-course perspective considers the individual's lifetime trajectory and the interplay of factors, such as genetics, environment, life experiences, and social systems. Its application to pregnancy suggests that determinants of maternal and infant health begin far before conception and prenatal care, possibly extending to even the health and experiences of previous familial generations. A growing base of scientific data supports the life-course model in maternal health, including epigenetics, studies of adaptive development, and allostatic load. Application of the framework may inform a better understanding of some of the seemingly intractable disparities in maternal and infant health.[1]

▶ Female Reproductive Physiology and Management

Menstrual Cycle

Historically, the biologic process of menstruation assumes a significant role in values of gender distinction throughout the world. Across diverse religious, cultural, and social contexts, menstruation-specific practices and beliefs are commonplace. Although varied, many are based on constructs of menstruation as an unhygienic, secretive, or even shameful process. These beliefs are often echoed in modern western advertising, which frequently promotes menstruation as a problem that requires treatment; examples include medications for menstrual discomforts and scented tampons or douches for concealment and cleanliness.[2]

The menstrual cycle is a highly complex and regulated process that results in the physiologic capacity to achieve fertilization and pregnancy. In general, the time from **menarche**, the first menstruation, until **menopause**, the absence of menstruation for 1 year, comprises the fertile period of a woman's lifetime.

In pubertal development, menarche occurs approximately 2–3 years after breast bud development. In the United States, the average age of menarche has remained stable for 3 decades, except among non-Hispanic black females, for whom the median age has decreased by 5.5 months.[3] Across all races in the United States, there exist significant variations in the average age of menarche, occurring at age 12.06 years among African American females, 12.25 years among Hispanic females, and 12.55 years among Caucasian females.[4] Potential modifiers of menarche onset include socioeconomic conditions, genetics, nutrition, and body composition, preventive health care, prenatal conditions, light exposure, exposure to endocrine-disrupting chemicals, and psychologic stress.[3,5] Although recent research suggests an association between higher childhood body mass index (BMI), weight gain, and earlier pubertal onset, there is at present no identified association between BMI and age of menarche.[3,5]

During each menstrual cycle, hormonal interactions between the hypothalamus of the brain, the pituitary organ, and the ovaries (the HPO axis) coordinate two concurrent cycles of growth: the ovarian cycle in the ovaries, and the endometrial cycle in the lining of the uterus. The typical length of a menstrual cycle, counted from the first menstrual day to the final day without menstruation, is 28 ± 7 days.[6]

The orchestration of the **hypothalamic–pituitary–ovarian (HPO) axis** primarily depends on a negative feedback loop. A **negative feedback loop** is among the most common form of feedback control in human physiology and functions to maintain a desired range of hormone level by decreasing the secretion of one substance in response to the rise of another.

The basic pathway of the HPO axis begins with the **hypothalamus**, a portion of the base of the brain, and the **anterior pituitary**, a small endocrine organ located just below the hypothalamus. The hypothalamus secretes pulses of **gonadotropin-releasing hormone (GnRH)**, a neurohormone, which then travel to the anterior pituitary and signal the secretion of follicle-stimulating hormone (FSH) and luteinizing hormone (LH). FSH and LH belong to a group of glycoprotein polypeptide hormones, known as **gonadotropins**, which target the gonads and serve important endocrine roles in sexual development and reproductive function.[7] In the menstrual cycle, FSH and LH act on the ovaries, stimulating the secretion of the gonadal hormones estrogen and progesterone. The hypothalamus subsequently responds to circulating levels of estrogen and progesterone by either increasing or decreasing secretion of GnRH and consequently, closing the HPO axis loop.

The **ovarian cycle** describes ova maturation and consists of three phases: follicular, ovulation, and luteal. The follicular phase is the most variable in length, ranging from 10 to 17 days, and accounts for major differences in overall menstrual cycle length among women.[8]

At the beginning of the follicular cycle, corresponding to day 1 of menstruation, the HPO axis responds to low levels of circulating estrogen by increasing FSH secretion from the anterior pituitary and consequently promoting estrogen secretion from the ovary. Increasing levels of estrogen in this stage promote follicular recruitment and growth in the ovary. A **follicle** is a structural and functional group of cells on the ovary responsible for housing a single oocyte and releasing gonadal hormones. Although several follicles are recruited with each cycle, only a *single* selected follicle will continue development and undergo ovulation. This follicle, referred to as the primary or dominant (graffian) follicle, is possibly primed in previous months and secretes a greater amount of estrogen than the other recruited follicles.

Around days 5–7 of the follicular cycle, LH and FSH levels begin to decline in response to the increased estrogen production by the ovaries and consequently cause the nondominant follicles to undergo atresia, or death. The dominant follicle, however, continues growing under the local influence of its own high estrogen production. Near the end of the phase, the achievement of a peak estrogen level causes the HPO axis to temporarily switch to a *positive feedback loop*, causing a surge of LH and FSH secretion. The LH surge is necessary for ovulation, and among many functions is also associated with increased sexual libido and resumption of meiosis in the oocyte. In addition, the LH surge consistently anticipates ovulation by approximately 36–44 hours and consequently is used as a clinical marker for determining time of ovulation.

During the ovulation phase, the influence of estrogen, prostaglandins, enzymes, and smooth muscle contractions contribute to follicle rupture and the release of a matured oocyte into the fallopian tube.[9] **Prostaglandins** are a group of physiologically active substances made from fatty acids. They are present in tissue throughout the body and assume numerous hormone-like functions, including dilation of blood vessels, inflammation, and smooth muscle contraction.[10] The remaining cells of the ruptured follicle form the **corpus luteum**, which literally translates to "yellow body." The corpus luteum is a temporary ovarian structure with a yellowish appearance from the cellular uptake of lutein pigment and steroid hormones after release of the ovum. Its principal function is the production of progesterone, which switches the menstrual cycle from an estrogen-high process in the follicular phase to a progesterone-high process in the luteal phase.[8]

The luteal phase begins with the pre-ovulatory LH surge and ends with the onset of menstruation. In contrast to the follicular phase, the luteal phase is consistently 13–15 days in length. The high progesterone production by the corpus luteum suppresses secretion of GnRH in the HPO axis and consequently suppresses follicular development. Progesterone levels also stimulate growth in the endometrium and initiate the secretory phase of the endometrial cycle. Approximately 7–8 days after the LH surge, progesterone levels peak to support implantation of a conceptus into the endometrium. In the absence of fertilization, the corpus luteum will degenerate, causing a drop in progesterone, and ending the menstrual cycle by day 14–15 of the luteal phase.[8]

The **endometrial cycle** pertains to the cyclical growth of the endometrial lining of the uterus and includes the proliferative, secretory, and menstrual phases. The proliferative phase occurs during the follicular ovarian phase and lasts from the end of menstruation until ovulation. As menstruation ceases, the endothelial cells of endometrium undergo hyperplasia in response to rising estrogen levels from the primary follicle. **Hyperplasia** refers to the growth of tissue due to cell proliferation, or an increased number of cells.[11] Under the influence of estrogen, the endometrial tissue becomes more vascular and increases to 3–5 mm in thickness.[9]

The secretory phase begins after ovulation and corresponds to the luteal phase of the ovarian cycle. Influenced predominately by the secretion of progesterone from the corpus luteum, the epithelial cells and blood vessels of the endometrium continue developing to prepare for implantation of a fertilized oocyte. The epithelial cells increase storage of glycogen, a primary source of cellular energy, the blood vessels coil and increase in permeability, and prostaglandins are produced.[9] If fertilization occurs, the endometrial tissue will continue growing and reach a thickness of 5–10 mm at time of implantation. If fertilization does not occur, the corpus luteum atrophies, causing a drop in progesterone and estrogen levels, and initiating the onset of the menstrual phase.

The menstrual phase lasts an average of 4 ± 2 days and marks the end of the endometrial cycle, as well as the onset of a new menstrual cycle. During menstruation, prostaglandin secretion contributes to uterine contraction, and the endometrial tissue degenerates and sloughs from the uterus with bleeding. Concurrently, the low circulating levels of ovarian hormones, resulting from degradation of the corpus luteum, signal the negative feedback loop of the HPO axis, initiating an increase in GnRH and the beginning of another cycle.[9] See **FIGURE 10-1**.

Conception

Conception, or fertilization, most often occurs in the outer third of the fallopian tube and refers to the entry of a sperm nucleus into the oocyte nucleus.[9,12]

Along the sperm's journey from the cervix to the fallopian tubes, the sperm undergoes cellular changes (capacitation) so that it can bind and enter the ovum. Although usually only one sperm is involved in fertilization, the presence of a thousand or so other sperm at the time of ovulation is essential. The additional sperm release enzymes that break down the outer layer of the oocyte cells (zona pellucida) and promote entry of a single sperm into the oocyte. To achieve fertilization, the single sperm must reach the traveling oocyte within a window of 12–24 hours from time of ovulation.[9] Sperm maintain fertility capacity for approximately 72 hours, and consequently, successful fertilization is often the result of intercourse occurring in the 2–3 days before ovulation.[8]

Within just hours of fertilization, the first cell of a human being, known as a **zygote**, develops. The zygote is a diploid cell, indicating a complete

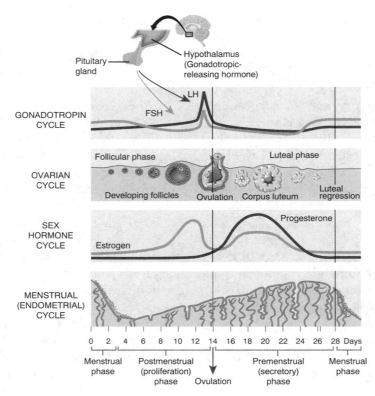

FIGURE 10-1 The Menstrual Cycle

set of 46 chromosomes and an equal contribution of 23 chromosomes from the oocyte and sperm.[4,9] The sperm determines the gender of the embryo by contributing either an X (female) or Y (male) sex chromosome, complementing the X sex chromosome from the oocyte.[9] The zygote then undergoes a series of mitotic cell divisions in which the zygote cell replicates and forms a mass of identical daughter cells.

During days 6–10 after conception, the cell mass, now containing 58 cells and known as a **blastocyst**, migrates into the uterus and begins the implantation process. The functions of the blastocyst in implantation are numerous. The blastocyst sheds its protective outer shell, secreting substances, such as **human**

chorionic growth hormone (hCG), to help prepare the endometrial lining for implantation. Clinically, hCG levels rise in pregnancy around day 9 after the LH surge and provide the chemical marker for urine and serum pregnancy tests. Physiologically, hCG is an important hormone throughout pregnancy. In the early pregnancy, hCG is responsible for maintaining the corpus luteum to ensure continued progesterone production until the placenta can take over production, around 6–8 weeks.[13]

In addition, the blastocyst releases enzymes that break down the endometrium and allow the blastocyst to adhere and embed itself in the uterine lining. If implantation is successful and the pregnancy continues, the inner layer of the blastocyst will develop into the embryo, and the outer layer, known as the trophoblast, will become the placenta. See **FIGURE 10-2**.

Contraception

Contraception describes the deliberate use of natural or artificial methods to prevent pregnancy.[8] Available methods range significantly in degree of intervention and level of efficacy. Natural contraception describes those methods that require no physical barrier or medical intervention, including abstinence, withdrawal, and natural family planning, which range in rate of failure from 0–25%, respectively.

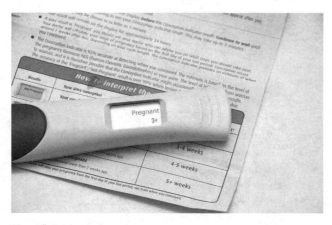

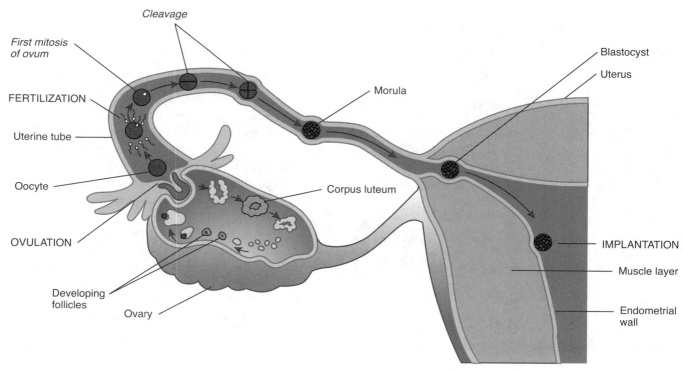

FIGURE 10-2 From Fertilization to Implantation

Barrier methods are those that utilize a physical and/or chemical barrier to prevent entry of sperm into the cervix. These include condoms (male and female), vaginal sponges, cervical caps, diaphragms, and spermicidal agents, and range from 14–50% in rates of failure. Except for the diaphragm, all barrier methods are available over the counter. Spermicidal agents may be used alone or in combination with physical barriers for added contraceptive protection and function by (1) physically blocking sperm entry, and (2) chemically reducing motility of sperm. Two methods, the diaphragm and cervical cap, require the addition of a spermicidal agent for efficacy. Lastly, male and female condoms are the only contraceptive methods that offer dual protection against sexually transmitted infections.

Hormonal methods of birth control are numerous. They include combination oral contraception, combination emergency oral contraception, progestin-only oral contraception, Depo-Provera (progestin only) injection, combination contraceptive patch, and combination hormonal vaginal ring; the failure rate ranges from 2–20%. In general, these methods rely on the administration of synthetic ovarian hormones to interrupt ovulation and the regulation of the menstrual cycle by the HPO axis. Due to their mechanism of action, some of these methods are also frequently used for noncontraceptive indications, such as cycle regulation, menstrual cramping, acne, premenstrual syndrome, premenstrual dysphoric disorder, and management of endometriosis.

The timing of intervention in the menstrual cycle is an important distinction between hormonal contraceptive methods and the medications used in abortion. Hormonal contraception (including emergency contraception) interrupts the menstrual cycle *before* fertilization occurs, whereas, abortion medications interfere with the hormones needed for continued development of an *existing* pregnancy. Except for emergency contraception, all types of hormonal contraception currently require a prescription in the United States. In contrast to natural and barrier methods, hormonal contraception is associated with both positive and negative side effects as well as a greater number of contraindications, all of which vary by dosage and route of method. The effect on menstrual

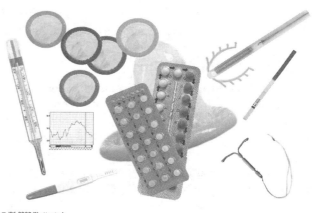

© JPC-PROD/Shutterstock

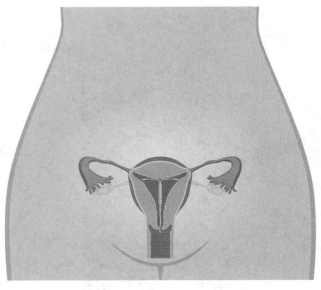

© Fancy Tapis/Shutterstock

bleeding also varies by person and formulation or type of method. However, any bleeding that occurs with use is due to variations in synthetic hormone levels and is *not* attributable to a true menstruation with shedding of the endometrial lining.

Long-acting reversible contraceptives (LARCs), including intrauterine devices (IUDs) and the progesterone-only implant, are the most effective nonpermanent forms of contraception. The two types of IUDs—progesterone-releasing and copper material—and progestin-only implant are associated with failure rates of < 1%. All LARC methods require an office visit for placement and removal. The length of efficacy ranges from 3–10 years, and all devices may be removed at any earlier point.

Lastly, female and male sterilization are permanent forms of contraception. These methods include the male vasectomy, female tubal ligation, and the female sterilization implant, and are associated with a failure rate range of 0.15–1%. Although subsequent procedures may be performed to attempt sterilization reversal, the success of these procedures is variable and should not be relied upon. Consequently, thorough, non-coerced consent is important with these procedures, which should be reserved for persons who desire permanent infertility.

Spontaneous Abortion

Spontaneous abortion, or miscarriage, is the demise of a pregnancy without medical or mechanical assistance.[4] The incidence is difficult to accurately ascertain; however, among clinically established pregnancies, the prevalence of miscarriage is 15%.[14] In general, data show an inverse relationship between increased gestational age and the relative risk of spontaneous abortion. Approximately 80% of spontaneous abortions occur

before 12 weeks' gestation, with only 2–3% occurring after clinical determination of cardiac activity.[4,14]

The etiology of spontaneous abortion varies by gestational age. In the first 2 weeks, most spontaneous abortions are attributed to unsuccessful embryo implantation or chromosomal abnormalities and overall, chromosomal abnormalities account for more than half of all cases in the first 12 gestational weeks.[15] Some of the risk factors for spontaneous abortion include increased maternal and paternal age, substance use or toxin exposure, autoimmune and endocrine disease, infection, psychosocial stress, genetics, and uterine or cervical abnormalities.[4,15]

In most cases, the uterus will expel the products of conception without complication. Depending on gestational age and maternal history, varying degrees of bleeding and cramping are common during miscarriage. If the products of conception do not expel spontaneously, or expel incompletely, medical or surgical management is required to evacuate the uterus and prevent infection.

Induced Abortion

In the United States, approximately one in four pregnancies results in an induced abortion.[16] An **induced abortion** is the termination of a pregnancy, by medical or surgical means, before the point of fetal viability. The term **fetal viability** purports to define the developmental age at which a fetus can survive the extrauterine environment. Historically, the determination of the viability has provoked significant debate regarding biologic, technologic, ethical, economic, social, religious, and medical issues. Currently there exists no universally accepted definition; however, in the United States, fetal viability is defined at 24 weeks' gestation.[17]

Induced abortion includes both **elective abortion**, which is performed at the request of the mother, and **therapeutic abortion**, which occurs for maternal medical indications or serious fetal anomalies.[4] The legal methods for induced abortion vary depending on gestational age. The **medication abortion** is approved for the first 10 weeks of pregnancy in the United States. The method approved by the U.S. Food and Drug Administration (FDA) consists of two medications, mifepristone and misoprostol, administered 24–48 hours apart. Mifepristone ends the pregnancy by blocking progesterone, while misoprostol stimulates uterine contractions and cervical softening. The products of conception typically pass within 24 hours of misoprostol administration and are associated with uterine cramping and bleeding. Overall, the medication abortion is most efficacious in early pregnancy, with a success rate of 98% among pregnancies less than 8 weeks' gestation and 93% among pregnancies less than 10 weeks' gestation.

A **surgical abortion** involves the mechanical removal of the pregnancy from the uterus. In the first 14–16 weeks, a procedure called dilation and curettage is performed, in which the cervix is mechanically dilated with dilator rods and the products of conception are removed by suction, using a curettage. After 16 weeks' gestation, a dilation and evacuation (D&E) procedure is performed. In addition to mechanical dilation with dilator rods, the cervix may be further prepared and softened with misoprostol or cervadil; these medications are also commonly used in labor induction. In the D&E, products of conception are removed using both suction and hand instruments, such as forceps. Both surgical abortion procedures can be performed in an outpatient setting, with the optional use of conscious sedation, and take approximately 5–10 minutes. The overall success rate of surgical abortion is 99%.

In general, the risks associated with legal medical and surgical abortions are significantly lower than the risks associated with pregnancy. According to data collected over 7 years in the United States, the risk of maternal death related to legal abortion was 14 times lower than the risk of death related to delivery of a live neonate. Similarly, associated rates of complications are lower with legal abortion, as compared with childbirth.[18]

In contrast, the practice of unsafe abortion, or those performed without the supervision of a licensed medical professional and/or by unapproved methods, is associated with significant medical risk and represents a major public health issue. Worldwide, deaths attributed to unsafe abortions are estimated at 47,000 per year, contributing to nearly 13% of all maternal deaths.[19]

▶ Physiology of Normal Pregnancy

The Embryo and Fetus

Developing human cells are referred to as an **embryo** from time of implantation to 8 weeks of pregnancy, and a **fetus** from 9 weeks of pregnancy to birth. On average, full fetal development occurs over 266 days, from the time of fertilization to birth. However, because pregnancy is traditionally measured from the first day of the last menstrual period (LMP), development is most often described as a 280- to 283-day process.[20]

In the second week after conception, an embryonic disc adjoined to a yolk sac and amniotic cavity develop within the implanted blastocyst. The yolk sac provides nutrients to the developing embryo in early pregnancy and the amniotic cavity encircles the growing embryo. The entire structure is connected to the outer blastocyst

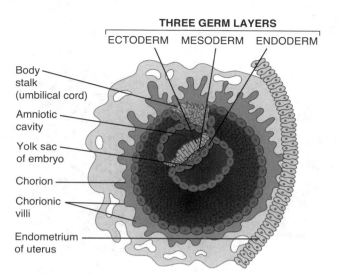

FIGURE 10-3 Embryonic Primary Germ Layers

cells by a connecting stalk. Later in pregnancy, the yolk sac disappears as placental function takes over, the connecting stalk develops into the umbilical cord, and the amniotic cavity forms the amniotic sac that surrounds the fetus, umbilical cord, and amniotic fluid.

The cells of the embryonic disc rearrange to develop from a bilayer cellular structure into three primary germ cell layers. The germ layers serve as the basis for development of fetal structure and all tissues and organs. The germ layers undergo a process of folding, resulting in a cylindrical embryo, followed by cellular differentiation into organ and tissue structures. The endoderm (inner germ layer) develops into the gastrointestinal, urinary, and respiratory tracts. The mesoderm (middle germ layer) becomes cartilage, bone, smooth muscle, blood, and lymph, as well as the heart, kidneys, reproductive organs, and adrenal glands. Finally, the outer ectoderm forms the nervous systems, muscle, mammary and pituitary glands, skin, hair, and nails.[20] See **FIGURE 10-3**. **Organogenesis** describes the period of embryo development from weeks 3–8 after fertilization, during which the major organ structures form.[21]

The cardiovascular system begins developing in the third week, becoming the first functional system of the embryo. Blood vessel formation begins and the connecting stalk associates with a small part of the forming umbilical vesicle, creating the fledgling structure of the umbilical cord, arteries, and vein. By day 22, the heart beats.[20]

The notochord is a rod-like structure that forms between the endoderm and ectoderm, and provides organization to development of the spine, nervous system, and surrounding skeleton. By the fourth week, the notochord degenerates and gives rise to the neural plate, from which the central nervous system and retina originate. By the eighth week, the cranial structure, brain,

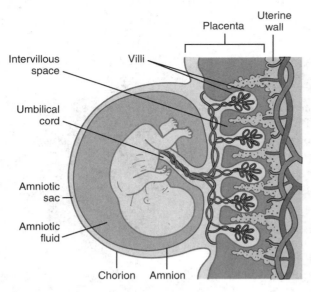

FIGURE 10-4 The Embryo at 8 Weeks

limbs, fingers, toes, and eyelids are distinctly developed, although not fully formed or functional. See **FIGURE 10-4**.

Fetal development begins after the eighth week. In general, major developmental landmarks are observed every 4 weeks during this period. In the first month of fetal development, the fetus doubles in length, and the intestinal and renal tracts mature. The fetus is capable of swallowing amniotic fluid, producing urine, and excreting waste into maternal circulation by week 11. In the second month, female reproductive organs are developed and fetal bones are visible by ultrasound. In the third month, growth is rapid and brown fat begins accumulating for heat production. Maternal sensation of fetal movements also occurs in this period.

At 24 weeks, fetal weight gain increases and the lungs begin production of surfactant. The presence of surfactant is critical to fetal adaptation to extra-uterine lung function and life, reducing surface tension and allowing the lungs to inflate when outside of the fluid-filled intrauterine environment. Clinically, this physiology informs the management of preterm labor, a common goal of which includes the reduction or cessation of contractions to allow for the delivery of maternal steroids, which stimulate fetal surfactant production and improve fetal respiratory outcomes.

By weeks 26–29 of pregnancy, the fetal nervous system is mature enough to direct breathing and internal temperature. However, although lung movement is visible on ultrasound, the lungs are not functional; the maternoplacental unit continues providing the fetus with oxygen and gas exchange until delivery. At this point in development, most neonates who receive intensive care unit assistance can survive extrauterine life. Throughout the last trimester, the fetus gains increased weight, acquires maternal antibodies, and develops fine motor skills, such as pupillary light and grasp reflexes. The fetal central nervous system and lungs continue maturing throughout the last weeks of pregnancy.

The Placenta and Amniotic Fluid

The placenta is a critical and complex organ of pregnancy. At term, the discoid placenta organ averages 450 grams—one-seventh of the total fetal weight.[13] Functionally, the placenta assumes many important roles for the immature fetus, including those of the lungs, liver, and kidneys. The placenta is responsible for (1) separation of maternal and fetal blood flow; (2) exchange of gases, nutrients, waste, and electrolytes; and (3) production of essential pregnancy hormones.[4,13] Notably, the placenta is responsible for 95% of maternal–fetal gas exchange in the second and third trimesters.[13]

Beginning with implantation of the blastocyst, the placenta develops from both maternal and fetal cells.[4,13] Structurally, the blastocyst is encircled by the outer trophoblast cell layer and within the blastocyst is the developing embryonic disc with adjacent amniotic and yolk sac structures. The trophoblast layer is

Human Embryonic and Foetal Development

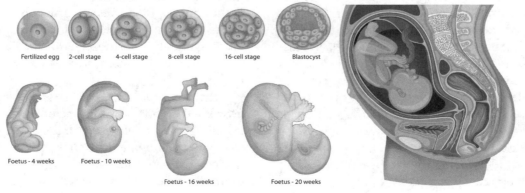

multinucleated and thicker directly below the embryonic pole. In placental development, the trophoblast cell layer differentiates into two layers, which invade the uterine lining toward maternal blood vessels.

The finger-like extensions of the outer trophoblast layer into the endometrium create a network of maternal serum filled cavities known as the intervillous space (IVS). The IVS is essential to pregnancy progression and allows for a system of steady, low-pressure, low-resistance circulation between the uterus and placenta.[13,20] Similar extensions of the inner trophoblast layer into the outer trophoblast layer and endometrium form the chorionic villi, which eventually develop into the fetal blood vessels of the placenta. Although these villi develop along the entire trophoblast, only those in the thicker area of the trophoblast, below the embryo, will remain after the first trimester. This vascular area of the trophoblast develops on the fetal side of the placenta, while the remaining trophoblast layer becomes the chorionic sac. High-resolution imaging reveals that significant fluid exchange in the IVS occurs around 10–12 weeks of pregnancy, coinciding with the functional demise of the yolk sac.[13]

Concurrently, the primed endometrium of the uterus undergoes cellular and vascular changes in response to implantation. In pregnancy, the endometrium has three distinct layers, the *decidua basalis*, *decidua capilaris*, and *decidua vera*.[4,20] The *decidua basalis* is the deepest layer, resting against the uterus, and located directly below the implanted blastocyst. The *decidua basalis* will form the maternal side of the placenta, as villi projections from the trophoblast extended into this layer of endometrium. As these projections repeat and branch, they create the characteristic "lobed" appearance of the maternal side of the placenta. Structurally, each lobule is a projection of the trophoblast with an epithelial covering and a core containing branches to the umbilical artery and vein. Functionally, each lobule is a point of exchange between the mother and fetus.[13] The *decidua capilaris* and *decidua vera* are superficial to the *decidua basalis* and located above the trophoblast. As embryo development progresses, the superficial *decidua capilaris* will disappear and the *decidua vera* will become fused with the chorionic sac.

Around week 12, the amniotic sac surrounding the embryo adheres to the chorionic sac.[20] Within the amniotic sac, the fetus is surrounded and protected by amniotic fluid. The volume of amniotic fluid is maintained within a normal range by the balance of fluid production and fluid reabsorption. The principal source of fluid production is fetal urination and lung liquid production, while fluid reabsorption is mostly due to fetal swallowing and membrane diffusion.[22] Amniotic fluid serves numerous functions essential to normal fetal development, including protection from trauma and bacterial infection, facilitation of growth and movement, promotion of gastrointestinal maturation, and temperature regulation.[20] Clinically, abnormally low or high levels of amniotic fluid may be associated with maternal dehydration or conditions affecting the fetal kidneys or gastrointestinal tract.

Basics of Fetal Circulation

As described previously, the fetus depends on the placenta and umbilical cord for its source of oxygenated blood and nutrients. In utero, the fetal lungs are fluid-filled organs, which exhibit intermittent movements but do not participate in fetal oxygenation or gas exchange. Gas exchange in the placenta provides the only source of well-oxygenated blood, while the umbilical cord functions to transport blood to and from the placental unit. The umbilical cord is comprised of two arteries and one vein. In contrast to blood flow in the developed human, the umbilical vein carries oxygenated blood toward the fetus, while the two umbilical arteries carry deoxygenated blood away from the fetus.[22] Structurally, the fetal heart maintains unique shunts to allow for blood exchange with the placenta, as well as reduced blood flow to the underdeveloped fetal liver and lungs. In utero, the fetus must also depend on the maternoplacental unit for the functions of the liver, including elimination of fetal waste products.

Major Maternal Adaptations of Pregnancy

The female body undergoes significant anatomic, endocrine, and physiologic changes to establish and accommodate pregnancy.[23,24] Over the course of pregnancy, the uterus grows from a small pelvic organ into a large abdominal organ. To fit the growing gravid uterus, the diaphragm rises by 4 cm, and the bladder, intestines, and liver are all displaced.[23] In a term pregnancy, average total gestational weight gain ranges from 22 to 37 lbs for women with a normal pre-pregnancy BMI (18.5–24.9). The placenta, fetus, and amniotic fluid contribute to 35–59% of this gestational weight.[23]

Hormonal regulation assumes a major role in the healthy development of pregnancy. In comparison to nonpregnant states, in which the menstrual cycle fluctuates between estrogen and progesterone dominance, pregnancy is characterized by persistently elevated progesterone levels. Among its numerous functions, progesterone promotes smooth muscle relaxation and maintains the quiescence of the uterus during pregnancy, allowing the fetus to adequately grow and mature within the organ for an extended period. This same relaxation effect throughout the body, however, contributes to many of the discomforts of pregnancy, including

TABLE 10-1 Select Maternal Adaptations in Pregnancy	
System	**Adaptation**
Immunologic	Immune system suppression; including suppression of T-helper cells and T-cytotoxic cells
Musculoskeletal	Lordosis of spine and change in center of gravity with growing uterus/fetus Relaxation of the joints and increased mobility due to progesterone Increased elasticity and relaxation of ligaments due to relaxin and estrogen
Cardiovascular	Heart is displaced up and to the left Cardiac output increases 30–50% (peak 25–30 weeks) Decrease in blood pressure due to decreased peripheral vascular resistance
Hematologic	Blood volume increases by 30–50% Red blood cell mass increases by 20–30% White blood cells increase by 8% (primarily neutrophils) Plasma volume increases by 45–50% (peak 32 weeks) Hemoglobin, hematocrit, serum ferritin decrease (physiologic anemia) Increased coagulopathy (i.e., increased clotting ability)
Metabolic	Metabolic rate increases 8× the normal rate by end of pregnancy Daily caloric needs increase by 300 calories in second and third trimesters
Respiratory	More efficient respiratory exchange and increased oxygen demands Reduced pulmonary resistance, increased respiratory rate, and increased sensitivity to CO_2 chemoreceptors
Renal	Kidneys grow in volume and length Kidney blood flow increases 60–80% (peak mid-pregnancy)
Hepatic	Liver is displaced up and back with gravid uterus Liver produces increased coagulation and fibrinogen factors
Gastrointestinal	GI system is displaced up and back Slowed peristalsis and intestinal transit time due to progesterone

constipation, acid reflux, sinus congestion, and varicose veins.

The fetoplacental unit, which describes the interactions of the fetus, placenta, and mother, is principally responsible for hormonal regulation.[25] The complete role of the fetal unit is still largely unknown. However, a major function is the production of androgens by the fetal adrenal glands. **Androgens** are a group of hormones that include testosterone and serve as precursors to estrogen production. In the fetoplacental unit, circulating levels of androgens are subsequently utilized by the placenta to create estriol, which is a weak form of estrogen and commonly referred to as "the estrogen of pregnancy." Estriol is responsible for increasing uterine blood flow, which promotes growth, and preparing the breasts for lactation.[25] To maintain estriol levels, the placenta secretes corticotropin-releasing hormone

(CRH), which stimulates the production of androgens by the fetus.

TABLE 10-1 outlines some of the major physiologic adaptations of the maternal body in pregnancy. Most often, these physiologic adaptations occur without incident and confer a normal pregnancy trajectory. However, it is important to consider the unique potential risks and vulnerabilities associated with these physiologic adaptations as they may inform many clinical and public health measures.

Labor and Parturition

Parturition, or childbirth, is achieved through the physiologic process of labor.[25,26] The initiation of labor is still not thoroughly understood; however, the fetoplacental unit is widely considered a major influencer. Most significantly, data from human and animal studies reveal that the fetus is principally responsible for regulation of the hormones associated with the onset of labor. Consequently, the fetus may also be a primary director of the gestational length of pregnancy.

The four physiologic phases of labor include: (1) quiescence (phase 0); (2) activation (phase 1); (3) stimulation (phase 2); and (4) involution (phase 3). The quiescence phase refers to the uterine state before labor, when uterine activity is suppressed by the influence of progesterone, relaxin, and other hormones.[25] The initiation of phase 1, activation, is hypothesized to result from fetal signaling mechanisms. Increased fetal production of CRH, corresponding to increasing fetal maturity, results in greater production of androgens and cortisol by the fetal adrenals. This, in turn, results in a higher yield of estriol by the placenta.

It is widely accepted that rising estrogen levels, or the change in the estrogen to progesterone ratio, influences the end of quiescence. Estrogen affects the uterine muscle by promoting the expression of uterine smooth muscle receptors, which in turn activate molecular signaling pathways involved in muscle contraction.[26] Additional hypotheses, based on recent data, include: (1) a signaling pathway between the fetal lungs and the fetoplacental unit near time of labor onset in term gestations,[25] and (2) a fetoplacental effect on maternal circadian rhythm (sleep cycle) that contributes to labor onset.[26]

The stimulation phase, which may take days to weeks in humans, involves the progressive onset of regular uterine contractions. The process largely occurs under the influence of prostaglandins and oxytocin, both of which are powerful uterotonics and used in synthetic forms to artificially augment labor. **Oxytocin** is a hormone produced in the hypothalamus of the brain and secreted by the posterior pituitary organ. Functionally, the hormone provokes uterine contractions directly, by binding to receptors on the uterus; and indirectly, by stimulating placental and amnion production of prostaglandins. During pregnancy, circulating maternal levels of oxytocin remain relatively consistent and are largely inactivated by the liver and kidneys. However, throughout pregnancy, the number of oxytocin receptors on the uterus increases by 200–300 times the normal concentration, causing an effective increase in uterine sensitivity to the hormone. At the onset of the first stage of labor, fetal circulation of oxytocin increases three-fold and in the second stage, maternal secretion increases significantly.[26]

During the stimulation phase, labor is further differentiated into three stages relating to the imminent event of parturition. Clinically, these stages are utilized as references for assessing normal progression

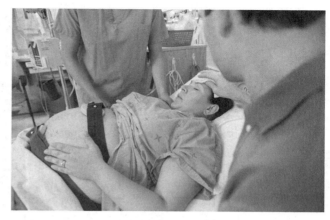
© Tyler Olson/Shutterstock

and alternatively, identifying complications. In respect to stages of labor, the term **labor** describes the occurrence of regular, effective contractions that are accompanied by progressive cervical change.[26] The **cervix**, also described as the "neck of the uterus," is cylindrical tissue that connects the lowermost portion of the uterus to the vagina. The inner tube of the cervix, known as the endocervical canal, serves as a passageway between the internal uterus and vagina. Structurally, the cervix is 2–3 cm in length, approximately 2.5 cm in width, and capable of changing shape under mechanical and chemical influence. Apart from a small amount of dilation during menstruation, the cervical os generally remains closed. However, in labor, cervical change is progressive and marked, reaching a final dilation of 10 cm width, with a barely palpable thickness (referred to as *complete effacement*). This substantial change in structure is largely achieved by the presence of prostaglandins and regular uterine contractions, which cause biochemical and mechanical breakdown of the cervical tissue connections.[26]

The first stage of labor comprises the onset of labor to complete dilation (10 cm) of the cervix. The stage is further differentiated into two phases, latent and active, which are characterized by slower and faster rates of cervical change, respectively. The average length of the first stage varies by a woman's obstetric history; women in their first delivery (*nulliparas*) average 6–13.3 hours in the first stage of labor, versus women with prior deliveries (*multiparas*), who average 5.7–7.5 hours. Often, women may also experience prodromal or "false" labor in the days or weeks prior to latent labor. During these transient periods, the body produces uterine contractions, often irregular, that are insufficient to cause progressive cervical change. Not surprisingly, these periods can be very exhausting and frustrating for women.[26]

The second stage of labor is the period from full dilation to the delivery of the infant. During this stage, the fetal head navigates and descends through the passageway of the pelvis via a series of seven distinct cardinal movements. Successful expulsion of the fetus through the vaginal canal depends on multiple factors, including maternal effort, adequacy of uterine contractions, fetal position, and adequacy of the maternal pelvis for fetal size. The length of the second stage similarly varies by obstetric history; nulliparous women average 36–57 minutes, versus multiparous women, who average 17–19 minutes. In addition, the use of an epidural is associated with a significant increase in the length of the second stage.

The rupture of membranes, or "breaking of waters," may occur at any point in the activation or stimulation phases. Most often, membrane rupture occurs *after* the onset of regular contractions and before the second stage. However, the membranes may also rupture *before* the onset of contractions, known as *premature rupture of membranes*, during the second stage, or even after delivery of the fetus. Membrane rupture results from the activation of structural and chemical changes in the maternal placenta and fetal membranes during the last weeks of pregnancy.[27] After membrane rupture, amniotic fluid production by the fetus and placenta continues, causing a constant leaking of fluid through the vagina.

The final phase of labor, uterine involution, begins immediately after the delivery of the infant and includes the third stage of labor, which comprises delivery of the infant to delivery of the placenta. The phase similarly depends on oxytocin and prostaglandins to mediate continued uterine contractions, resulting in detachment and expulsion of the placenta, immediate reduction in uterine size, and occlusion of the uterine blood vessels.[28]

Clinically, the third stage and the involution phase represent a critical point in maternal adaptation to the post parturition state. In the absence of adequate uterine contraction and involution, the mother is at significant risk for postpartum hemorrhage (PPH). PPH is defined as blood loss greater than 500 mL in a vaginal birth. Worldwide, PPH is the greatest cause of maternal morbidity and mortality; associated morbidities are frequently related to anemia, blood transfusion, kidney failure, blood-clotting disorders, and surgical removal of the uterus (hysterectomy).[28]

The physiology of this phase has informed global public health efforts to reduce associated maternal morbidity and mortality. The World Health Organization (WHO) currently recommends active management of the third stage, which includes biochemical promotion of uterine contraction via immediate postpartum administration of synthetic uterotonics (i.e., oxytocin), controlled cord traction during placental delivery, and mechanical promotion of uterine contraction by external uterine massage (*fundal massage*)

after placental delivery.[26,29] The implementation of active management is associated with a significant reduction in postpartum hemorrhage. A recent randomized control trial revealed that subjects were 66% less likely to experience PPH if active management was implemented.[26]

Historically, nipple stimulation is also utilized as physiologic management of the third stage, particularly in low-resource or low-intervention settings. The act of breastfeeding or manual nipple stimulation causes secretion of oxytocin from the posterior pituitary, leading to increased blood level values and uterine contractility.[28] However, despite evidence showing a measurable increase in intrauterine pressure associated with 15 minutes of immediate breastfeeding, the evidence on postpartum hemorrhage reduction is inconclusive. In 2016, a Cochrane review of available evidence concluded that the data on nipple stimulation and PPH are of poor quality and overall insufficient to determine any relationship.[28]

Preterm Birth

In 2005, preterm birth represented an estimated 9.6% of births worldwide. Defined as birth occurring between 20 and 37 completed weeks gestation, preterm birth is associated with significantly higher infant morbidity and mortality. Infant outcomes vary by gestational age at birth and include both acute and chronic conditions. The premature infant is particularly vulnerable to circulatory, heart, lung, and brain problems related to immature development, as well as severe infection.[27]

Despite increasing research and public health efforts, there remain few options for effectively identifying and reducing maternal risk of preterm delivery. The strongest indicator of preterm birth is a prior history of preterm birth, conferring a 1.5- to 2-fold increase in risk.[27] However, nearly half of women who deliver preterm have no identified risk factors.

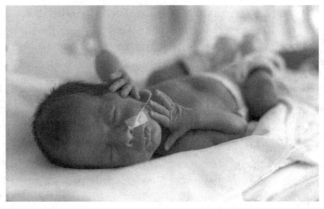

Additional maternal risk factors include: Black race, history of genital tract infection, bleeding of unknown cause in pregnancy, uterine structural anomaly, use of assisted reproductive technology, multiple fetal gestation, cigarette smoke and/or substance use, pre-pregnancy BMI classified as underweight (BMI < 18.5 kg/m²) or overweight (BMI > 30 kg/m²), periodontal disease, limited education, low income, low social status, late entry into prenatal care, and high levels of personal stress.[27]

The etiology of preterm birth is complex and variable across gestational age. Apart from those preterm births that occur as the result of artificial induction for maternal or fetal condition, the physiologic process of parturition in preterm birth is the same as in term birth. However, in preterm birth, a pathologic process is responsible for labor activation. In general, common identified causes of pathology include: (1) early cervical shortening, (2) uterine infection, (3) increased uterine contractility, (4) early rupture of membranes, (5) reduced oxygenation between the placenta and uterus, and (6) maternal endocrine disorders that affect progesterone levels.[27]

The rate of preterm birth in the United States fell from 12.8% in 2006 to 11.4% in 2013.[27] However, significant racial disparities persist, and the rate among non-Hispanic black women is nearly twice that of non-Hispanic white women. Moreover, 80% of the difference in black/white infant mortality is attributable to preterm birth.[30] Early research on the disparity focused on possible biologic etiologies across races; however, these investigations were largely fruitless and failed to identify any racially linked biologic mechanisms associated with preterm birth. In contrast, there exists strong biologic plausibility for an association between the biologic pathway provoked by stress and pathologic pathway of preterm labor. Increasingly, researchers are investigating the role of social structure and lived experience, including experiences of structural and overt racism, as well as chronic stress, in the etiology of preterm birth disparities.[30]

Cesarean Delivery

Cesarean delivery is the surgical birth of a fetus through an incision in the maternal abdomen. Worldwide, cesarean delivery rates vary substantially, ranging from excessively high to inadequately low. In the United States, the cesarean rate has risen from less than 5% in 1960 to 32% in 2015.[31,32] Undoubtedly, cesarean delivery represents a significant achievement in obstetric care; however, it is also associated with increased maternal morbidity and risk in future pregnancies, as compared to vaginal delivery. The common indications for cesarean delivery include: (1) failure

for labor to progress (30%), (2) prior cesarean delivery (30%), (3) nonreassuring fetal heart rate monitoring patterns (10%), and (4) an undesirable presentation of the fetus (i.e., fetal malpresentation) in the pelvis.[32] Although frequently discussed, a macrosomic fetus, or those weighing more than 4,000 g, accounts for only 4% of cesareans, while maternal request for cesarean delivery accounts for only 3% of cesarean deliveries.[32]

As compared with a vaginal delivery or unplanned cesarean, a planned cesarean is associated with a decreased risk of hemorrhage and transfusion, surgical complications, and urinary incontinence in the first year postpartum.[33] The potential short-term risks of planned cesarean delivery are relatively low in developed countries but include a longer hospital stay, uterine infection, wound infection, development of a life-threatening blood clot, and an increased risk of transient infant respiratory problems.[32,33]

Most notably, cesarean delivery is associated with substantial risks in subsequent pregnancies. After each cesarean, the relative risks of uterine rupture and abnormal placentation increase significantly, conferring an increased risk of infant and maternal morbidity and mortality. Uterine rupture is the separation of the uterus, usually at the site of a previous scar, and denotes a potentially fatal medical emergency for the woman and fetus. The incidence of rupture among women laboring is 0.7–0.9% after one cesarean, and 0.9–1.8% after two cesareans.[34]

Corresponding to the rising trend of cesareans in the United States, the rate of placenta accreta has increased from 1 in 30,000 births in 1960, to estimates of 1 in 333 births today.[32,34] **Placenta accreta** is the growth of placental tissue into one or more layers of the uterine muscle (versus decidua). The condition interferes with complete placental separation after birth, and subsequently results in a significantly higher risk of hemorrhage, large blood volume transfusion, intensive care unit admission, and hysterectomy.[34] The two leading risk factors for placenta accreta are history of prior cesarean delivery and the presence of placenta previa. The risk of accreta increases with each subsequent cesarean delivery; recent estimates show a risk of 3%, 11%, 40%, and 67%, among women with a history of no cesarean, one prior cesarean, two prior cesareans, and four or more prior cesareans, respectively.[32,34] See **FIGURE 10-5**.

Placenta previa is another condition of abnormal placentation associated with prior cesarean deliveries. In previa, the placenta grows in front of, or immediately next to, the cervical os, creating a condition incompatible with safe vaginal delivery and requiring a planned cesarean delivery before spontaneous onset of labor. The risk of previa similarly increases by

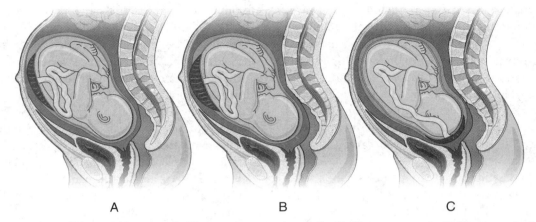

FIGURE 10-5 Disorders of Placental Position. **A.** Placenta in normal position. **B.** Placenta accreta. **C.** Placenta previa.

number of prior cesareans, ranging from 0.9% among women with one prior cesarean to 10% among women with four or more cesarean deliveries.[32]

In a 2013 opinion, The American College of Obstetricians and Gynecologists (ACOG) concluded that vaginal delivery should be recommended for all women in the absence of maternal or fetal indications for cesarean.[33] Moreover, ACOG specifies that cesarean by maternal request is not appropriate among women who desire future fertility due to the increased risk of complications in subsequent pregnancies.[33]

In 2015, the WHO revised its longstanding opinion that population-level cesarean rates should range from 10–15% and moreover discouraged countries and/or hospitals from utilizing a "target cesarean rate" to direct care. In contrast, this recommendation, which remains current today, advises that utilization of cesarean delivery be guided by medical indication alone. The data reveal that population-level cesarean rates less than 10% are associated with poorer infant and maternal mortality, while rates greater than 10% are not associated with any improvement in maternal and infant mortality.[35]

Vaginal Birth After Cesarean

The safety of vaginal birth after cesarean (VBAC) delivery has been a much-disputed topic among obstetric practitioners for nearly six decades in the United States. In 2010, ACOG publicly affirmed that most women with a history of one cesarean delivery are eligible for VBAC and consequently should receive such counseling.[36] It is difficult to ascertain a national estimate, but data available from the revised birth certificate program in 48 states reveal a VBAC rate of 11.2% in 2015.[37] In comparison, estimated trial of labor after cesarean (TOLAC) rates in other developed countries are between 50–70%.[38] Fluctuations in

the trend of VBAC rates in the United States since the 1960s largely reflect the changing clinical guidelines on VBAC, which affected access and practice. Currently, access to healthcare providers who perform VBACs remains unequal throughout the country and a primary topic among birth advocates.

Clinically, it is important that women are carefully screened for the appropriateness of attempting a VBAC, otherwise known as a TOLAC. According to ACOG, maternal eligibility criteria include: (1) one or two previous, low-transverse cesarean deliveries, (2) a clinically adequate pelvis, and (3) absence of other uterine scars of history of rupture.[33] Similar to repeat cesarean deliveries, the primary risk associated with VBAC is uterine rupture, which also increases with a greater number of prior cesarean deliveries.

Although the risk of uterine rupture increases significantly with greater number of past cesarean deliveries, the magnitude of risk remains relatively small. Data from large studies reveal estimated rates of uterine rupture during VBAC ranging from 0.6–0.9% among women with one prior cesarean delivery, and 0.9–3.7% among women with two or more previous cesarean deliveries.[38] In addition, a recent large multicenter study of 13,617 women showed that success rates are statistically similar—approximately 75%—among women with a history of one versus two prior cesarean deliveries.[38]

Newborn Transition to Extrauterine Life

The fetus undergoes many adaptations in order to successfully transition to life in the extrauterine environment. Notably, the occlusion of the umbilical cord demarks the cessation of oxygenation and nutrients from the maternoplacental unit, and consequently, the lungs must undergo a major physical and functional change. The lungs change from a fluid-filled to an air-filled organ and assume responsibility for gas exchange and oxygenation of the body. All mechanisms by which the lungs make this transition are not completely known. However, the presence of fetal surfactant, as well as chest compression by the maternal pelvis in delivery, are well-known contributors to successful clearance of fetal lung fluid at birth. With the initial compression and subsequent recoil of the fetal chest with vaginal delivery, the lungs both expel fluid and fill with air, aiding in the pressure gradient shift that supports lung function as the infant takes its first breaths. Premature infants, who lack sufficient lung surfactant, as well as infants born by cesarean delivery who do not receive the benefits of passage through the maternal pelvis, are at higher risk of delayed lung clearance.[39]

Accompanied with the occlusion of the umbilical cord at birth, as well as the shift in pressure gradient with air filling the fetal lungs, the circulatory system must also concurrently adapt in order to maintain extrauterine survival. From the first breaths to weeks after delivery, the heart subsequently undergoes functional and structural adaptations to accommodate the loss of the maternoplacental blood supply and redirect complete blood flow through the newly functional lungs and liver.[39]

Postpartum Physiology and Breastfeeding

The postpartum period describes the time from expulsion of the placenta to 6–8 weeks after delivery. In general, the major maternal adaptations to pregnancy return to the pre-pregnancy state by 6 weeks postpartum. Approximately 2 days after birth, the uterus begins the process of involution and returning to pre-pregnancy size. Involution is complete by 14 days postpartum, at which time the uterus is again a pelvic organ and no longer palpable in the abdomen. As the uterus cramps, blood and debris from the conceptus are expelled. Typically, vaginal discharge evolves from a bright red color, in the immediate days postpartum, to a pinkish-yellow color, which indicates regeneration of the endometrial lining and lasts up to 4 weeks.[4]

Major postpartum cardiac adaptations include the return to pre-pregnancy cardiac output and blood volume levels within 1 week, and the return to pre-pregnancy blood pressure within 4 days. The return to pre-pregnancy cardiac output levels denotes a major maternal adaptation, as the body must suddenly manage a high volume of blood circulation with loss of the fetoplacental unit. In the first postpartum week, when cardiac output is still elevated, the mother remains vulnerable to pregnancy-induced hypertension problems. In addition, the mother is also at higher risk of life-threatening blood clots (deep vein thrombosis or pulmonary embolism) during the early postpartum period.

Female breast development is not complete or fully functional until pregnancy and lactation.[4] Under the influence of progesterone, prolactin, and other hormones, the breasts begin developing and preparing for breastfeeding early in pregnancy. As early as 12–16 weeks, the mammary glands are capable of producing colostrum. Colostrum is a yellowish milk, rich in nutrients and maternal antibodies, that provides the infant with initial nutrition until mature milk comes in. The onset of copious mature milk supply does not typically occur until days 3–7 post-delivery.

Breast milk production occurs via a positive feedback loop involving the secretion of prolactin hormone in response to nipple stimulation and the subsequent ejection of milk. This physiology is important to consider in regard to breastfeeding promotion and support. Initially, a newborn requires a breastfeed every 2–3 hours (8–12 times/day), providing adequate nipple stimulation for milk production. However, when formula is introduced early, and/or as mixed feeding, the newborn is not stimulating the breast as frequently, because (1) not every feeding occurs by breast, and (2) neonatal satiation is longer with formula due to slower digestion. In addition, the newborn does not utilize the same exertion with sucking from an artificial nipple and consequently may lose interest in breastfeeding.[40]

The benefits of breastfeeding are numerous. Many properties of breastmilk are not replicable in formula, including nutritional properties that adapt to the developmental needs of the infant; and immune supportive properties, including maternal antibodies, powerful antioxidants, and proteins for supporting gut health. Moreover, data reveal numerous positive

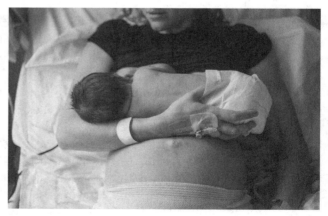

outcomes associated with breastfeeding, as compared to formula feeding. These include:

- Reduced infant risk of developing childhood obesity and type 2 diabetes
- Reduced maternal risk of developing heart disease and type 2 diabetes
- Reduced neonatal risk of developing infection and allergic disease[40]

▶ Maternofetal Transmission

The transport of substances across the placental barrier occurs by four mechanisms: simple diffusion, facilitated diffusion, active transport, and pinocytosis. Simple transfusion is the movement of a substance down a concentration gradient (high to low) and relates to oxygen, carbon dioxide, water, steroids, electrolytes, anesthetic gases, and most drugs. Facilitated diffusion utilizes a transport molecule, without additional energy input, to move a substance across the placental membrane. Facilitated diffusion is the transport mechanism of glucose, cholesterol, triglycerides, and phospholipids. Active transport utilizes energy to move a substance against or up a concentration gradient (low to high) and pertains to the transport of amino acids (basic units of proteins), vitamins, iodine, and calcium. Finally, pinocytosis describes when the substance is enveloped by another molecule for transport across the membrane. Maternal to fetal transmission of antibodies, as well as some larger-sized drugs, occurs via pinocytosis.[20]

The ability of a substance to cross the placental barrier depends on the interplay of many factors. In general, substances that are likely to cross the placental membrane are small, un-ionized (vs. ionized); lipid soluble (vs. water soluble); and/or described by a high protein-binding capacity. In addition, substances present in high concentrations in the maternal blood have a greater likelihood of transport, as more substance is available.[20]

Teratogens

In pregnancy, drugs associated with adverse fetal outcomes are described by one or more of the following terms: (1) *embryocidal*, if causing fetal death, (2) *teratogenic*, if causing *irreversible* damage to fetal structure or function, and (3) *fetotoxic*, if causing impairment to fetal growth or development in the second or third trimesters.[21] The term **teratogen** similarly applies to non-drug agents, or exposures, that are associated with such fetal harm; these may be "chemical, physical, infectious, or environmental in nature."[21]

It is well established that the timing of exposure is a major determinant of fetal outcome. In general,

anticipated effects of harmful substances, as related to time of exposure in fetal development, include (1) "all or none"—either no effect or destruction of the blastocyst, with exposure occurring before implantation; (2) major congenital abnormalities (teratogenic outcomes) or abortion with exposure during organogenesis; and (3) minor congenital abnormalities or growth impairment (fetotoxic outcomes) with exposure during the fetal period.[20,21] Organogenesis, weeks 3 through 8 of pregnancy, is the period of greatest fetal vulnerability to teratogens, as it encompasses the initial development of all organ systems.

The teratogenic pathway is governed by several principles, which were outlined in the late 1970s by James Wilson. The six principles of teratology are listed in **BOX 10-1**.

Largely summarized, these principles describe that the teratogenic effect depends on fetal genetics, timing of the teratogenic exposure, the teratogenic mechanism of action, the type of teratogenic agent, and the dosage of the teratogen.

Pharmacokinetics, or the process of drug absorption, distribution, metabolism, and excretion in the body, also plays an important role in determining the potential fetal effect of a drug. Maternal adaptations in pregnancy, particularly those affecting the gastrointestinal tract, blood circulation, hormone levels, and kidney filtration rate, have varying effects on the pharmacokinetics of different drugs and consequently may decrease or increase the amount of drug available to cross the placental barrier.[21] In addition,

---

BOX 10-1   Wilson's Six Principles of Teratology

1. Susceptibility is dependent on the genetic make-up (genotype) of the conceptus and the manner in which it interacts with environmental factors.
2. Susceptibility varies with the developmental stage at the time of exposure.
3. Teratogenic agents act in specific ways (mechanisms) on developing cells and tissues to initiate abnormal embryogenesis (pathogenesis).
4. The fetal manifestations of abnormal development are death, malformation, growth retardation, and functional disorder.
5. The access of adverse environmental influences to developing tissues depends on the nature of the influences (agent).
6. Manifestations of deviant development increase in degree as the dosage increases from the no-effect level to the totally lethal level.

Modified from Wilson J. Current status of teratology, general principles and mechanisms derived from animal studies. In: Wilson J, Fraser F, eds. *Handbook of Teratology*. New York: Plenum Press; 1977:47-74.

the rate of placental blood flow factors into assessment of drug exposure and fetal risk. Pathologic conditions that reduce placental blood flow, and consequently decrease placental clearance of the substance, contribute to an increased time of the substance in fetal circulation and greater fetal exposure.[20]

Assessment of Drug Exposure Risk in Pregnancy

The determination of drug safety in pregnancy presents significant challenges. It is generally considered unsafe or unethical to conduct research on pregnant human subjects, and consequently, quality data on drug use in pregnancy are limited; information is largely reliant on rodent or animal studies and retrospective data. Currently, the FDA, which is responsible for drug approval and safety regulation, requires animal studies on fetal drug effects for all drug proposals and oversees the classification of drug safety in pregnancy. However, this was not always the case.

Historically, the years following the international thalidomide tragedy marked a major public health shift in the national approach to drug safety in pregnancy. In the late 1950s, thalidomide, a sedative drug used commonly for a wide variety of ailments, became marketed in 48 countries for the management of nausea and insomnia in early pregnancy. The outcome was disastrous. In the following years, reports of infants born with severe physical deformities increased. It was not until 1961 that the first report asserting an association with use of thalidomide in pregnancy was published by a researcher in Australia. By 1962, most countries had banned the drug. Tragically, the exposure from just those few years of use was profound. Worldwide, more than 10,000 infants were affected by intrauterine thalidomide exposure. The range of birth defects included absent limbs, abnormally short or long limbs, incomplete limbs, and malformations of the internal organs.[41]

In 1962, the U.S. Congress responded by passing the Kefauver-Harris Amendments. Notably, the amendments required that drug sponsors perform *monitored* clinical studies to prove safety, as opposed to efficacy alone, in the application of a new drug. The sponsors were also required to now wait for drug approval before manufacturing and dispensing a drug to the market. In addition, the FDA responded by developing a letter-grade classification system for drug safety in pregnancy. The system classified the drug's safety in pregnancy by the evidence of associated fetal harm and the quality of available research.[41]

In 2014, the FDA announced the adoption of a new system for classifying drug use risk and safety in pregnancy.[42] The new system abandons the letter grades and utilizes a narrative text to provide more specific details on risks of use across trimesters and in breastfeeding, addressing prior criticism about the fact that the letter system oversimplified the risks. Although the letter-grade system is still widely used, the new system is planned to completely replace the letter system by 2018.

▶ Maternal–Perinatal Infection

TORCHH

As mentioned, some maternal infections similarly have the capacity to cross the placental barrier and adversely affect the developing fetus. The acronym TORCHH is commonly utilized to recall those infections identified as transmissible and particularly deleterious to the fetus (**TABLE 10-2**). TORCHH stands for **T**oxoplasmosis, **R**ubella, **C**ytomegalovirus, **H**erpes simplex, and **H**uman immunodeficiency virus (HIV). Among these infections, current guidelines only recommend routine screening for rubella immunity and HIV (opt-out testing). Consequently, public health and prenatal education on risk reduction, as well as the use of diagnostic testing for suspected maternal infection, are crucial.

In the case of rubella, the United States achieved successful eradication status in 2004, after years of vaccination programs targeted at preventing congenital rubella syndrome (CRS). However, endemic rubella transmission persists in areas outside of the United States; worldwide, CRS is estimated to affect 100,000 infants annually. In order for the United States to maintain elimination status, given the frequency of international travel and immigration, it is important to continue high rates of vaccination and population immunity.[43]

Among women identified as non-immune, it is important to not only advise exposure reduction in pregnancy but also recommend immediate postpartum vaccination for protection in future pregnancies. Although there is no case of fetal infection following accidental administration of the vaccine in pregnancy, the combined measles, mumps, and rubella vaccine is a live-attenuated virus and consequently is contraindicated in pregnancy due to its potential for fetal harm.[43,44]

Given the diversity in infectious agents, the management and treatment of TORCHH infections in pregnancy vary greatly. In the case of acute or symptomatic toxoplasmosis infection, maternal and neonatal treatment with combination therapy is indicated.

TABLE 10-2 TORCHH Infections in Pregnancy

Agent	Characteristics of Infection	Fetal Infection	Risk Reduction Education
Toxoplasmosis *Protozoan*[45]	Lives in the intestines of domestic and wild cats; excreted in cat feces. Common source(s) and route of maternal infection: Cat feces, raw meat; ingestion of infected meat Individuals with increased risk of infection: Immunocompromised, HIV +	Prevalence: 1 in 8,000 pregnancies in the United States Fetal Risk: Highest risk of fetal injury with primary maternal infection in first trimester; fetal injury occurs in approximately 40% of these cases. Highest risk of fetal infection with maternal infection in third trimester. Fetal Outcomes: Rash, enlarged liver, ascites, fever, calcification and/ or enlargement of brain ventricles, seizures, mental retardation	1. Avoid cat litter or wear gloves and wash hands after exposure. 2. Avoid raw meat consumption and wash hands after touching raw meat.
Rubella *Viral*[43,44]	Single-stranded RNA virus. Common source(s) and route of maternal infection: Exposure to crowded conditions; transmitted via respiratory droplets and close contact Individuals with increased risk of infection: Non-immune, living in crowded conditions	Prevalence: Four reported cases of congenital rubella syndrome during the years 2005 to 2011 in the United States. Fetal Risk: Fetal outcomes are worst when maternal infection occurs in first 12 weeks of pregnancy. Approximately 80% of infections acquired in first 12 weeks of pregnancy result in fetal infection. Risk of fetal transmission and infection decreases with increasing gestational age. Fetal Outcomes: Miscarriage, stillbirth, growth restriction, hearing loss, cardiac abnormalities, microcephaly, cerebral palsy, mental retardation *Long-term*: Type 1 diabetes, panencephalitis	1. Avoid individuals who are ill during pregnancy and perform regular hand hygiene. 2. If non-immune, educate on symptoms and transmission of virus and advise care to prevent exposure. Advise postpartum vaccine to provide immunity in future pregnancies.
Cytomegalovirus (CMV) *Viral*[44]	Large, double-stranded DNA virus; herpes simplex virus Common source(s) and route of transmission: Contact with infected bodily fluids (saliva, urine, blood); includes sexual contact. Children and infants with subclinical symptoms are a major source of infection in United States; approximately 50% of children in daycare shed the virus in their urine/saliva. Individuals with increased risk of infection: Immunocompromised, daycare workers	Prevalence: 0.2–2.0% of infants in United States are born with congenital CMV infection. Fetal Risk: Fetal outcomes are worst when maternal infection occurs in the first trimester. However, the highest risk of fetal transmission occurs with maternal illness in the third trimester. Fetal Outcomes: Jaundice, petechiae, thrombocytopenia, enlarged spleen, growth restriction, non-immune hydrops *Long-term:* Developmental delay, seizures, neurologic impairment, hearing loss (leading cause in children)	1. Avoid sharing utensils and food. 2. Avoid contact with potentially infected items (diapers, toys) and perform regular hand hygiene.

<u>H</u>erpes Simplex Virus (HSV) *Viral*[44,46]	Large, double-stranded DNA virus; two strains: HSV-1 and HSV-2. Both HSV-1 and -2 can cause genital herpes; HSV-2 is responsible for most recurrent cases. Common source(s) and route of transmission: Personal contact with viral shedding; includes oral and sexual contact. Individuals with increased risk of infection: Sexual partner with HSV, high number of sexual partners, history of other STI, HIV positive status, men who have sex with other men, low socioeconomic status	Prevalence: 25–65% of U.S. population is positive for HSV-2 antibodies; 1 in 3,500 births in United States Fetal Risk: Fetal infection is most likely to occur via exposure to a primary maternal infection (genital outbreak) during vaginal delivery. Maternal infection earlier in pregnancy (primary or recurrent) rarely harms the fetus. Fetal Outcomes: Skin scarring and/or lesions, eye disease, microcephaly, brain deformity (hydranencephaly), and disseminated infection (extending to multiple organs and associated with increased morbidity and mortality)	1. STI risk reduction with condom use and routine testing. 2. If orolabial HSV-positive partner (or suspected), education on avoidance of oral sex during third trimester. 3. If genital HSV-positive partner (or suspected), education on avoidance of vaginal intercourse during third trimester.
<u>H</u>uman Immunodeficiency Virus (HIV) *Viral*[44]	Retrovirus; two strains: HIV-1, HIV-2 (endemic in Africa, Portugal, France) Common source(s) and route of transmission: Exchange of bodily fluids; most often via sexual contact or injection drug use. Individuals with increased risk of infection: High number of sexual contacts, high-risk sexual behavior, receptive anal intercourse, sexual contact with uncircumcised male, past or present IV drug and/or crack cocaine use, residing in "inner city," presence of other STIs drug transfusion between 1978–1985	Prevalence: 2.6 infants per 100,000 live births in 2013 in the United States.[44,46] Globally, an estimated 540,000 children were infected with HIV in 2005; mostly due to perinatal transmission.[29] Fetal Risk: Most transmission occurs during delivery (intrapartum period). In the United States, risk of perinatal transmission without antiretroviral therapy (ART) is 16–25% across the period of pregnancy, delivery, and postpartum breastfeeding. Risk of transmission is < 1% with combination ART in pregnancy/delivery.[47] Globally, risk of transmission in untreated mothers is 15–45%.[48] Fetal Outcomes: HIV infection; Globally, 25–30% of infants infected in utero die before age 1 (WHO) *ART-related outcomes:* possible association with preterm birth[47]	1. HIV risk reduction: condom use, routine testing, identification of high-risk behavior, injection drug use risk-reduction methods, and substance use treatment options. 2. If HIV-positive partner (HIV-discordant couple): risk reduction with patient use of PreP (ART prophylaxis), condoms, plan for HIV testing. Encourage patient to discuss risk reduction with partner via medication compliance, viral load testing, and regular care.

In comparison, there is no available treatment for perinatal infection with rubella or cytomegalovirus, and medical management entails supportive care.

Both herpes and HIV are viruses that can be treated, but not cured, to reduce risk of perinatal transmission. Regarding herpes, it is recommended that the woman take an appropriate retroviral medication for the management of outbreak in pregnancy, as well as daily from weeks 34–36 until time of delivery to reduce the likelihood of outbreak at birth. If evidence of an outbreak is present at time of labor onset, then a cesarean delivery is indicated to reduce risk of vertical transmission and adverse fetal outcomes.

HIV treatment in pregnancy involves maternal treatment with an appropriate combination therapy of three retroviral drugs, from at least two drug classes.[44] Clinical management also involves ensuring patient compliance and monitoring for drug resistance, viral load (level of HIV RNA copies in blood), and CD4 counts. If the CD4 count falls below 200 cells/mm^3, then prophylaxis for opportunistic infections may likely also be initiated. Early initiation of combination antiretroviral therapy (ART) is critical, as studies show that prior to 28 weeks of pregnancy, each additional week of therapy confers a 10% reduction in perinatal transmission.[44] However, independent of the point in pregnancy or the viral load, combination ART remains a mainstay of perinatal risk reduction and should be strongly encouraged. A large recent study reveals that use of ART for at least 14 days is associated with less than 0.8% risk of perinatal transmission.[44]

Historically, zidovudine (ZDZ) was the first drug used to manage maternal HIV and perinatal transmission in pregnancy. The classic regimen included daily maternal oral dosing in the prenatal period, maternal intravenous dosing during labor, and daily oral infant dosing for 6 weeks postpartum.[44] However, with the development of more effective and tolerable ART drugs, as well as the emergence of better clinical research, ZDZ is no longer recommended as a prenatal regimen or universal intrapartum treatment. Subsequent clinical research revealed that ZDZ is associated with a risk of toxicity and does not significantly reduce HIV transmission in women who are already receiving combination ART. Moreover, combination ART is more effective at reducing perinatal transmission, as compared to ZDZ.[44]

In the intrapartum setting, during time of labor and delivery, women are recommended to continue the same prenatal ART combination therapy. In the setting of a woman who presents in labor with viral loads > 1,000 copies and/or a positive rapid HIV test at time of labor admission (i.e., HIV status likely unknown in pregnancy), intravenous ZDZ *is* indicated for reduction of perinatal transmission; the infant should also receive subsequent prophylaxis and monitoring. Among women with viral loads identified as greater than 1,000 copies in the third trimester, an elective cesarean delivery is recommended at 38 weeks. In this setting, intravenous ZDZ is again recommended as prophylaxis before the cesarean. A scheduled cesarean is *not* recommended among women with viral loads less than 1,000 copies/mL, as risk of perinatal transmission is less than 1%. In addition, there is an increased risk of maternal morbidity and mortality, and neonatal morbidity, among HIV-positive women who undergo cesarean delivery.[44]

Other Viral Infections

Apart from infections included in TORCHH, there are numerous other infections with known risks of maternofetal transmission and adverse fetal consequences. Additional maternal perinatal viral infections associated with adverse fetal consequences include hepatitis (B, C, D, E), parvovirus, rubeola (measles), and varicella (chickenpox). Although not associated with direct fetal outcomes, maternal infection with influenza virus is also a primary concern in pregnancy, as it is associated with increased maternal risk of pneumonia and mortality. Consequently, the influenza vaccine is recommended for all women during pregnancy.[44]

Other Sexually Transmitted Infections

In addition, other sexually transmitted infections (STIs) such as untreated gonorrhea, chlamydia, and syphilis in pregnancy are associated with harmful fetal effects. All are caused by bacterial agents, which are treatable with appropriate and adequate antibiotic coverage. Currently, the Centers for Disease Control and Prevention (CDC) recommends testing for gonorrhea and chlamydia in pregnant women less than 25 years of age, and in those older than 25 years who are described as having an increased risk of infection.[46] However, due to the prevalence of asymptomatic infection, universal screening at initiation of prenatal care is standard of care in many practices. Routine testing for chlamydia and gonorrhea in the third trimester is also recommended for persons less than 25 years of age or at increased risk. According to the CDC, *all* pregnant women should receive testing for syphilis in early pregnancy, and women should not leave the hospital after delivery without documentation of a negative syphilis test during pregnancy or at time of delivery. Currently, most states mandate syphilis screening in early pregnancy.[46]

Gonorrhea and chlamydia infections are asymptomatic in most women and, if left untreated, are associated with a perinatal transmission risk of 30–50%, and 50–75%, respectively, during vaginal delivery.[49] Gonorrheal infection is associated with neonatal conjunctivitis (eye infection), arthritis, gonococcemia, and genital infection.[49] Chlamydial infection is also associated with neonatal conjunctivitis, as well as pneumonia. Infants routinely receive antibiotic eye ointment after delivery to treat possible infection related to maternal gonorrhea and chlamydia. In regard to maternal health, timely and adequate treatment of infection is also important in the reduction of pelvic inflammatory disease and infertility complications.[49]

In the United States, 8.4 infants per 100,000 live births had congenital syphilis in the years from 2009 to 2012. Congenital syphilis also remains a major global maternal health problem, and consequently, its eradication is included in the WHO millennial goals. Untreated syphilis in pregnancy is associated with a 52% risk of adverse fetal outcomes, including miscarriage, stillbirth, prematurity, low birth weight, and neonatal infection. Penicillin remains the mainstay of treatment for all individuals with syphilis.[50]

Group Beta Streptococcal Infection

Group beta streptococcal (GBS) infection is an asymptomatic bacterial infection that lives in the lower gastrointestinal and urogenital tract of approximately 20–25% of women in pregnancy.[45] Although harmless to the mature host, vertical transmission to the neonate is associated with adverse outcomes. In the United States, GBS infection of the neonate represents the leading cause of meningitis and sepsis[4]; neonatal GBS infection occurs in approximately 0.5 per 10,000 live births, with 10,000 cases of neonatal sepsis occurring per year.[45] The risk of transmission is highest during delivery; approximately 80–85% of neonatal GBS infections result from vertical transmission.[45]

The CDC recommends universal screening for GBS infection in pregnancy. Screening includes a urine culture in the first trimester and vaginal–rectal culture in weeks 35–37 of pregnancy. In the setting of a positive screening test at either point in pregnancy, or maternal history of a GBS-septic infant, maternal intravenous antibiotic treatment is recommended during delivery.[4,45]

▶ Management of Normal Pregnancy

Antenatal Care: Goals & Considerations

Overall, the three primary goals of antenatal care are: (1) risk assessment, (2) health promotion, and (3) medical and psychologic intervention and follow-up.[51] According to ACOG, prenatal care should be initiated prior to 12 weeks of pregnancy and include 12–14 visits, occurring at specified points throughout the pregnancy; a minimum of 9 prenatal visits must be attended to consider care adequate.[51]

The first prenatal visit is often the most exhaustive and lengthy visit, with the following educational goals:

- Nutrition, supplementation, exercise, and weight gain recommendations
- Promotion of healthy behaviors, preventive healthcare measures (oral health, mental health), and avoidance of teratogens (illicit, prescribed, environmental, infectious)
- STI risks and safe sex practices
- Common psychologic and physical changes in pregnancy
- Safe management of pregnancy discomforts
- Maternal infection risk reduction measures and immunization recommendations
- Typical structure of anticipated prenatal care and review of common screening tests
- Risk factors associated with genetic conditions and available screening tests
- Indications of problems in pregnancy

In addition, a thorough history, physical assessment, and laboratory panel are completed at the initial visit to identify patient-specific risks and needs in the pregnancy. Finally, an estimated delivery date (EDD) is determined by either measuring from a certain date of the first day of LMP or by ultrasound. In case of uncertainty regarding the LMP, an ultrasound is recommended to confirm accuracy of the EDD. The accuracy of EDD is important, as it informs gestational-specific care and risks throughout the pregnancy.

In subsequent visits, many educational components of the initial visits remain, such as promotion of healthy behaviors, weight, nutrition, and avoidance of teratogens, as well as management of normal pregnancy discomforts. Additional components vary by trimester and patient-specific needs but at a minimum include education on anticipated fetal growth and development (i.e., fetal movement), preparation for labor and parenthood, psychologic and emotional changes, breastfeeding, infant care, postpartum changes and expectations, and contraceptive or family planning.[51]

Beginning with the initial visit, maternal blood pressure is routinely monitored for early indications of pregnancy-related hypertension. Around 12–14 weeks, when the uterus becomes an abdominal organ, fetal viability and development are also routinely assessed through fetal heart tones and uterine size; both are measured externally from abdominal examination. Maternal weight gain is also monitored with each visit. Inadequate weight gain is associated with preterm birth, intrauterine growth restriction, and hypertension.[52] Conversely, obesity and excessive weight gain are associated with the postpartum weight retention and denotes a risk factor for subsequent obesity.[53] The Institute of Medicine currently recommends varying amounts of pregnancy weight gain for U.S. women, depending on the pre-pregnancy BMI; among women with an average pre-pregnancy BMI, a 25- to 35-lb weight gain is recommended.[52]

Additionally, routine assessment of safety should occur throughout pregnancy. Pregnancy represents a period of heightened risk for intimate partner violence (IPV), with some estimated 3–8% of pregnancies affected.[52] According to the recent Maternal Mortality Report on IPV, nearly 15% of IPV among reproductive-aged women occurs during pregnancy or in the 6 weeks postpartum.[52,54] Moreover, homicide represents one of the leading causes of death among women aged 44 years or younger. In pregnancy, the frequency of regular visits and assessments provides a unique opportunity for public health and medical practitioners to develop patient trust, identify IPV risk factors, and offer support. Routine screenings by trimester are listed in **TABLE 10-3**.[51]

The indications for screening of STIs, GBS, and rubella immunity, as well as the administration of influenza immunization in pregnancy, are reviewed in the previous section on perinatal infection. The CDC currently recommends that all pregnant women receive the tetanus, diphtheria, and pertussis (Tdap) vaccine during weeks 27–36 of pregnancy, regardless of prior vaccination history. Data show that the maternal antibody response to Tdap is passed to the fetus and consequently offers the neonate some protection against pertussis (whooping cough) from the immediate post-delivery though the first weeks of life; pertussis in newborns is a potentially life-threatening respiratory infection.[55]

TABLE 10-3 Routine Screenings by Trimester	
First Trimester: 0–13 weeks	Complete blood count (blood type, Rh factor, hemoglobin, hematocrit, white blood cell count, platelets) RBC antibody screen Syphilis test HIV test (opt out) Hepatitis B antigen test Rubella titer Gonorrhea & chlamydia test Urine culture (assess for urinary tract infection) Urine dipstick (assess for glucose and protein) *If clinically indicated:* HSV antibodies Tuberculosis screen Varicella antibody screen Toxoplasmosis Hemoglobinopathies Genetic screening (opt-in) Urinalysis (assess drug use) Pap smear
Second Trimester: 14–27 weeks	1-hour glucose challenge test (gestational diabetes screen) Hemoglobin and hematocrit (assess for anemia) Syphilis test Genetic screening (opt-in)
Third Trimester: 28–40 weeks	Group B Strep culture *If clinically indicated:* Rhesus antibody screening Hemoglobin and hematocrit Gonorrhea & chlamydia test

Data from Kilma C. Prenatal care: Goals, structure, and components. In: Jordan RG, Engstrom JL, Marfell JA, Farley CL, eds. *Prenatal and Postnatal: A Woman-Centered Approach*. Ames, IA: Wiley-Blackwell; 2014:73-97.

Lastly, Rh (D) immune globulin (RhoGAM) immunization represents a landmark development in obstetrics research. RhoGAM was first available in 1968, approximately 29 years after the Nobel prize-winning discovery by Landsteiner on Rhesus factor in pregnancy. Its administration is indicated in every pregnancy of women with Rh-negative blood type regardless of pregnancy outcome. RhoGAM administration effectively prevents isoimmunization, or the development of maternal antibodies in response to Rh-positive fetal blood exposure. In the absence of RhoGAM immunization, the woman is at significant risk of developing anti-D antibodies and complications in subsequent pregnancies. Anti-D antibodies easily pass the placental barrier and are associated with hemolytic disease of the newborn; outcomes related to hemolytic disease include anemia, hydrops fetalis, jaundice, kernicterus, and death.[21] Currently, RhoGAM is recommended at 28 weeks of pregnancy and also immediately postpartum, if the fetus has a positive Rh blood type.

Postpartum and Newborn Care: Goals and Considerations

Routine postpartum care in the United States most often includes a 6-week postpartum visit for all women, with an additional 2-week postpartum visit for women with cesarean sections or special concerns. In comparison, the postpartum care in all northern and western European countries includes home-care visits by healthcare professionals, regardless of birthplace.[56]

The postpartum period, often described as the fourth trimester, represents a major period of maternal adjustment and adaptation in the life-course. Consequently, the goals of care in this time are numerous but often include (1) physical and emotional adjustment since delivery, including issues or concerns, (2) the maternal experience in birth, (3) family adaptation, (4) return of menstruation, contraception and future fertility desires, and (5) infant health and feeding.

Physical assessment varies by maternal history and concerns but likely includes an assessment of vital signs, heart and lungs, breasts, abdomen, vagina, perineal area, uterus, and lower extremities.[4] Additionally, a nonphysical component of the exam is a screening for postpartum depression and safety. It is recommended that women receive a screening for postpartum depression *at every health visit encounter* following delivery. An estimated 10–20% of women are affected by postpartum depression in the United States.[4]

Breastfeeding is the gold standard in infant nutrition throughout the world. Currently, consensus among the major maternal and child health medical organizations in the United States recommends exclusive breastfeeding until 6 months of age and continued nonexclusive breastfeeding until at least 12 months of age.[40] It is important that practitioners offer thorough education on the benefits of breastfeeding and explore any associated fears, misperceptions, previous challenges, and any special circumstances. Data from 2011 reveal that the United States falls short of the recommendations; at 3 months, 40.7% of infants are exclusively breastfeeding, and at 6 months, 18.8% of infants are breastfeeding.[40] Increasingly, the issue of breastfeeding initiation is being addressed in the labor and delivery setting; efforts include the promotion of immediate skin-to-skin contact after delivery, the provision of lactation support, and reducing the visibility of formula.

In general, there are only a few contraindications to breastfeeding: (1) infants with galactosemia, (2) mothers who have active tuberculosis, a herpes outbreak on the nipple, or human T-cell lymphotropic virus, (3) mothers receiving radiation therapy or chemotherapy, and (4) report of maternal substance abuse. Due to adequate access to clean, potable water (which makes use of formula safe), U.S. women with HIV-positive status are also advised against breastfeeding due to risk of perinatal transmission. This recommendation includes women using combination ART and/or undetectable viral loads.[4]

Preconception and Interconception Care: Goals and Considerations

As previously mentioned, the determinants of maternal and infant health are not isolated to the period of pregnancy. In accordance with the life-course theory framework, prenatal care ideally extends beyond pregnancy, including periods of preconception, the first year postpartum, and interconception.[51,52] Provision of regular and adequate care in the time *before conception* offers the opportunity to address numerous important health concerns that may impact maternal and infant health. Among others, these include: health promotion, identification and management of chronic disease and mental illness, identification and treatment of infection, and individual-specific pregnancy risk assessment and planning.

Specific recommendations for low-risk women in the preconception period may include folic acid supplementation with a prenatal vitamin, immunizations, infection risk reduction, avoidance of teratogenic medications and exposures (e.g., alcohol, nicotine, etc.), and adequate nutrition. Folic acid supplementation is shown to significantly reduce the risk of neural tube defects (e.g., spina bifida) in pregnancy, and the maximum benefit is observed when taken from at least 1 month prior to pregnancy, through the first trimester.[4]

In the postpartum and interconception period, counseling on pregnancy spacing (via natural family planning or other contraceptive method) is among the primary goals. Data show that deliveries spaced closer than 18 months are associated with increased risk of adverse maternal and infant outcomes, including preterm birth and low birthweight infants.

▶ Maternal Health in the World

The state of maternal health worldwide is tragic. An estimated 303,000 women die in childbirth-related causes every year.[57] The maternal mortality rate is commonly employed as a measure of maternal health comparison across populations. According to WHO, the **maternal mortality rate (MMR)** is the number of direct and indirect maternal deaths per 100,000 live births during pregnancy or up to and including 42 days after the end of pregnancy.[58] The global estimate of MMR in 2013 was 210 deaths per 100,000 live births.

The distribution of poor maternal health measures is not equal throughout the world. Countries described as "low and middle income" bear the greatest burden, accounting for nearly 99% of maternal and newborn deaths worldwide.[58] Sub-Saharan Africa has an MMR of 520 deaths per 100,000 live births, as compared to an average of 12 deaths per 100,000 live births among developed countries.

The leading causes of maternal death globally include hemorrhage (27%), hypertension in pregnancy (14%), infection (11%), and unsafe abortion (3%).[58] Deaths related to HIV and acquired immune deficiency syndrome remain a major contributor to global MMR, accounting for more than half of maternal mortality in some sub-Saharan African countries.[58]

In general, women are dying from largely preventable and treatable causes. WHO estimates that in the setting of universal access to basic maternity care, the maternal death rate would decrease by two-thirds, to an estimated 96,000 women per year. Similarly, infant deaths would fall from 3 million to approximately 660,000 per year. Nearly 54 countries are characterized by cesarean rates that are too low for safety, and among low-income countries, more than 50% of births occur without assistance from any skilled provider, midwife, or doctor.[58]

Associated with the topic of access to care, access to contraception and safe abortion represent major determinants of maternal health outcomes. In 2012, the global rate of unintended pregnancy was 53 per 1,000 reproductive-aged women (15–44 years of age).[59] Increased access to contraception and family

planning is directly related to improved health outcomes, as well as possible socioeconomic outcomes.[58] Lastly, unsafe abortion remains one of the top five leading causes of maternal death, worldwide. Conversely, in areas where safe, legal abortions are offered, associated death is rare.[58]

Maternal Health in the United States

In comparison to other developed countries, WHO finds that the United States fares the worst in maternal mortality. According to WHO, the MMR more than doubled from the years 1990 to 2013, with an estimated 28 deaths per 100,000 live births in 2013, classifying the United States as the only developed country with an *increasing* MMR trend.[60] In contrast, the CDC utilizes a **pregnancy-related mortality ratio** to describe maternal health in the United States. The pregnancy-related mortality ratio is the number of deaths directly attributable to pregnancy, or caused by a condition aggravated by pregnancy that occur during pregnancy or within the first year after pregnancy, per 100,000 live births. The CDC similarly finds a rising trend in this rate; however, it estimates an increase from 10.0 deaths per 100,000 live births in 1990 to 17.3 deaths per 100,000 live births in 2013.[61] Utilizing the CDC's estimates of MMR, the U.S. fares somewhat better in overall maternal health. Among public health practitioners, there remains debate as to which estimate is a more accurate reflection of maternal health in the United States.

Moreover, maternal and child health in the United States is characterized by significant disparities. Like preterm birth, the risk of maternal mortality is nearly four times higher among African American women, as compared to white women—a risk that persists even when women are compared by type of complication.[61] In addition, women who lack insurance in the United States are three times more likely to die in pregnancy than their counterparts.[60]

The leading causes of maternal death in the United States include heart conditions, infection, bleeding, and blood clots.[61] Many of the issues contributing to poor maternal health and outcomes globally also apply to the United States. The WHO identifies the following three contributors: (1) inconsistent obstetric practices, (2) increased prevalence of chronic comorbidities among women presenting for care in pregnancy, and (3) lack of quality data and reporting.[60]

Additionally, access to reproductive education and liberty is similarly an issue in the United States. United States. Nearly half of all U.S. pregnancies are unintended. Although contraception became available to unwed women in 1972, it remains highly controversial and inaccessible for many women. Regarding abortion, the U.S. Supreme Court decision in the case of *Roe v Wade* (1973) established the legality of abortion and determined that the decision to electively terminate, or bear children, is protected under a woman's constitutional (and fundamental) right to privacy. However, four decades after this landmark ruling, abortion remains highly controversial and largely inaccessible for many women.[16] Its proponents and opponents continue to actively engage over recurrently emerging legislation which restricts women's physical access on the state level, as well as financial access to funding and insurance coverage at the federal level.

Key Terms

Androgens
Anterior pituitary
Blastocyst
Cervix
Contraception
Corpus luteum
Elective abortion
Embryo
Endometrial cycle
Fetal viability
Fetus
Follicle
Gonadotropin-releasing hormone (GnRH)

Gonadotropins
Human chorionic growth hormone (hCG)
Hyperplasia
Hypothalamic–pituitary–ovarian (HPO) axis
Hypothalamus
Induced abortion
Labor
Maternal mortality rate (MMR)
Medication abortion
Menarche
Menopause
Negative feedback loop

Organogenesis
Ovarian cycle
Oxytocin
Placenta accreta
Placenta previa
Pregnancy-related mortality ratio
Prostaglandins
Spontaneous abortion
Surgical abortion
Teratogen
Therapeutic abortion
Zygote

Discussion Questions

1. Approximately 50% of pregnancies in the United States are unintended.[59,62] In thinking about embryology, why is this a significant public health concern?

2. Fetal alcohol exposure is the leading cause of mental retardation in the United States.[63] The data reveal a direct dose–response relationship between amount of maternal alcohol consumption and severity of adverse fetal outcomes; however, they do not identify a minimum threshold of effect.

    a. Discuss how these data inform the opinions of the CDC, ACOG, the American College of Nurse-Midwives, and other major health organizations that assert *there is no safe level of alcohol consumption in pregnancy.*

    b. How would you explain these data in simple terms to a friend who asks you if it is safe to have a few drinks in pregnancy?

3. In February 2016, the CDC provoked significant controversy with the release of the following recommendations in the *Morbidity and Mortality Weekly Report*, 2011-2013.[62]

    Three in four women who wanted to get pregnant as soon as possible reported drinking alcohol, putting them at risk for an alcohol-exposed pregnancy.

    Any sexually active woman of reproductive age who is drinking alcohol and not using birth control is at risk for an alcohol-exposed pregnancy.

    To help prevent adverse consequences of alcohol consumption during pregnancy, health care providers should discuss and recommend, as appropriate, available contraception methods to women who are sexually active and drink alcohol.[62 (p96)]

    a. What was the likely intent of this public health message?

    b. Discuss some of the possible sources of controversy. What assumptions did the CDC make about its target audience? What might have been some effects of these assumptions?

    c. One of the major challenges in public health is to develop and disseminate messages that address risky health behaviors, while also not infringing on an individual's sense of personal freedom or choice. Given your knowledge of pregnancy, embryology, and prenatal care, discuss alternative public health strategies for addressing fetal alcohol syndrome in the United States.

References

1. Hobel CJ, Gambone JC. A life-course perspective for women's health care: safe, ethical, value-based practice with a focus on prevention. In: Hacker N, Gambone J, Hobel C, eds. *Hacker & Moore's Essentials of Obstetrics and Gynecology*. Philadelphia, PA: Elsevier; 2016:2-11.

2. Society for Menstrual Cycle Research. *The menstrual cycle: a feminist lifespan perspective* [Fact Sheet]. Available from http://www.socwomen.org/wp-content/uploads/2010/05/fact_4-2011-menstruation.pdf. Accessed October 31, 2017.

3. American College of Obstetricians and Gynecologists. Committee Opinion No. 651. Menstruation in girls and adolescents: using the menstrual cycle as a vital sign. *Obstet Gynecol*. 2015;126:e143-e146.

4. Durham RF, Chapman L. *Maternal-Newborn Nursing: The Critical Components of Nursing Care*. 2nd ed. Philadelphia, PA: F. A. Davis; 2014.

5. Bratke H, Bruserud IS, Brannsether B, et al. Timing of menarche in Norwegian girls: associations with body max index, waist circumference and skinfold thickness. *BMC Pediatr*. 2017;17(138):1-6. doi: 10.1186/s12887-017-0893-x.

6. Hoffman BL, Schorge JO, Bradshaw KD, Halvorson LM, Schaffer JI, Corton MM. Reproductive endocrinology. In: *Williams Gynecology*. 3rd ed. New York, NY: McGraw-Hill; 2016:334-368.

7. Fritz M, Speroff L. Neuroendocrinology. In: *Clinical Gynecologic Endocrinology and Infertility*. Philadelphia, PA: Lippincott Williams & Wilkins; 2011:193-197.

8. Hatcher RA. *Contraceptive Technology*. New York, NY: Ardent Media, Inc.; 2004.

9. Jordan RG, Engstrom JL, Marfell JA, Farley CL. *Prenatal and Postnatal: A Woman-Centered Approach*. Ames, IA: Wiley-Blackwell; 2014.

10. Utiger RD. *Prostaglandin: chemical compound*. Encyclopedia Britannica. Available at https://www.britannica.com/science/prostaglandin. Revised and updated December 21, 2009. Accessed October 31, 2017.

11. Caudle P. Reproductive tract structure and function. In: Jordan RG, Engstrom JL, Marfell JA, Farley CL, eds. *Prenatal and Postnatal: A Woman-Centered Approach*. Ames, IA: Wiley-Blackwell; 2014:5-18.

12. Gambone J. Female reproductive physiology. In: Hacker N, Gambone J, Hobel C, eds. *Hacker & Moore's Essentials of Obstetrics and Gynecology*. Philadelphia, PA: Elsevier; 2016:37-49.

13. Burton G, Sibley CP, Jauniaux ERM. Placental anatomy and physiology. In: Gabbe SG, Niebyl JR, Simpson JL, et al., eds. *Obstetrics: Normal and Problem Pregnancies*. 7th ed. Philadelphia, PA: Elsevier, Inc.; 2017:2-25.

14. Richards D. Obstetric ultrasound: imaging, dating, growth, anomaly. In: Gabbe SG, Niebyl JR, Simpson JL, et al., eds. *Obstetrics: Normal and Problem Pregnancies*. 7th ed. Philadelphia, PA: Elsevier, Inc.; 2017:160-192.

15. Hobel C, Williams J. Antepartum care: preconception and prenatal care, genetic evaluation and teratology, and antenatal fetal assessment. In: Hacker N, Gambone J, Hobel C, eds. *Hacker & Moore's Essentials of Obstetrics and Gynecology*. Philadelphia, PA: Elsevier; 2016:76-95.

16. Annas GJ, Elias S. Ethical and legal issues in perinatology. In: Gabbe SG, Niebyl JR, Simpson JL, et al., eds. *Obstetrics: Normal and Problem Pregnancies*. 7th ed. Philadelphia, PA: Elsevier, Inc.; 2017:1183-1212.

17. Pignotti MS, Donzelli G. Perinatal care at the threshold of viability: an international comparison of practical guidelines for the treatment of extremely preterm births. *Pediatrics*. 2008;121(1):e193-e198. doi: 10.1542/peds.2007-0513.

18. Raymond E, Grimes D. The comparative safety of legal induced abortion and childbirth in the United States. *Obstet Gynecol*. 2012;119:215-219. doi: 10.1097/AOG.0b013e31823fe923.

19. Department of Reproductive Health and Research, World Health Organization. *Unsafe Abortion: Global and Regional Estimates of the Incidence of Unsafe Abortion and Associated Mortality in 2008*. 6th ed. Geneva, Switzerland: World Health Organization.

20. Caudle P. Conception, implantation, and embryonic and fetal development. In: Jordan RG, Engstrom JL, Marfell JA, Farley CL, eds. *Prenatal and Postnatal: A Woman-Centered Approach*. Ames, IA: Wiley-Blackwell; 2014:19-32.

21. Lassiter N, Manns-Jones L. Pregnancy. In: Brucker MC, King TL, eds. *Pharmacology for Women's Health*. Burlington, MA: Jones & Bartlett Learning; 2017:1025-1064.

22. Ross M, Ervin M. Fetal development and physiology. In: Gabbe SG, Niebyl JR, Simpson JL, et al., eds. *Obstetrics: Normal and Problem Pregnancies*. 7th ed. Philadelphia, PA: Elsevier, Inc.; 2017:26-37.

23. Antony K, Racusin D, Aagaard K, Dildy G. Maternal physiology. In: Gabbe SG, Niebyl JR, Simpson JL, et al., eds. *Obstetrics: Normal and Problem Pregnancies*. 7th ed. Philadelphia, PA: Elsevier, Inc.; 2017:38-63.

24. Koos B, Hobel C. Maternal physiologic and immunologic adaptation to pregnancy. In: Hacker N, Gambone J, Hobel C, eds. *Hacker & Moore's Essentials of Obstetrics and Gynecology*. Philadelphia, PA: Elsevier; 2016:61-75.

25. Gambone J, Hobel C. Endocrinology of pregnancy and parturition. In: Hacker N, Gambone J, Hobel C, eds. *Hacker & Moore's Essentials of Obstetrics and Gynecology*. Philadelphia, PA: Elsevier, Inc.; 2016:52-60.

26. Kilpatrick S, Garrison E. Normal labor and delivery. In: Gabbe SG, Niebyl JR, Simpson JL, et al., eds. *Obstetrics: Normal and Problem Pregnancies*. 7th ed. Philadelphia, PA: Elsevier, Inc.; 2017:246-270.

27. Simhan H, Iams J. Preterm labor and birth. In: Gabbe SG, Niebyl JR, Simpson JL, et al., eds. *Obstetrics: Normal and Problem Pregnancies*. 7th ed. Philadelphia, PA: Elsevier, Inc.; 2017:615-646.

28. Abedi P, Jahanfar S, Namvar F, Lee J. Breastfeeding or nipple stimulation for reducing postpartum haemorrhage in the third stage of labour. *Cochrane Database Syst Rev*. 2016;1:CD010845. doi: 10.1002/14651858.CD010845.pub2.

29. International Confederation of Midwives and International Federation of Gynaecology and Obstetrics. *Prevention and Treatment of Postpartum Haemorrhage: New Advances for Low Resource Settings Joint Statement by ICM and FIGO*. The Hague and London, UK: International Confederation of Midwives and International Federation of Gynaecology and Obstetrics; 2006.

30. Borders A, Wolfe K, Qadir S, Kim K, Holl J, Grobman W. Racial/ethnic differences in self-reported and biologic measures of chronic stress in pregnancy. *J Perinatol*. 2015;35(8):580-584. doi: 10.1038/jp.2015.18.

31. Hamilton B, Martin J, Osterman M. Births: preliminary data for 2015. *Natl Vital Stat Rep.* 2016;65(3). Hyattsville, MD: National Center for Health Statistics. Available at https://www.cdc.gov/nchs/data/nvsr/nvsr65/nvsr65_03.pdf. Accessed October 24, 2017.

32. Berghella V, Mackeen A, Jauniaux E. Cesarean delivery. In: Gabbe SG, Niebyl JR, Simpson JL, et al., eds. *Obstetrics: Normal and Problem Pregnancies.* 7th ed. Philadelphia, PA: Elsevier, Inc.; 2017:425-443.

33. American College of Obstetricians and Gynecologists. Committee Opinion No. 559. Cesarean delivery on maternal request. *Obstet Gynecol.* 2013;121:904-907.

34. Silver RM. Implications of the first cesarean: perinatal and future reproductive health and subsequent cesareans, placentation issues, uterine rupture risk, and mortality. *Semin Perinatol.* 2012;36:315-323. doi: 10.1053/j.semperi.2012.04.013.

35. World Health Organization. WHO statement on cesarean section rates. Geneva, Switzerland: World Health Organization. Available at http://www.who.int/reproductivehealth/publications/maternal_perinatal_health/cs-statement/en/. Published April 2015. Accessed October 24, 2017.

36. American College of Obstetricians and Gynecologists. Practice Bulletin No. 115. Vaginal birth after previous cesarean delivery. *Obstet Gynecol.* 2010;116(2 pt 1):450-463. doi: 10.1097/AOG.0b013e3181eeb251.

37. National Partnership for Women & Families. Cesarean trends in the United States, 1989-2015. *Childbirth Connection.* Available at http://www.nationalpartnership.org/research-library/maternal-health/cesarean-section-trends-1989-2014.pdf. Published March 2017. Accessed October 24, 2017.

38. Landon M, Grobman W. Vaginal birth after cesarean delivery. In: Gabbe SG, Niebyl JR, Simpson JL, et al., eds. *Obstetrics: Normal and Problem Pregnancies.* 7th ed. Philadelphia, PA: Elsevier, Inc.; 2017:444-455.

39. Rozance P, Rosenberg A. The neonate. In: Gabbe SG, Niebyl JR, Simpson JL, et al., eds. *Obstetrics: Normal and Problem Pregnancies.* 7th ed. Philadelphia, PA: Elsevier, Inc.; 2017:468-498.

40. Newton E. Lactation and breastfeeding. In: Gabbe SG, Niebyl JR, Simpson JL, et al., eds. *Obstetrics: Normal and Problem Pregnancies.* 7th ed. Philadelphia, PA: Elsevier, Inc.; 2017:517-548.

41. Tantibanchachai C. US Regulatory Response to Thalidomide (1950-2000). *Embryo Project Encyclopedia.* Available at http://embryo.asu.edu/handle/10776/7733. Updated April 1, 2014. Accessed October 24, 2017.

42. Gaffney A. FDA scraps pregnancy labeling classification system in favor of new standard. Regulatory Affairs Professionals Society. Available at http://www.raps.org/Regulatory-Focus/News/2014/12/03/20893/FDA-Scraps-Pregnancy-Labeling-Classification-System-in-Favor-of-New-Standard/. Posted December 3, 2014. Accessed October 24, 2017.

43. McLean H, Redd S, Abernathy E, Icenogle J, Wallace G. Rubella. *VPD Surveillance Manual.* 5th ed. Available at https://www.cdc.gov/vaccines/pubs/surv-manual/chpt14-rubella.pdf. Accessed October 24, 2017.

44. Bernstein H. Maternal and perinatal infection in pregnancy: Viral. In: Gabbe SG, Niebyl JR, Simpson JL, et al., eds. *Obstetrics: Normal and Problem Pregnancies.* 7th ed. Philadelphia, PA: Elsevier, Inc.; 2017:1099-1129.

45. Duff P, Birsner M. Maternal and perinatal infection in pregnancy: Bacterial. In: Gabbe SG, Niebyl JR, Simpson JL, et al., eds. *Obstetrics: Normal and Problem Pregnancies.* 7th ed. Philadelphia, PA: Elsevier, Inc.; 2017:1130-1147.

46. Centers for Disease Control and Prevention. 2015 Sexually Transmitted Disease Treatment Guidelines. *Clin Infect Dis.* 2015;61(8). Available at https://www.cdc.gov/std/tg2015/syphilis-pregnancy.htm.

47. Centers for Disease Control and Prevention. HIV among pregnant women, infants, and children. Available at https://www.cdc.gov/hiv/group/gender/pregnantwomen/index.html. Updated September 14, 2017. Accessed January 12, 2018.

48. World Health Organization. Mother-to-child transmission of HIV. Available at http://www.who.int/hiv/topics/mtct/about/en/. Updated 2017. Accessed October 24, 2017.

49. Garland M, Brennan B. Sexually transmitted infections and common vaginitis. In: Jordan RG, Engstrom JL, Marfell JA, Farley CL, eds. *Prenatal and Postnatal: A Woman-Centered Approach.* Ames, IA: Wiley-Blackwell; 2014:608-619.

50. Nyholm J, Ramin K, Landers D. Maternal and perinatal infection: chlamydia, gonorrhea, and syphilis in pregnancy. In: Gabbe SG, Niebyl JR, Simpson JL, et al., eds. *Obstetrics: Normal and Problem Pregnancies.* 7th ed. Philadelphia, PA: Elsevier, Inc.; 2017:1089-1098.

51. Kilma C. Prenatal care: goals, structure, and components. In: Jordan RG, Engstrom JL, Marfell JA, Farley CL, eds. *Prenatal and Postnatal: A Woman-Centered Approach.* Ames, IA: Wiley-Blackwell; 2014:73-97.

52. Gregory K, Ramos D, Jauniaux E. Preconception and prenatal care. In: Gabbe SG, Niebyl JR, Simpson JL, et al., eds. *Obstetrics: Normal and Problem Pregnancies.* 7th ed. Philadelphia, PA: Elsevier, Inc.; 2017:102-121.

53. Catalano P. Obesity in pregnancy. In: Gabbe SG, Niebyl JR, Simpson JL, et al., eds. *Obstetrics: Normal and Problem Pregnancies.* 7th ed. Philadelphia, PA: Elsevier, Inc.; 2017:899-909.

54. Petrosky E, Blair JM, Betz CJ, Fowler KA, Jack SP, Lyons BH. Racial and ethnic differences in homicides of adult women and the role of intimate partner violence — United States, 2003–2014. *MMWR Morb Mortal Wkly Rep.* 2017;66:741-746. doi: http://dx.doi.org/10.15585/mmwr.mm6628a1.

55. Centers for Disease Control and Prevention. *Get the Whooping Cough Vaccine While You Are Pregnant.* National Center for Immunization and Respiratory Diseases, Division of Bacterial Diseases. Available at https://www.cdc.gov/pertussis/pregnant/mom/get-vaccinated.html. Updated July 24, 2017. Accessed October 24, 2017.

56. Chen C, Fowles E, Walker L. Postpartum maternal health care in the United States: a critical review. *J Perinat Educ.* 2006;15(3):34-42. doi: 10.1624/105812406X119002.

57. World Health Organization. *Maternal mortality: Fact sheet.* Available at http://www.who.int/mediacentre/factsheets/fs348/en/. Updated November 2016. Accessed October 24, 2017.

58. Lewis G, Regan L, Morroni C, Jauniaux E. Improving global maternal health: Challenges and opportunities. In: Gabbe SG, Niebyl JR, Simpson JL, et al., eds. *Obstetrics: Normal and Problem Pregnancies.* 7th ed. Philadelphia, PA: Elsevier, Inc.; 2017:1196-1213.

59. Sedgh G, Singh S, Hussain R. Intended and unintended pregnancies worldwide in 2012 and recent trends. *Stud Fam Plann.* 2014;45(3):301-314. doi:10.1111/j.1728-4465.2014.00393.x.

60. Agrawal P. Maternal mortality and morbidity in the United States of America. *Bull World Health Org.* 2015;93:135. Available at http://dx.doi.org/10.2471/BLT.14.148627.

61. Centers for Disease Control and Prevention. *Pregnancy Mortality Surveillance System.* Atlanta, GA: Centers for Disease Control and Prevention. Available at https://www.cdc.gov/reproductivehealth/maternalinfanthealth/pmss.html. Updated June 29, 2017. Accessed October 24, 2017.

62. Green P, McKnight-Eily L, Tan C, Mejia R, Denny C. *Vital Signs: Alcohol-Exposed Pregnancies—United States, 2011–2013. Morbid Mortal Wkly Rep.* 2016;64(4):91-97. Available at https://www.cdc.gov/mmwr/volumes/65/wr/pdfs/mm6504a6.pdf.

63. Maeir S, West J. Patterns and alcohol-related birth defects. *Alcohol Res Health.* 2001;25(3):169-174. Available at https://pubs.niaaa.nih.gov/publications/arh25-3/168-174.pdf.

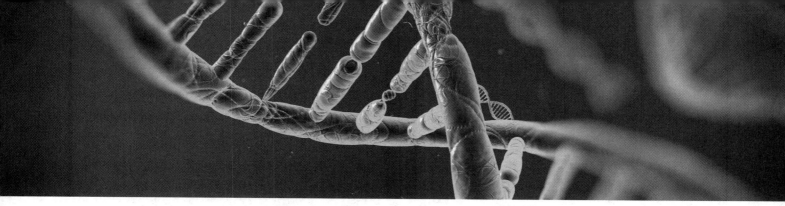

CHAPTER 11

Aging

Loretta DiPietro

LEARNING OBJECTIVES

By the end of this chapter, the student will be able to:

- Describe demographic trends in aging in the United States and globally
- Differentiate between mandatory and facultative models of aging
- Define the "Compression of Morbidity" and provide two examples
- Describe the physiologic changes occurring with aging over several systems
- Define "successful aging" and provide examples of such
- Explain how lifestyle-related behaviors can attenuate aging-related functional decline across multiple systems
- Discuss the impact of current aging demographics on public health and on the global economy
- Describe several Healthy People 2020 Objectives for older people and justify the need for these objectives

---

CHAPTER OUTLINE

▶ Introduction

Public health and healthcare advances are lengthening people's lives, "and consequently, the proportion of older people in the global population is increasing rapidly."[1] In the United States, 13% of the population is persons aged 65 years and older, and by 2030 that percentage is projected to be 19% of the total population (72.1 million).[2] By the year 2060, the number of Americans aged 65 years and older will more than double, from approximately 40 million in 2010 to a projected 98 million. By the year 2050, the global population of people over age 60 years is projected to reach 2 billion (**FIGURE 11-1**). Perhaps of greatest interest in aging research is the rise in the segment of the population that is aged 85 years and older. Since 1930, this demographic subgroup has doubled in number every 30 years and is projected to be the fastest-growing sector of the older population well into the 21st century. In fact, by 2040 this sector is projected to rise to 14.6 million.[2]

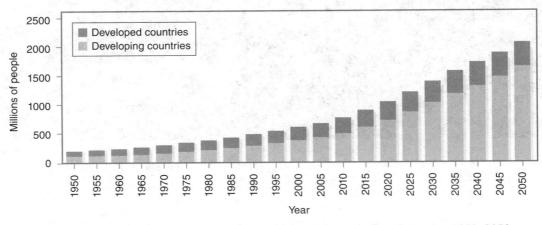

FIGURE 11-1 Number of People Aged 60 or Older: World, Developed, and Developing Countries, 1950–2050

Reproduced from United Nations Population Fund, HelpAge International. *Ageing in the Twenty-First Century: A Celebration and A Challenge*. New York, NY and London, UK: United Nations Population Fund and HelpAge International; 2012.

Of concern is the fact that in many developed countries, the population of older people has surpassed that of the 12- to 24-year-old age group, resulting in a shrinking workforce population relative to the growing older population. For example, data from the Japanese Ministry of Health indicate that in 1950, the proportion of the population older than 65 years in rural Japan was approximately 5%, relative to the workforce population (15–64 years) of 60%; the projected estimates for 2050 are 39% relative to 52%. Current census data show that those 65 and over now account for 26.7% of Japan's population.[3] These shifting demographic trends have substantial political, social, medical, and economic implications for most of the world and underscore the importance of keeping people healthy and functional for as long as possible across the life span.

▶ Theories of Aging

The exact mechanisms of how people age have not been defined fully. Theories of how people age generally fall into major categories of social and biologic. Prominent among the social theories are the Activity/Disengagement and the Continuity theories.[4] The Activity Theory is related to Role Theory and proposes that there is a positive relation between activity of any sort and life satisfaction. Those people who are more active in older age can better withstand the consequences of life changes that result in loss, such as the death of a spouse or relocation. This theory has received criticism for discounting individual preferences and social/economic inequalities.[5] In contrast, the Disengagement Theory posits that there is a mutually agreeable withdrawal between older people and others in their social network in accepting their

impending death. The Continuity Theory proposes that those people who can continue in their perceived social roles and activities, as well as their psychologic characteristics, across the life-course into older age are most likely to age successfully.[6]

Biologic theories of aging can be divided into **mandatory aging** and **facultative aging**.[7] Mandatory (or true biologic) aging is outside of our control and involves the interaction between error build-up in the cell and genetic programming. The first hypothesis proposes that random environmental events, such as oxygen free-radical damage, cell gene mutations, or cross-linkage among macromolecules preclude the cell from acting normally. Normally, the cell will synthesize protein by transferring information from deoxyribonucleic acid to ribonucleic acid; however, with error build-up, the genetic foundation of the cell is altered, thereby impairing the expression of essential protein.

A telomere is a sequence of repetitive nucleotide sequences at each end of a chromosome, which protects

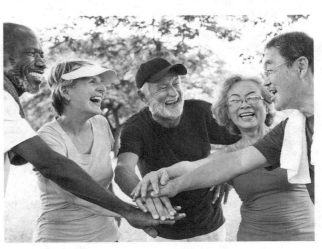

© Rawpixel.com/Shutterstock

the end of the chromosome from losing important information. Telomere shortening is associated with aging, mortality, and aging-related diseases, and there is evidence that those with longer telomeres lead longer lives than those with short telomeres.[8] It is not known, however, whether short telomeres are just a sign of cellular age or actually contribute to the aging process. In any case, individual cell loss is not vital to tissue or organ function until a significant number of cells fails. We can therefore think of "aging" as a result of the lifetime accumulation of errors in cell function due to the inability of the cell's repair process to maintain itself. The second of these hypotheses proposes that the aging process is genetically programmed by the cell. Although there is evidence that certain cell lines die during development and maturation, it is not clear how this affects aging *per se*.

In contrast, facultative aging is that which is under our control and can be attributable to social conditions (such as poverty and low access to health care) and lifestyle factors such as poor diet, cigarette smoking, alcohol intake, obesity, and most notably, low physical activity. In 1982, Walter Bortz[9] first noted that many of the physiologic changes that occur with aging (muscle atrophy, insulin resistance, orthostatic intolerance) are similar to those induced in young people by enforced inactivity or microgravity, such as during bed rest or prolonged space flights. He proposed that the common factor in the dysregulation of several systems under these conditions was the absence of gravitational force, and that regular physical activity could attenuate, or even reverse, these age-related impairments.

Even among the most healthy individuals, physiologic function declines as one ages. As stated previously, the degree to which this decline is attributable to true biologic aging and the degree to which it is attributable to social or lifestyle factors that accompany older age are not entirely clear.[1] There is considerable variability in patterns of aging, with some older people showing expected patterns of decline in health and function, while others appear more resilient to various physiologic (e.g., infection), emotional (e.g., bereavement), or environmental challenges (**FIGURE 11-2**).

"Plasticity" is the ability of a cell, tissue, organ, or system to adjust to a challenge in a timely manner (e.g., increased blood flow to working muscles during exercise) and "resiliency" is the ability to return to the homeostatic state in a timely manner once the challenge has ceased. Plasticity and resiliency to various challenges or perturbations can be considered an underlying hallmark of "**successful aging**."

Rowe and Kahn[10] first developed a model to characterize those very robust and independent older

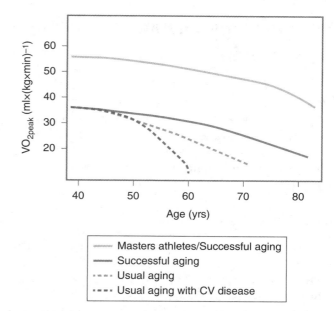

FIGURE 11-2 Hypothetical Trajectory of Functional Decline in Four Distinct Groups of Older People

Reproduced from DiPietro L, Seals DR. Introduction to exercise in older adults. In: Lamb DR, Gisolfi CG, Nadel ER, eds. *Perspectives in Exercise and Sports Medicine*. Vol. 8. Carmel, IN: Cooper Publishing Group; 1995:1-10.

BOX 11-1 Measures of Successful Aging

- Not hospitalized in last 6 months
- No days in bed in last 2 weeks
- Life satisfaction score of 1–4
- Life-view score of 1–3
- Center for Epidemiologic Studies Depression (CES-D) Scale score < 10
- No reported ADLs impairment
- Intact extremity strength
- Self-rated health of good to excellent
- Mini Mental Status score > 89
- Timed 15-foot walk < 15 seconds
- Ambulation – reported walking > 4 blocks/day

Data from Rowe JW, Kahl RL. Successful aging. *Gerontologist*. 1997;37:433-440.

persons according to three domains: (1) disease risk; (2) physical or cognitive capacity; and (3) engagement with life. Most newer models of successful aging now expand these domains to include additional measures of physical (e.g., self-rated health; days in bed; extremity strength; timed 15-foot walk; report of **activities of daily living [ADLs]** or **instrumental activities of daily living [IADLs]** limitations), cognitive (e.g., Mini-Mental Status score), psychosocial function (e.g., life satisfaction score, depression score; life-view score; perceived economic status) and spirituality.[1,11] See **BOX 11-1**.

▶ Physiologic Changes Occurring with Aging

As stated previously, physiologic function declines with age even among the most robust sectors of the population. The role of public health practitioners is to deliver strategies that can attenuate this slope of functional decline, in order to compress or delay the state of disease and frailty as close to the end of life as possible.

Endocrine Changes

One of the precursors to older age is a drop in sex hormones among both men and women. In women, menopause occurs anywhere from age 45 to 55 years, when estrogen and progesterone levels begin to decline rapidly, leaving relatively greater circulating concentrations of testosterone. As women transition through menopause and lose many of the protective effects of estrogen, their risk for diseases such as cardiovascular disease and **osteoporosis** increases dramatically. For example, whereas women experience a lower risk for cardiovascular disease compared with their male peers in middle age, once this "estrogen advantage" is lost in older age, that risk gap begins to get smaller.

Growth hormone concentrations also decline in late middle age in both men and women, and this has consequences for muscle growth and strength, and along with declining sex hormone levels, influences the preferential deposition of body fat toward the deep abdominal (visceral) depot. Visceral belly fat lies underneath the abdominal muscles and around the organs, while subcutaneous belly fat lies on top of the abdominal muscle wall. Indeed, this deep abdominal fat depot, comprising hypertrophied (enlarged) adipocytes, is much more metabolically active compared with subcutaneous abdominal fat and fat deposited in the lower body (hips and thighs). Because the portal vein drains directly into the liver, excess lipolysis (fat mobilization into the blood) from the visceral depot can lead to fat build-up in the liver, which will impair insulin action at that site. In addition, excess **visceral adiposity** has been linked to increased amounts of inflammatory factors in the blood, and this is especially so in older people.

Insulin secretion begins to decline with older age due to a loss of beta cell function in the pancreas. Insufficient insulin secretion is an important contributor to impairments in glucose homeostasis following a meal. Potentiation refers to a phenomenon that is time varying and appears to modulate the dose–response relationship between circulating glucose concentrations and insulin secretion. This system appears to be blunted and delayed in older people, especially later in the day, thereby exposing older people to large glucose excursions after the evening meal and into the night. Fortunately, muscle contractions will clear glucose from the bloodstream independent of endogenous insulin secretion, as these contractions will stimulate the GLUT-4 transporter proteins up to the cell membrane so that they can escort the glucose molecules into the cell. Post-meal walking has demonstrated an effective strategy for maintaining daily glycemic control in older people.

Body Composition Changes

Some of the more noticeable physiologic changes occurring with older age involve body composition. After age 65 years, body weight begins to decrease due to a loss of muscle and bone. Lean (muscle) mass declines about 3–6% per decade, while fat-free mass decreases by about 15% between the third and eighth decades.[12] **Sarcopenia** refers to the distinct loss of muscle *quantity* and *quality* in older age. This loss of muscle mass, along with accompanying increase in the proportion of body fat, has negative consequences for maintaining resting metabolic rate and metabolic function, as well as for maintaining strength, balance, reaction time, and flexibility—all important factors for maintaining physical function and independence in older age.

FIGURE 11-3 displays the relationship between body mass index [BMI = (weight (kg)/height (m)^2] and mortality among 313,047 older men within several different age groups from the National Institutes

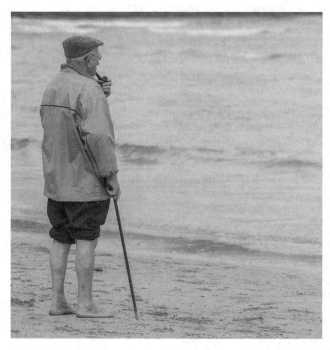

© Marco Antonio/Shutterstock

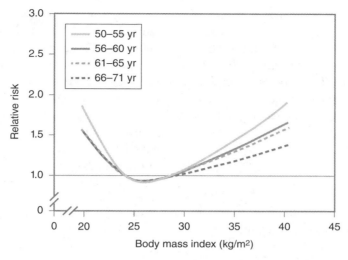

FIGURE 11-3 The Relation Between Body Mass Index and Mortality in Older Men: The NIH-AARP Cohort Study

Data from Adams KF, Schatzkin A, Harris T, et al. Overweight, obesity, and mortality in a large prospective cohort of persons 50–71 years old. *N Engl J Med*. 2006;355:763-778.

of Health (NIH)–AARP Diet and Exercise Study.[13] As indicated, this relationship is J-shaped, with the lowest mortality risk occurring for all age groups at a BMI of about 26 kg/m², which is one unit higher than the cut-point used to define overweight in younger adults (i.e., 25 kg/m²). Compared with those men having a BMI between 23.5 and 24.9 kg/m² (the reference group), mortality risk increases with a BMI greater than 29 kg/m², and this was especially so among men aged 50–55 years. Relative risk also appears to increase among those men considered to be of normal body weight (i.e., 20–24 kg/m²), with those men aged 50–55 years experiencing an accelerated curve compared with the older age groups of similar BMI. Importantly, these data included men who were smokers and those with pre-existing disease and therefore, the greater relative mortality risk (especially among men aged 50–55 years) at a lower BMI may be confounded by these two factors, because both smoking and disease are related to low BMI and to mortality.

Also, the relative mortality risk at higher or lower BMIs is attenuated as one becomes older—indeed, the youngest age group experienced a curvilinear (or exponential) increase in mortality risk. This attenuated relative risk with increasing age may be due in part to the issue of **selective survival**, with those least susceptible to the punitive effects of low or high body weight able to survive to older ages, thus presenting a more robust physiologic profile. In any case, these data suggest that the "ideal" BMI for older people may be slightly higher than for younger adults, and they underscore the importance of maintaining muscle mass and body weight in older age.

Childhood and adolescence is the time for bone accrual, and women reach the point of peak bone mass at about age 25 years. The next 20 years is characterized by a relative stability in bone growth, until the time of menopause when, due to the drop in estrogen, bone mass begins to decline irreversibly. Indeed, by age 70, there is a decrease in maximal skeletal mass weight of about 40%. The stimulus for bone growth is the physical deformation of bone cells, which is accomplished via ground-reaction forces produced during weight-bearing exercise. Site-specific overloading forces on the bone will stimulate an adaptive response at the specific site and continued adaptations requiring a progressively increasing overload. There is now ample evidence that girls who participate in high levels of weight-bearing and high-impact activity have greater bone accrual compared with their inactive counterparts. Similar to having a greater amount of money in one's retirement account, those with greater peak bone mass have a greater bone reserve during the period of bone mass decline. Moreover, those women who remain physically active in older age will have a slower and blunted slope of decline relative to older women who are sedentary.

Cardiovascular Changes

Loss of both plasticity and resiliency in the arterial walls also comes with aging. Consequently, maximal heart rate declines, as does **stroke volume** and **cardiac output**. Arterial venous oxygen difference (AV-O_2 diff; the difference in oxygen content between arterial and venous blood) also declines with age. As the AV-O_2 difference declines, so does maximal aerobic capacity (VO_{2max}). Maximal VO_2, defined as the body's ability to extract and utilize oxygen in response to a physical demand, declines approximately 15–55% per decade after age 25 years[12]—obviously, those people who maintain an active lifestyle will experience a smaller decline, relative to those who are sedentary. The reason that most amateur road races and marathons have different age classes for competition is to "adjust" for the biologic decline in the cardiorespiratory system with age. Athletic performance notwithstanding, it is important for older people to maintain an adequate level of aerobic capacity in order to do things like climb stairs, carry groceries, and carry out ADLs.

Sensory Changes

Accompanying the physical changes that occur with older age are the neurosensory changes in vision, hearing, touch, taste, and smell. The changes have important consequences for health and safety, especially if older people are living alone. For example, anorexia and loss of interest in eating result in malnutrition; losses in vision and hearing increase the risk of injury when driving an automobile or crossing the street; a diminished sense of smell may prevent recognition of a gas leak or of smoke (as well as potentially diminishing interest in food); and a loss of touch may result in burns from hot surfaces. Reaction time also declines with age due to changes in cognitive processing, and therefore an older person may not be able to compensate in a timely manner to a given perturbation. For example, unintended falls are a major source of injury in older people, as they may not be able to catch their balance as a result of a stumble or slip.

All humans will also develop some degree of decline in cognitive function as they age due to the deterioration of the biologic framework that underlies the ability to think and to reason. This decline begins as early as young adulthood and includes a drop in regional brain volume, loss of myelin integrity, cortical thinning, impaired serotonin, acetylcholine, and dopamine receptor binding and signaling, accumulation of neurofibrillary tangles, and altered

concentrations of various brain metabolites.[14-16] Cumulatively, these changes result in a variety of symptoms associated with aging, such as short-term memory loss, decreased ability to maintain focus, and decreased problem-solving capability. If left unchecked, symptoms oftentimes progress into more serious conditions, such as dementia and depression, or even Alzheimer disease (more on Alzheimer disease later). Fortunately, aspects of cognitive decline are modifiable, with lifestyle changes such as regular physical activity, cognitive training, and nutritional intervention demonstrating effectiveness in minimizing the rate of intellectual decay in older age.

Taken together, diminished neurosensory and cognitive function can be very stressful for older people with regard to maintaining their daily interactions with their environment and their independence. Many older people respond to this stress by isolating and decreasing contact with their environment, which can exacerbate these neurosensory and cognitive losses further, as people who maintain an active lifestyle and continue to interact with environmental challenges experience a far better maintenance of sensory function compared with those who do not. See **BOX 11-2** about phenotype of frailty.[17]

▶ Public Health Challenges

About 80% of older people have at least one chronic health problem.[18] Chronic conditions in older adults exact a markedly disproportionate toll on the economy. For example, older adults comprised about 13% of the U.S. population in 2010; however, they consumed 34% of total U.S. personal healthcare expenses.[19] The average healthcare expense in 2010 was $18,429 per year for older people, but only $6,125 per year for working-age people (ages 19–64).[20] Similar differences among age groups are reflected in the data on the top 5% of healthcare spenders. People aged 65–79 years (9% of the total population) represented 29% of the top 5% of spenders. Similarly, people 80 years and older (about 3% of the population) accounted for 14% of the top 5% of spenders.[21] Healthcare expenditures, as well as the older adult population, have increased considerably since 2002, resulting in even greater disparities in healthcare spending among older, relative to younger people.

TABLE 11-1 displays the chronic diseases of greatest prominence in older age, along with the attributable risk factors for these conditions. It is important to note that these diseases, to some extent, are modifiable; that is, lifestyle-related behaviors such as a poor diet, sedentary living, tobacco use, excessive alcohol intake,

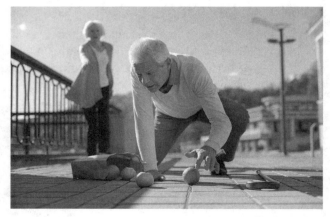

© Dmytro Zinkevych/Shutterstock

BOX 11-2 Phenotype of Frailty

The phenotype of frailty is characterized by the presence of three or more attributes of unintentional weight loss, weakness, loss of physiologic reserve, fatigue, slow motor performance, or low physical activity. The prevalence of frailty tends to be higher in older women than men and is highest among minority populations. The underlying cause of frailty is an aggregate loss of function among multiple interconnected and mutually adapted physiologic systems (cardiovascular, musculoskeletal, inflammatory, and endocrine) resulting in the inability of these systems to maintain homeostasis. When the number of dysregulated systems reaches a critical threshold, frailty becomes clinically evident. Among older women especially, the prevalence of frailty increases in a curvilinear manner with the number of dysregulated systems (**FIGURE 11-4**).

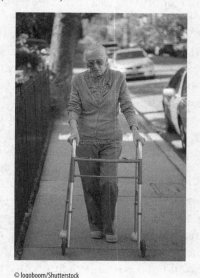

© logoboom/Shutterstock

Data from Fried LP, Xue QL, Cappola AR, et al. Nonlinear multisystem physiological dysregulation associated with frailty in older women: implications for etiology and treatment. *J Gerontol A Biol Sci Med Sci.* 2009;64:1049-1057.

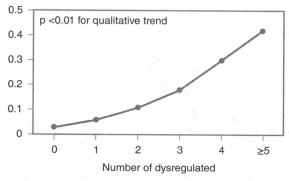

FIGURE 11-4 Frailty as a Function of Dysregulated Systems in Women Aged 70–79 Years

Data from Fried LP, Xue QL, Cappola AR, et al. Nonlinear multisystem physiological dysregulation associated with frailty in older women: implications for etiology and treatment. *J Gerontol A Biol Sci Med Sci.* 2009;64:1049-1057.

TABLE 11-1 Prominent Chronic Diseases of Older Age

Chronic Disease	Risk Factor
Cardiovascular disease	Hypertension, dyslipidemia, obesity
Type 2 diabetes	Insulin resistance, glucose, intolerance, dyslipidemia, obesity
Cancer	Obesity, bowel immotility, sex hormone profile
Osteoporosis	Low bone density
Physical disability	Sarcopenia, musculoskeletal weakness, poor balance, neuromuscular defects, arthritis

and overweight contribute heavily to their etiology and their progression. There is now ample evidence that positive changes in these aforementioned lifestyle risk behaviors are quite effective in preventing, minimizing, and (in some cases) reversing the course of disease even in older age.

Ideally, successful aging begins *in utero* with the promotion of a healthy and active lifestyle, equal access to education and income, as well as to health services across the life course. Clearly, if the onset of chronic conditions could be postponed or eliminated altogether, the public health benefits would be enormous. With a delay in the onset of chronic disease, the maintenance of physical function could be extended closer to the life expectancy. This "**compression of morbidity**" would no doubt improve quality of life and preserve autonomy for older people, as well as reduce health-related costs to the individual and to society. The compression of morbidity[22] refers to the delay of chronic disease and frailty until the end of life, or as close to the end of life as possible. Unlike life extension, this compression would maintain physical function, autonomy, and quality of life for a greater proportion of the life span.

▶ Health Promotion Initiatives for Older People

In 1979, the U.S. Department of Health and Human Services published the document, *Healthy People: The Surgeon General's Report on Health Promotion and Disease Prevention.*[23] This important document then set the stage for fostering subsequent health promotion initiatives throughout the nation. A call-to-action document in 1980, *Promoting Health/Preventing Disease: Objectives for the Nation*, set health objectives for the nation over the next 10 years. In 1990, *Healthy People 2000* was initiated by the U.S. Public Health Service in order to address preventable causes of death and disability.[24] Every decade since then, a new set of health objectives has been issued. Interestingly, however, is the fact that these objectives are not supported by federal funds. **BOX 11-3** lists selected measurable objectives for this current decade that specifically address the health of older people.

Separate from medical expenditures is the impact of a growing older population on community resources, and this is especially true with regard to transportation, building, and community design. In the United States, age-friendly initiatives are part of the international effort started by the World Health Organization (WHO) in response to two significant demographic trends: urbanization and population aging. As of 2015, just over half of the world population lived in cities, and by 2030 that population will increase to about three in every five people in the world.[25] At the same time, improvements in public health have led to more people living longer. In preparation for these two trends, the WHO created the Global Age-Friendly

Cities project. The Project comprises eight domains (the District of Columbia has 10 domains) that influence the health and quality of life of older people living all around the world. These domains are: (1) outdoor spaces and buildings; (2) transportation; (3) housing; (4) social participation; (5) respect and social inclusion; (6) civic participation and employment; (7) communication and information; (8) community support and health services; (9) emergency preparedness; and (10) elder abuse and fraud.[26]

The "village movement" refers to the formation of a nonprofit organization by a group of older residents within a specific community designed to foster access to services that support their goal of living at home, rather than in senior housing or assisted living, for as long as possible ("**aging in place**"). A village can range from a few blocks in an urban or suburban neighborhood to a rural area with a 20-mile radius. Each village is autonomous, and its members determine which services it will offer. Typical offerings shared by all members include: (1) home-safety modifications; (2) transportation; (3) meal delivery; (4) dog walking; (5) technology training and support; (6) health and wellness programs; (7) social activities; and (8) the services of visiting nurses and care managers. Most of these services are under the purview of an administrator (paid or volunteer) who serves to connect members with services as needed, as well as to coordinate village-wide programs and activities. Many villages recruit and rely on local volunteers to help deliver services to their members as well. For example, if a member needs modification to his or her home, the member would contact the village administrator, who then would make arrangements with a contractor who is either a volunteer or works at a discount for the village. Materials are then purchased using the village's group discount for materials (the member would have to pay for the goods), and the renovations are performed by the contractor or other volunteers.

BOX 11-3 Selected Health Objectives for Older Adults: Healthy People 2020

Objective: Increase the proportion of older adults who are up to date on a core set of clinical preventative services.

Baseline: 47.3% in 2008
Target: 52.1% in 2020

Objective: Reduce the proportion of older people who have moderate to severe functional limitations.

Baseline: 28.3% in 2007
Target: 25.5% in 2020

Objective: Increase the proportion of older adults with reduced physical or cognitive function who engage in light, moderate, or vigorous leisure-time physical activities.

Baseline: 33.7% in 2008
Target: 37.1% in 2020

Objective: Reduce the rate of emergency department visits due to falls among older adults.

Baseline: 5,235/100,000 in 2007
Target: 4,711/100,000 in 2020

Reproduced from U.S. Office of Disease Prevention and *Health Promotion. Healthy People 2020: Objectives.* Available at https://www.healthypeople.gov/. Accessed November 1, 2017.

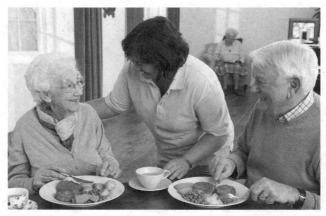

These aforementioned examples of global, federal, and local health promotion efforts are key to helping older people to take charge of the determinants of their health in order to maintain their independence and quality of life for as long as possible. Environmental interventions are those performed at the community level, rather than at the individual level. These types of interventions can affect everyone equally and target risk conditions rather than individual risk factors or behaviors. Many of the most innovative public health interventions and policies have little to do with health *per se* but rather with altering the barriers that prevent people from maintaining control over their lives. As with any environmental action, an informed and active public takes the lead in influencing public health policy. Similarly, multiple community agencies need to work together to ensure a health-promoting environment for older people to thrive within.

🔍 CASE REPORT

Alzheimer Disease in Nuns

In 1986, a scientist named David Snowdon studied an unusual population of 678 nuns and produced one of the world's most comprehensive neurologic research projects that gives insight into the types of people who might eventually develop Alzheimer disease. The School Sisters of Notre Dame, a religious congregation in Minneapolis, Minnesota, allowed Snowdon to test them each year, and each nun agreed to donate her brain to scientific research. The nuns provided a valuable research group because of their relatively homogeneous background: nonsmokers, same marital and reproductive history, who lived in similar housing, held similar jobs, and had similar access to preventive medical care. Snowdon discovered that when the women entered the order between the approximate ages of 18 and 22, they filled out a 3- by 5-inch index card upon which they were asked to answer two questions: (1) Why did you become a nun; and (2) What is your vision for what you hope to do?

Snowdon observed that the women with strong writing skills, syntactical and grammatical complexity, and strong vocabulary fared much better in contrast with those with poor writing skills, etc., who developed Alzheimer disease. Snowdon's study also revealed that a college education and an active intellectual life may protect one from Alzheimer disease. After analyzing autobiographies, he observed that sisters who had expressed the most positive emotions in their writings lived longest and those on the road to Alzheimer disease expressed fewer and fewer positive emotions as their mental functions declined.

1. Why study nuns?
2. What are the definite risk factors for Alzheimer disease? What are some suspected risk factors?
3. Briefly describe the pathophysiology of Alzheimer disease.
4. What are the symptoms of Alzheimer disease?
5. How might a college education, an active intellectual life, and a positive outlook on life protect someone from Alzheimer disease?
6. If one lives past age 80 years, the odds of developing Alzheimer disease increase to about 50%. Given current aging demographic trends, describe the economic burden associated with this disease (include medical costs, medication, and caretaking costs).
7. How should public health practice respond to this impending crisis?

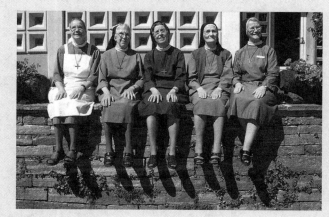
© Alexandre Zveiger/Shutterstock

Key Terms

Activities of daily living (ADLs)
Aging in place
Cardiac output
Compression of morbidity
Facultative aging

Instrumental activities of daily living (IADLs)
Mandatory aging
Osteoporosis
Sarcopenia

Selective survival
Stroke volume
Successful aging
Visceral adiposity

Discussion Questions

1. List several political, social, and economic consequences of having a shrinking workforce population (aged 18–64 years) relative to a growing population of older adults (≥ 65 years) in developed countries.

2. Let's assume a marathon runner maintained exactly the same training regimen through middle age and after menopause. Describe the trajectory over 10 years in her marathon times and her body weight and why this might be so.

3. Discuss the pros and cons of compressing morbidity within a set life expectancy vs. extending the life expectancy without attempting to compress morbidity.

4. How can you help an older parent or relative to "age in place"? What would need to happen?

5. Create your own 2020 Health Objectives for older people.

References

1. DiPietro L, Singh MF, Fielding R, Nose H. Successful aging. *J Aging Res*. 2012;2012:438537. doi: 10.1155/2012/438537.

2. Administration on Aging and U.S. Department of Health and Human Services. *A Profile of Older Americans: 2016.* Washington, DC: Department of Health and Human Services; 2016. Available at https://www.giaging.org/documents/A_Profile_of_Older _Americans__2016.pdf. Accessed November 1, 2017.

3. Yoshida R. Japan census report shows surge in elderly population, many living alone. *Japan Times*. June 29, 2016. Available at https://www.japantimes.co.jp/news/2016/06/29/ national/japan-census-report-shows-surge-elderly- population-many-living-alone/. Accessed November 1, 2017.

4. Howe CZ. Selected social gerontology theories and older adult leisure involvement: a review of the literature. *J Appl Gerontol*. 1987;6:448-463.

5. Bengtson VL, DeLiema M. Theories of aging and social gerontology: explaining how social factors influence well-being in later life. In: Harrington Meyer M, Daniele EA, eds. *Gerontology: Changes, Challenges, and Solutions*. New York, NY: Praeger Publishers; 2016:25-56.

6. Atchley RC. A Continuity Theory of normal aging. *Gerontology*. 1989;29(2):183-190.

7. DiPietro L, Seals DR. Introduction to exercise in older adults. In: Lamb DR, Gisolfi CG, Nadel ER, eds. *Perspectives in Exercise and Sports Medicine*. Vol. 8: Exercise in Older Adults. Carmel, IN: Cooper Publishing Group; 1995:1-10.

8. Shammas MA. Telomeres, lifestyle, cancer, and aging. *Curr Opin Clin Nutr Metab Care*. 2011;14(1):28-34.

9. Bortz WM. Disuse and aging. *JAMA*. 1982;248:1203-1208.

10. Rowe JW, Kahn RL. Successful aging. *Gerontologist*. 1997;37:433-440.

11. Crowther MR, Parker MW, Achenbaum WA, Larimore WL, Koenig HG. Rowe and Kahn's model of successful aging revisited: positive spirituality – the forgotten factor. *Gerontologist*. 2003;42(5):613-620.

12. American College of Sports Medicine. Exercise and physical activity for older adults. *Med Sci Sports Exerc*. 2009;41:1510-1530.

13. Adams KF, Schatzkin A, Harris T, et al. Overweight, obesity, and mortality in a large prospective cohort of persons 50-71 years old. *N Engl J Med*. 2006;355:763-778.

14. Piperhoff P, Hömke L, Schneider F, et al. Deformation field morphometry reveals age-related structural differences between the brains of adults up to 51 years. *J Neurosci*. 2008;28(4):828-842.

15. Del Tredici K, Braak H. Neurofibrillary changes of the Alzheimer type in very elderly individuals: neither inevitable nor benign: Commentary on "No disease in the brain of a 115-year-old woman." *Neurobiol Aging*. 2008;29(8):1133-1136.

16. Kadota T, Horinouchi T, Kuroda C. Development and aging of the cerebrum: assessment with proton MR spectroscopy. *Am J Neuroradiol*. 2001;22(1):128-135.

17. Fried LP, Xue QL, Cappola AR, et al. Nonlinear multisystem physiological dysregulation associated with frailty in older women: implications for etiology and treatment. *J Gerontol A Biol Sci Med Sci*. 2009;64:1049-1057.

18. National Council on Aging. Chronic Disease Management. Available at https://www.ncoa.org/healthy-aging/chronic -disease/. Accessed June 17, 2017.

19. Stanton MW. The high concentration of US health care expenditures. Agency for Healthcare Research and Quality. *Research in Action* 2006;19. Available at https://archive.ahrq .gov/research/findings/factsheets/costs/expriach/expendria .pdf. Accessed June 17, 2017.

20. Leatherby L. Medical spending among the U.S. elderly. Journalist's Resource. February 22, 2016. Harvard Kennedy School/Shorenstein Center on Media, Politics and Public Policy. Available at https://journalistsresource.org/studies /government/health-care/elderly-medical-spending -medicare. Accessed November 1, 2017.

21. Federal Interagency Forum on Aging Related Statistics. *Older Americans, 2004: Key Indicators of Well-Being*. Washington, DC: Federal Interagency Forum on Aging-Related Statistics; 2004.

22. Fries JF. Aging, natural death and the compression of morbidity. *N Engl J Med*. 1980;303:130-135.

23. U.S. Department of Health and Human Services. Healthy people: the surgeon general's report on health promotion and disease prevention. Washington, DC: DHHS USGPO; 1979.

24. U.S. Office of Disease Prevention and Health Promotion. Healthy People 2020: Objectives. Available at https://www .healthypeople.gov/. Accessed November 1, 2017.

25. World Health Organization. Global Health Observatory data: Urban population growth. Available at http://www.who.int /gho/urban_health/situation_trends/urban_population _growth_text/en/. Accessed June 17, 2017.

26. Advisory Neighborhood Commission. Resolution. Available at http://www.anc3g.org/wp-content/uploads/2014/09 /Senior-Wellness-Center-resolution-2016.pdf. Accessed February 20, 2018.

Additional Reading

Haber D. *Health Promotion and Aging: Practical Applications for Health Professionals*. 6th ed. New York, NY: Springer Publishing Co.; 2013.

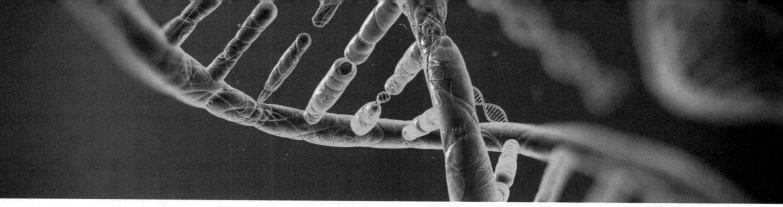

CHAPTER 12

Mental Illness and Addiction

Sean D. Cleary, Loretta DiPietro, and Amy E. Seitz

LEARNING OBJECTIVES

By the end of this chapter, the student will be able to:

- Describe the public health burden associated with mental illness and addiction
- Differentiate among different types of mental illness
- List four of the most prevalent mental illnesses worldwide
- Compare differences in occurrence of mental illness by age and sex
- Describe the midbrain reward pathway
- Identify several hormones and neurotransmitters that play a role in mental health
- Define epigenetics and explain how it relates to depression
- Summarize the interplay between genetics, biology, and environment in mental illness
- Justify the prevention and treatment of mental illness and addiction as a way to lower the global economic burden

CHAPTER OUTLINE

▶ Introduction

Mental health as defined by the World Health Organization (WHO) is "a state of well-being in which an individual realizes his or her own abilities, can cope with the normal stresses of life, can work productively and is able to make a contribution to his or her community."[1] Specifically, a state of mental health requires a multifaceted state of well-being. Mental illnesses, or mental health disorders, are the "health conditions that are characterized by alterations in thinking, mood, or behavior (or some combination thereof) associated with distress and/or impaired functioning."[2] Differences in cultural interpretations of mental health and mental illness should also be considered, complicating the task of classifying mental health and disorder.

TABLE 12-1 The Four Humours with Their Corresponding Elements, Seasons, Sites of Formation, and Resulting Temperaments

Humour	Season	Element	Organ	Qualities	Ancient Name	Temperament	Temperament Characteristics
Blood	spring	air	heart	warm and moist	*sanguis*	sanguine	courageous, hopeful, playful, carefree
Yellow bile	summer	fire	liver	warm and dry	*kholé*	choleric	ambitious, leader-like, restless, easily angered
Black bile	autumn	earth	spleen	cold and dry	*melaina kholé*	melancholic	despondent, quiet, analytical, serious
Phlegm	winter	water	brain	cold and moist	*phlégma*	phlegmatic	calm, thoughtful, patient, peaceful

Data from Keirsey D. *Please Understand Me II: Temperament, Character, Intelligence*. Del Mar, CA: Prometheus Nemesis Book Company; 1998:26; Lewis-Anthony J. *Circles of Thorns: Hieronymus Bosch and Being Human*. London, UK: Bloomsbury; 2008:70.

The first classification system for all illnesses, including mental illness, originated in ancient Greece by Hippocrates and was based on the proposed imbalance of the four humours: black bile, yellow bile, phlegm, and blood. Each of these humours corresponded to one of the traditional four temperaments of *melancholic* (black bile; gloomy, depressed), *choleric* (yellow bile; ill-tempered), *phlegmatic* (phlegm; calm, unemotional), and *sanguine* (blood; courageous, hopeful) (**TABLE 12-1**).

Since that time, elaborate classifications of mental illnesses have evolved over centuries in order to group them according to their proposed origin or cause (**etiology**). The introduction of operationalized criteria to define various mental disorders in the late 1970s and their subsequent incorporation into the **Diagnostic and Statistical Manual of Mental Disorders (DSM)** represented a key development in our ability to define, diagnose, and track these illnesses.[3] The DSM is a comprehensive classification system for mental disorders that is maintained and updated by the American Psychiatric Association through participation of workgroups formed by experts in the field of mental health. Since the first publication in 1952, the DSM has been revised and updated multiple times in order to be consistent with current mental health knowledge. The current version of the DSM, the DSM-5, was released in May 2013.[4] Mental illnesses are also classified in the International Classification of Diseases, currently in its tenth edition.

The classification schemes commonly used are based on separate, but possibly overlapping, categories of disorder schemes. These classification schemes have achieved some widespread acceptance in psychiatry and other fields and include: (1) anxiety disorders, (2) attention deficit/hyperactive disorders, (3) autism spectrum disorders, (4) eating disorders, (5) mood disorders, (6) personality disorders, and (7) schizophrenia. Some approaches to classify mental illness do not use categories with single cut-points to define those with illness from those who are healthy. Such classification may instead be based on broader underlying "spectra," where each spectrum links together a range of related categorical diagnoses and nonthreshold symptom patterns.[5]

▸ The Descriptive Epidemiology of Mental Illness and Addiction

On average, about 30% of adults worldwide experience some type of mental disorder over their lifetime, with about 18% reporting a common mental disorder in the past 12 months.[3] Globally, women are more likely to report a mood or anxiety disorder over the previous 12 months, whereas men more commonly report alcohol or substance use disorders. The global lifetime prevalence of mental disorders among low- and middle-income countries (LMIC; 22.7%) is lower compared with that of high-income countries (HIC; 33.2%). Overall, the LMIC of the East Asia and Pacific region experience the lowest prevalence of mental disorders (8.6%), whereas the HIC English-speaking regions report the highest prevalence (39.7%). In an effort to increase mental health services globally, there has been a call for action through the recent global mental health movement; however, some critics emphasize the need for mental health issues to be interpreted in the context of local cultures rather than imposing Western ideas of mental health and mental illness.[6]

Anxiety and Depressive Disorders

Anxiety disorders such as phobias, separation anxiety disorder, generalized anxiety disorder (GAD), obsessive-compulsive disorder (OCD), and post-traumatic stress disorder (PTSD) are among the most common class of mental disorders.[5,7] They are characterized by excess fear stemming from an impending threat (actual or perceived) or excess or persistent anxiety from a future threat. Behavioral disturbances can be a component, as avoidance behaviors may be used to reduce fear and anxiety. The DSM outlines nine specific anxiety disorders, as well as three "other" or "unspecified" anxiety-disorder categories.[4]

The lifetime prevalence of such disorders is about 28.8% in the United States and about 13% globally,[3]

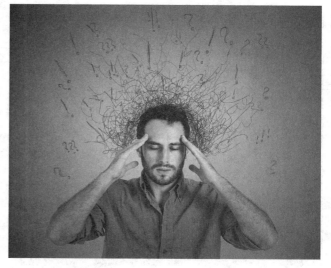

© SIphotography/iStock/Getty Images Plus

while the 12-month period prevalence is approximately 18% among adults in the United States[5] and 6.7% globally (**FIGURE 12-1**).[3] Women are about 60% more likely than men to report an anxiety disorder over their lifetime, and in the United States, non-Hispanic Blacks are 20% less likely and Hispanics are 30% less likely than non-Hispanic whites to experience an anxiety disorder over their lifetime. The age of onset for anxiety disorders is about 11 years; however, onset varies depending on the specific type. Separation anxiety disorder and

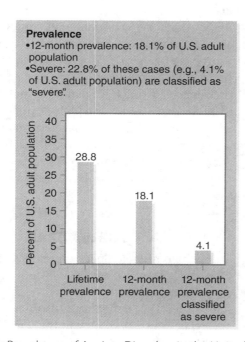

Prevalence
- 12-month prevalence: 18.1% of U.S. adult population
- Severe: 22.8% of these cases (e.g., 4.1% of U.S. adult population) are classified as "severe."

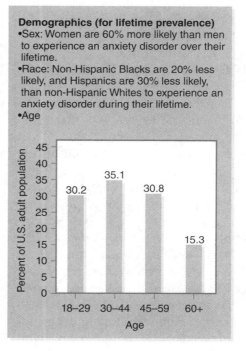

Demographics (for lifetime prevalence)
- Sex: Women are 60% more likely than men to experience an anxiety disorder over their lifetime.
- Race: Non-Hispanic Blacks are 20% less likely, and Hispanics are 30% less likely, than non-Hispanic Whites to experience an anxiety disorder during their lifetime.
- Age

FIGURE 12-1 The Prevalence of Anxiety Disorders in the United States

Reproduced from National Institute of Mental Health. Any anxiety disorder Among Adults. Available at https://www.nimh.nih.gov/health/statistics/prevalence/any-anxiety-disorder-among-adults.shtml. Data from Kessler RC, Chiu WT, Demler O, Walters EE. Prevalence, severity, and comorbidity of twelve-month DSM-IV disorders in the National Comorbidity Survey Replication (NCS-R). *Arch Gen Psychiatry*. 2005;62: 617-627; Kessler RC, Berglund P, Demler O, Jin R, Merikangas KR, Walters EE. Lifetime prevalence and age-of-onset distributions of DSM-IV disorders in the National Comorbidity Survey Replication. *Arch Gen Psychiatry*. 2005;62:593-602.

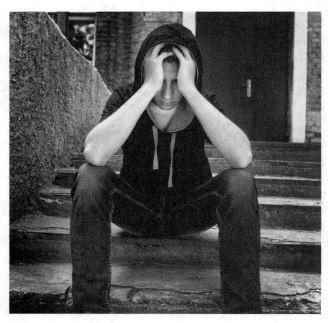

© Sabphoto/Shutterstock

phobia have a median age of onset ranging from 7 to 14 years, whereas GAD and PTSD have a later median age of onset distributions (25–53 years).[5]

Depressive disorders as defined within the DSM-5 include disorders with the common features of "sad, empty, or irritable mood, accompanied by somatic or cognitive changes that significantly affect the individual ability to function."[4] Distinguishing features include etiology and length and timing of the disorder. Examples of depressive disorders include disruptive mood dysregulation disorder, major depressive disorder, and persistent depressive disorder.

The global lifetime prevalence for mood disorders (such as dysphoric, **bipolar**, or major depressive disorders) is 9.6%, with a 12-month period prevalence of 5.4%.[3] In the United States, the lifetime and period prevalence is about 20.8% and 9.5%, respectively.[7] Similar to anxiety disorders, women are 50% more likely to report a mood disorder over their lifetime than are men, while Black and Hispanic Americans report a lower prevalence compared with non-Hispanic whites. These sex differences are not observed, however, among children under age 14 years,[8] and additional studies have described an inverse relationship among men and women over age 55 years.[9,10] The median age of onset for mood disorders is between 25 and 45 years, with age distribution curves demonstrating a low prevalence until the early teenage years, followed by a linear increase through late middle-age and a declining trend thereafter.[11]

One type of mood disorder is major depressive disorder, which affects about 16.5% of the U.S.

population over their lifetime and has a 12-month period prevalence of 6.7%. Approximately 2% of the U.S. population suffers from "severe" major depression. Women are 70% more likely to experience major depression over their lifetime compared with men, with African Americans being about 40% less likely than their white counterparts to report major depression.[7] The highest prevalence of major depression in the United States occurs among adults between the ages of 30 and 44 years. Indeed, compared with U.S. adults over age 60 years, adults 18–29 years are 70% more likely to experience major depression over their lifetime, while those 30–44 years are 120% more likely, and those ages 45–59 years are 100% more likely to experience the same. In contrast, compared with those age 60 years and older, adults aged 18–29 years are 200% more likely to experience depression over a 12-month period, with adults 30–44 years about 80% more likely.[7] The average age of onset for major depression is about 32 years (**FIGURE 12-2**).

Post-Traumatic Stress Disorder

PTSD describes a long-term psychologic reaction to a traumatic event such as serious injury, sexual violence, or exposure to death (threatened or actual).[4] It was initially included in the DSM-III in 1980 after recognition of specific symptoms among Vietnam war veterans and other persons who have experienced trauma.[12] The disorder often co-occurs with mood disorders, substance abuse, and risky behavior and the prevalence is especially high among persons with combat-related exposures, as well as people whose work has a higher risk of exposure to traumatic experiences, such as police and firefighters. The 12-month prevalence in the U.S. general population has been identified as 1–3.5%[13] and lifetime prevalence as 6.8%,[7] whereas 12-month prevalence estimates among military combat veterans, and specifically military veterans serving in the infantry, have been described as ranging from 6–13% with lifetime prevalence as high as 15–18.7%.[14,15]

Psychosis and Schizophrenia

The Schizophrenia Spectrum and Other Psychotic Disorders chapter of the DSM-5 contains information on psychotic disorders, such as schizophrenia and schizotypical (personality) disorder. Schizophrenia and related disorders vary in the length of the symptoms (e.g., brief psychotic disorder lasts between 1 day to 1 month and schizophrenia lasts at least 6 months) and severity of symptoms.[4] Persons with schizophrenia are more likely to be unemployed and have

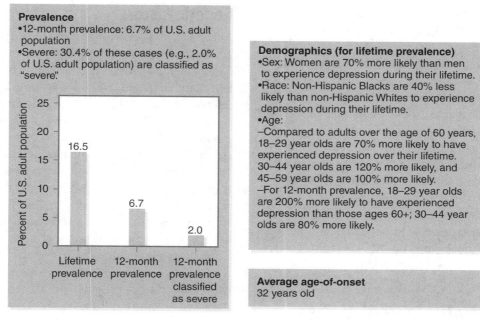

FIGURE 12-2 The Prevalence of Major Depression in the United States

Reproduced from Kessler RC, Berglund P, Demler O, Jin R, Merikangas KR, Walters EE. Lifetime prevalence and age-of-onset distributions of DSM-IV disorders in the National Comorbidity Survey Replication. *Arch Gen Psychiatry*. 2005;62:593-602.

a decreased life span.[16] Symptoms usually become apparent in late adolescence or early adulthood and are categorized as positive symptoms, such as hallucinations, thought insertion, or general disconnect from reality; negative symptoms, such as decreased motivation, poverty of speech, or social withdrawal; and cognitive impairment.[16]

McGrath et al. identify variations in the epidemiology of schizophrenia for different populations and an overall lifetime risk of 4/1,000 persons.[17] In their meta-analysis, McGrath et al. identified no significant sex differences in the schizophrenia standardized mortality ratio or in prevalence; however, the incidence was higher for men.

Addiction

Substance-related and addictive disorders can take the form of mild, moderate, or severe substance use disorders or behavioral addictions. Substance use disorders are identified by the particular substance and defined as a disorder when their recurrent use results in functional or clinical impairment, potentially resulting in health problems and/or repercussions in work and home life. Determination of mild, moderate, or severe disorder is defined based on the number of diagnostic criteria met. The DSM-5 includes over 50 specific addictive disorders, all with the commonality of potentially activating the brain's reward pathway in such an intense manner as to result in the neglect of normal activities.[4]

The global lifetime prevalence of substance use disorders is 3.4%, with a 12-month prevalence of 3.8%.[3] Among the U.S. population, approximately 15% report a substance use disorder over their lifetime.[7] Among the substance use disorders, alcohol abuse is by far the most prevalent (13.2%). Globally, men are over three times more likely to suffer from substance use disorders compared with women. Substance use disorders are relatively uncommon prior to the mid-teenage years; however, thereafter there is an accelerated increase in prevalence in late adolescence and early adulthood.[11]

Behavioral addictions are being increasingly described in the literature, and similarities have been noted with substance use disorders. For example, the clinical presentation, physiology, and treatment aspects of gambling disorder are similar to those of substance-related disorders. Gambling disorder was recently added to the DSM-5 as a diagnosable condition within addictive disorders, although it is the only non-substance-related disorder within the substance-related and addictive disorders category. Examples of other behavioral addictions described in the literature (but not defined as diagnosable conditions in the DSM) include sex, pornography, compulsive buying, and internet use.

In all, untreated mental disorders account for approximately 13% of the total global burden of disease.[18] In fact, **unipolar depressive disorder** is the third-leading cause of disease, accounting for 4.3% of the global disease burden. WHO predicts that by the year 2030, the leading cause of disease burden across the world will be attributable to depression. People suffering from mental disorders experience higher mortality than the general population, both all-cause and suicide mortality. In fact, some mental illnesses have all-cause mortality rates comparable to heavy smoking.[19] For instance, those with schizophrenia and major depression have an overall mortality risk of 60%—40% higher than those without mental illness—due to myriad comorbid conditions such as diabetes, cancer, and human immunodeficiency virus infection.[18] Substance abuse disorders and anorexia nervosa have the highest all-cause mortality rates. Suicide mortality risk is increased with occurrence of mental illness, as 90% of those who commit suicide (globally) have a diagnosed mental illness at time of death.[20]

▶ The Psychobiology of Mental Illness and Addiction

Mental illness is a chronic disease, and all chronic diseases have biologic components. The only difference is that the organ of interest in mental illness is the brain, rather than the heart, liver, or pancreas. In recent years, scientists have made numerous discoveries about the function—and dysfunction—of the human brain. Several gene mutations linked to specific mental illnesses have been identified, along with specific structural defects in the brain that may increase the risk of developing a mental disorder in response to environmental stress. Other research has identified neurologic impairments that are associated with mental illness, including neurologic defects and under-connectivity among brain regions. Neurotransmitters are naturally occurring brain chemicals that carry signals to other parts of your brain and body. An impairment to the neural networks involving these chemicals alters the function of nerve receptors and nerve systems, leading to a chemical imbalance and increasing the likelihood of experiencing a mental illness.

Certain disorders such as schizophrenia, bipolar disorder, and autism fit the biologic model of disease, because structural and functional abnormalities are evident in imaging scans or during postmortem dissection. Yet for other conditions, such as depression or anxiety, the biologic foundation is less certain.[21] In fact, mental illnesses are likely to have multiple causes, including genetic, biologic, and environmental factors that interact in a way that may increase or decrease one's susceptibility to one or more mental disorders over the life span.

Genetic Factors

Many psychiatric disorders tend to run in families, suggesting potential genetic variations to their origin. In the case of major depression, family studies have suggested a heritability of about 40%,[22,23] while case-control studies have implicated several specific genes that appear to regulate pathways in the development of depressive disorders. These genes include brain-derived neurotrophic factor, which regulates neural plasticity and connectivity, as well as serotonin receptor, serotonin transporter, and catechol-o-methyltransferase, which regulate neurotransmitter signaling.[24,25] Interestingly, none of these genes has been consistently identified in any large genome-wide association studies (GWAS). In fact, despite the number of GWAS performed, very few genetic variants have been robustly identified in the etiology of depression,[26-29] thereby underscoring the complex and multifactorial origins of depression. Indeed, it is possible that numerous genes, each with a relatively small effect, contribute to this common disorder.[30]

Other disorders having a genetic origin include autism, attention deficit hyperactivity disorder, bipolar disorder, and schizophrenia. Differentiating among these major psychiatric syndromes can be difficult because their symptoms often overlap. Shared symptomatology may thus indicate a shared biology. Recent studies have reported some evidence of shared genetic risk factors for: (1) schizophrenia and bipolar disorder; (2) autism and schizophrenia; and (3) depression and bipolar disorder. Evidence also suggests that several major mental disorders, traditionally thought to be distinct, actually share certain genetic characteristics.[31] A recent GWAS of over 33,000 patients, diagnosed with at least one of the five psychiatric disorders listed above, indicated genetic variations significantly associated with all five disorders. These included variations in two genes responsible for regulating the flow of calcium into neurons (CACNA1C and CACNB2), which were linked to bipolar disorder, schizophrenia, and major depression. In addition, the investigators reported illness-linked gene variations for all five disorders that occurred in certain regions of chromosomes 3 and 10. It is important to note that while all of these genetic associations are statistically significant, they account for only a small amount of risk for mental illness. Nonetheless, this information may be useful in providing more accurate diagnoses of mental illness.

The Toxic Mind Theory

There is now considerable accumulated evidence that most nervous and mental disorders are linked to disturbances in **noradrenergic function**. Physical symptoms of mental illness (such as excessive mental activity, heart palpitations, and blood pressure spikes) often reflect an exaggerated *fight or flight* response due to enhanced activity of the noradrenergic and sympathetic nervous systems. The catecholamine hypothesis of mental illness states that behavioral depression may be related to a deficiency in catecholamine (usually, **norepinephrine**) at functionally important central adrenergic receptors, whereas mania results from excess catecholamine (usually **epinephrine**).[32] A newer theory proposes that a primary biologic factor in the etiology of mental illness is *endogenous toxicosis*.[33]

Symptoms of most diseases represent the body's attempts to eliminate toxins.[34] As we discussed in a previous chapter, any substance that cannot be utilized by the cells is recognized as toxic and eliminated. When elimination is impaired, toxins accumulate until the body can initiate a detoxification process. Toxicosis is widespread in nerve cells and the idea that the symptoms of mental illness result from the body trying to eliminate these toxins is not new.[34,35]

The cornerstone of this theory is the idea that mental illness is caused by the continual suppression of emotions—namely, anger—that begins in early childhood and sets a pattern throughout adulthood. The continued suppression of emotions (such as fear and anger during fight or flight reactions) results in atrophy and endogenous toxicosis in noradrenergic neurons. Diminished levels of norepinephrine within the synapses are associated with depression. During periodic detoxification crises (i.e., a "meltdown"), excess norepiphrine and other metabolites flood the synapses, causing post-synaptic neurons to become overexcited and resulting in symptoms ranging from mild anxiety to violent behavior. According to this theory, recovery from nervous and mental disease is a process of detoxification, facilitated by therapy and self-help measures that involve the releasing and redirecting of repressed emotions.

The Midbrain Reward Pathway

The role of biology in addiction is becoming increasingly clearer. Agents such as nicotine, opiates, "comfort foods," or alcohol become addictive because they bind to specific neurotransmitter receptors or transporters in the brain to activate what is termed the midbrain reward pathway (**FIGURE 12-3**). Morphine and heroin bind to opiate receptors, cocaine binds to **dopamine** receptors, and nicotine binds to nicotinic receptors. The normal role of these receptors and transporters in the reward pathway is to reinforce certain beneficial behaviors, such as eating and sexual activity. Addictive agents, however, artificially enhance activity in the reward pathway by increasing the release

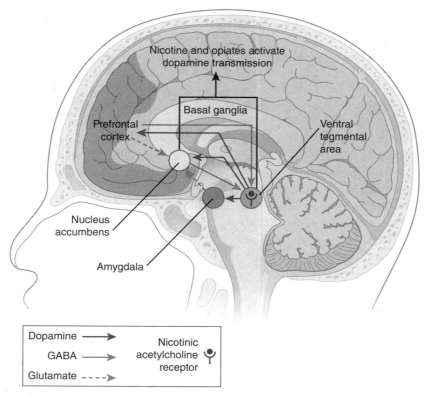

FIGURE 12-3 The Midbrain Reward Pathway

TABLE 12-2 Selected Year 2020 Objectives for Substance Abuse (SA)

SA 2.4	Increase the proportion of high school seniors never using substances—illicit drugs to 58.6% from a baseline of 53.3% in 2009 (10% improvement goal).
SA 8.2	Increase the proportion of persons who need alcohol and/or illicit drug treatment and received specialty treatment for abuse or dependence in the past year to 10.9% from a baseline of 9.9% in 2008 (10% improvement goal).
SA 13.2	Reduce the proportion of adolescents aged 12–17 years reporting use of marijuana during the past 30 days to 6.0% from a baseline of 6.7% in 2008 (10% reduction goal).
SA 14.2	Reduce the proportion of college students engaging in binge drinking during the past 2 weeks to 37% from a baseline of 41.1% in 2008 (10% reduction goal).
SA 18.3	Decrease the occurrence of alcohol-impaired driving (0.08+ blood alcohol content [BAC]) fatalities to 0.38 deaths per 100 million vehicle miles traveled from a baseline of 0.39 deaths per 100 million vehicle miles traveled in 2008.
SA 19.1	Reduce the past-year nonmedical use of pain relievers from 4.8% in 2008 among persons aged 12 years and older.
SA 20	Reduce the number of deaths attributable to excessive alcohol to 71,681 deaths/year from a baseline frequency of 79,646 deaths occurring in 2001–2005 (average annual number) (10% reduction goal).

Reproduced from Office of Disease Prevention and Health Promotion. Healthy People: 2020 Topics and Objectives: Substance Abuse. Washington, DC: DHHS. Available at https://www.healthypeople.gov/2020/topics-objectives/topic/substance-abuse. Accessed June 1, 2017.

of a neurotransmitter called dopamine within the brain nucleus. The hallmark of addictive agents is that once they are consumed for a period of time, abrupt cessation leads to a series of adverse effects that can be prevented only by consuming more of the agent (i.e., withdrawal effects). The mechanism underlying this withdrawal effect is that neurons adapt in response to chronic exposure of an addictive agent so that they become adjusted to their presence (i.e., tolerance) and begin to produce lower quantities of endogenous **endorphins**. After tolerance develops, a person has to take greater and greater quantities of the addictive agent to avoid unpleasant (or even lethal in the case of alcohol) withdrawal symptoms, a condition called dependence. Several federal agencies, working collaboratively, set specific Healthy People 2020 goals for substance abuse, including a reduction in college-age binge drinking and increase in people receiving alcohol and/or drug treatment (see **TABLE 12-2**).

Of recent public health interest are love/sex/pornography and gambling addictions—especially as the internet has made these activities so accessible. The nature of these addictions purportedly stems from the need to seek satisfaction from an external source to alleviate internal emotional pain due to childhood neglect or trauma. A significant problem with this unlimited accessibility of pornography is that children may be exposed to it at earlier ages and may begin to form unrealistic, unhealthy, and confusing expectations about love and sex. What happens in the brains of people with these types of addictions is exactly the same as for substance addictions—that is, dopamine receptors are activated during engagement in the activity and remain activated after the activity has ceased. These primed dopamine receptors crave more and more of the activity to get a similar level of thrill or to avoid the feelings of despair, depression, and rage. Thus, a dependency is set up biologically and psychologically.

▶ Epigenetic Modifications in Mental Illness

Environmental and Social Factors

As stated previously, mental illnesses are thought to be caused by a combination of biologic, genetic, environmental, and social factors. That is, certain biologic factors and genes may increase your risk of developing a mental illness (loading the gun); however, your life situation may trigger either episodic or chronic psychiatric impairment (pulling the trigger). Environmental

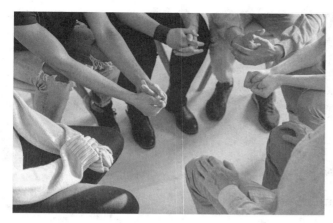

© Photographee.eu/Shutterstock

conditions such as chronic poverty, racism, physical or mental abuse (including bullying), or an occupation that offers an employee little control over his or her workday may be toxic for anyone, but may be especially so for those susceptible to mental illness due to their biology or family history. Prolonged feelings of deprivation, hopelessness, rejection, and anger can serve as triggers to anxiety and depressive disorders, due in part to excessive **cortisol** release from the adrenal cortex. A strong social support system often can mitigate the interaction between biology and environmental stressors, however, thus providing some "protection" against mental illness for those who may be vulnerable. A major social movement in public health is the organization of "self-help" groups. Indeed, these groups (usually peer-led) have been instrumental in providing social support for people struggling with or recovering from mental illness, addiction, bereavement, or abuse.

The Role of Epigenetics

"Epigenetics research examines the ways in which environmental factors change the way genes express themselves,"[36] thus providing a link between the biologic and other causes of mental illness. The theory behind this suggests that proper cellular function depends on the homeostatic regulation of the **epigenome**, and because this regulation is quite sensitive to environmental cues, small alterations in the environment may theoretically lead to long-term changes in gene expression. Change in deoxribonucleic acid (DNA) **methylation** is the most widely studied mechanism of epigenetic regulation.[37] One of the first classic epigenetics experiments, by researchers at McGill University, reported that pups of negligent rat mothers were more sensitive to stress in adulthood than pups that had been raised by doting mothers.[38] The differences could be traced to epigenetic markers, chemical tags that attach to strands of DNA and, in the process, turn various genes on and off. Those tags don't just affect individuals during their

lifetime, however; like DNA, epigenetic markers can be passed from generation to generation. More recently, these same investigators studied the brains of people who committed suicide and observed that those who had been abused in childhood had unique patterns of epigenetic tags in their brains.[39]

▶ The Economic Cost of Mental Illness and Addiction

Much of the economic burden associated with mental illness is not the cost of health care, but the loss of income due to unemployment, expenses for social supports, and myriad other costs associated with chronic disability that start early (rather than later) in life.[40] The WHO reports that mental illnesses are the leading causes of disability-adjusted life years worldwide, accounting for approximately 37% of healthy years lost from all noncommunicable disease (NCD).[18] A newer WHO report estimated the global cost of mental illnesses at nearly $2.5 trillion in 2010, with a projected increase to over $6 trillion by 2030.[18] For perspective, the gross domestic product for low-income countries is less than $1 trillion.[41]

Costs attributed to mental illness are greater than for cardiovascular disease, chronic respiratory disease, cancer, or diabetes. Globally, mental illness will account for more than 50% of the projected total economic burden from NCDs over the next two decades, as well as for 35% of global lost output.[41] Given that people with mental illness are at greater risk for other NCDs, the true costs of mental illness may be even higher.[40] This may be especially so as alcohol, nicotine, drug, and other addictions often accompany mental illness and add to the economic burden because of the additional costs of rehabilitation and of possible incarceration.

The disparity between the need for treatment for mental illness and its availability and accessibility is wide. Globally, annual spending in U.S. dollars on mental health prevention and treatment services is $2 per person.[42] Thus, among LMIC, between 76% and 85% of people with severe mental disorders receive no treatment; among HIC, treatment prevalence is between 35% and 50%.[42] Moreover, the social and economic impact of mental illness can be devastating, with marginalization, homelessness, human rights violations, unemployment, poverty, and incarceration being highly prevalent associated conditions. In 2011, the WHO recently issued a call for action and outlined a series of strategies for addressing this global burden with health and social sectors among member states.[42] The strategies are summarized in **BOX 12-1**.

BOX 12-1 WHO Strategies for Improving Outcomes Among Those with Mental Illness

Improve the provision of good-quality treatment and care for mental health conditions by:

- Including mental health in broader health policies
- Expanding evidence-based mental health interventions in general health services and including them in packages of care on the basis of cost-effectiveness, affordability, and feasibility

Improve access for people with or at risk for mental illness to social welfare services and opportunities for education and employment by:

- Actively supporting children and adolescents to receive an education
- Promoting preschool education for vulnerable children
- Including people with mental illness in employment and income-generating programs, introducing supported employment programs, and providing social protection grants
- Creating strong links between mental health services, housing, and other social services

Introduce human rights protection for people with mental illness by:

- Developing policies and laws that protect and promote human rights and establishing independent monitoring mechanisms
- Supporting the development of a strong civil society and promoting the full inclusion and participation of people with mental disabilities in public affairs, including policy-making

Data from World Health Organization. Global burden of mental disorders and the need for a comprehensive, coordinated response from health and social sectors at the country level. World Health Organization; 2012. Available at http://apps.who.int/iris/bitstream/10665/78898/1/A65_10-en.pdf. Accessed November 6, 2017.

Key Terms

Bipolar

Cortisol

Diagnostic and Statistical Manual of Mental Disorders (DSM)

Dopamine

Endorphins

Epigenome

Epinephrine

Etiology

Methylation

Noradrenergic function

Norepinephrine

Unipolar depressive disorder

Discussion Questions

1. Describe the possible link between childhood sexual abuse and alcohol addiction in adulthood. What are some mediating factors and conditions in this pathway?

2. As a public health practitioner, what advice would you give to a couple hoping to start a family when one of the couple has schizophrenia among four primary relatives (grandfather, father, and two paternal uncles) and the other has a family history of bipolar depression and substance addiction in the mother, brother, and maternal uncle?

3. Why are the various 12-step programs for alcohol, drug, sex, food, and gambling addictions so successful in helping people "recover" from their addictions?

4. Discuss the evolution of treatment programs for mental illness over the last 100 years.

5. Discuss the adequacy of mental health services in the United States and provide examples to support your viewpoint.

References

1. World Health Organization. *Mental Health: Strengthening Our Response.* Available at http://www.who.int/mediacentre/factsheets/fs220/en/. Updated April 2016. Accessed November 5, 2017.

2. U.S. Department of Health and Human Services. *Mental Health: A Report of the Surgeon General.* Rockville, MD: U.S. Department of Health and Human Services; Substance Abuse and Mental Health Services Administration, Center for Mental Health Services, National Institutes of Health, National Institute of Mental Health; 1999.

3. Steel Z, Marnane C, Iranpour C, et al. The global prevalence of common mental disorders: a systematic review and meta-analysis 1980–2013. *Int J Epidemiol.* 2014;43(2):476-493. doi:10.1093/ije/dyu038.

4. American Psychiatric Association (APA). *Diagnostic and Statistical Manual of Mental Disorders.* 5th ed. Available at https://www.psychiatry.org/psychiatrists/practice/dsm. Accessed November 5, 2017.

5. Maser JD, Akiskal HS. Spectrum concepts in major mental disorders. *Psychiatr Clin North Am.* 2002;25(4):11-13.

6. Whitley R. Global mental health: concepts, conflicts and controversies: *Epidemiol Psychiatr Sci.* 2015;24:285–291.

7. Kessler RC, Berglund P, Demler O, Jin R, Merikangas KR, Walters EE. Lifetime prevalence and age-of-onset distributions of DSM-IV disorders in the National Comorbidity Survey Replication. *Arch Gen Psychiatry.* 2005;62:593-602.

8. Blazer DG, Kessler RC, McGonagle KA, Swartz MS. The prevalence and distribution of major depression in a national community sample: The National Comorbidity Survey. *Am J Psychiatry.* 1994;151:979-986.

9. Bebbington PE, Dunn G, Jenkins R, et al. The influence of age and sex on the prevalence of depressive conditions: report from the National Survey of Psychiatric Morbidity. *Psychol Med.* 1998;28:9-19.

10. Patten SB, Williams JV, Lavorato DH, Wang JL, Bulloch AG, Sajobi T. The association between major depression prevalence and sex becomes weaker with age. *Soc Psychiatry Psychiatr Epidemiol.* 2016;51(2):203-210.

11. Kessler RC, Angermeyer M, Anthony JC, et al. Lifetime prevalence and age-of-onset distributions of mental disorders in the World Health Organization's World Mental Health Survey Initiative. *World Psychiatry.* 2007;6:168-176.

12. Helzer, JE, Robins LN, McEvoy L. Post-traumatic stress disorder in the general population. *N Engl J Med.* 1987;317:1630-1634.

13. Kessler RC, Chiu WT, Demler O, Merikangas KR, Walters EE. Prevalence, severity, and comorbidity of 12-month DSM-IV disorders in the National Comorbidity Survey Replication. *Arch Gen Psychiatry.* 2005;62:617-627.

14. Lee DJ, Warner CH, Hoge CW. Advances and controversies in military posttraumatic stress disorder screening. *Curr Psychiatry Rep.* 2014;16(9):467. doi: 10.1007/s11920-014-0467-7.

15. Terhakopian A, Sinaii N, Engel CC, Schnurr PP, Hoge CW. Estimating population prevalence of posttraumatic stress disorder: an example using the PTSD checklist. *J Trauma Stress.* 2008;21:290-300.

16. Owen MJ, Sawa A, Mortensen PB. Schizophrenia. *Lancet.* 2016;388(10039):86–97.doi:10.1016/S0140-6736(15)01121-6.

17. McGrath J, Saha S, Chant D, Welham J. Schizophrenia: a concise overview of incidence, prevalence, and mortality. *Epidemiol Rev.* 2008;30:67-76.

18. World Health Organization. Global status report on non-communicable diseases 2010. Geneva: WHO. Available at http://www.who.int/nmh/publications/ncd_report2010/en/. Accessed November 5, 2017.

19. McNally R. *What Is Mental Illness?* Cambridge, MA: Harvard University Press; 2011.

20. Chesney E, Goodwin GM, Fazel S. Risks of all-cause and suicide mortality in mental disorders: a meta-review. *World Psychiatry.* 2014;13(2):153-160. doi:10.1002/wps.20128.

21. Bertolote JM, Fleischmann A. Suicide and psychiatric diagnosis: a worldwide perspective. *World Psychiatry.* 2002;1(3):181-185.

22. Kendler KS, Gatz M, Gardner CO, Pedersen NL. A Swedish national twin study of lifetime major depression. *Am J Psychiatry.* 2006;163:109-114.

23. Sullivan PF, Neale MC, Kendler KS. Genetic epidemiology of major depression: review and meta-analysis. *Am J Psychiatry.* 2000;157:1552-1562.

24. Klengel T, Pape J, Binder EB, Mehta D. The role of DNA methylation in stress-related psychiatric disorders. *Neuropharmacology.* 2014;80:115-132.

25. López-León S, Janssens A, González-Zuloeta Ladd A, et al. Meta-analyses of genetic studies on major depressive disorder. *Mol Psychiatry.* 2008;13:772-785.

26. Wray NR, Pergadia ML, Blackwood DHR, et al. Genome-wide association study of major depressive disorder: new results, meta-analysis, and lessons learned. *Mol Psychiatry.* 2012;17:36-48.

27. Ripke S, Wray NR, Lewis CM, et al.; Major Depressive Disorder Working Group of the Psychiatric GWAS Consortium. A mega-analysis of genome-wide association studies for major depressive disorder. *Mol Psychiatry.* 2013;18:497-511.

28. Ripke S, Neale BM, Corvin A, et al. Biological insights from 108 schizophrenia-associated genetic loci. *Nature.* 2014;51:421-427.

29. Januar V, Saffery R, Ryan J. Epigenetics and depressive disorders: a review of current progress and future directions. *Int J Epidemiol.* 2015;1364-1387. doi: 10.1093/ije/dyu273.

30. Levinson DF. The genetics of depression: a review. *Biol Psychiatry.* 2006;60:84-92.

31. Cross-Disorder Group for Psychiatry Genomics Consortium. Identification of risk loci with shared effects on five major psychiatric disorders: a genome-wide analysis. *Lancet.* 2013;381:1371-1379.

32. Cooper JR, Bloom FE, Roth RH. *The Biochemical Basis of Neuropharmacology.* New York, NY: Oxford University Press; 1991.

33. Van Winkle E. The toxic mind: biology of mental illness and violence. *Med Hypotheses.* 2000;55:356-368.

34. Tilden JH. *Toxemia: The Basic Cause of Disease.* Bridgeport, CT: Natural Hygiene Press; 1974.

35. Shelton HM. *Human Life: Its Philosophy and Laws: An Exposition of the Principles and Practices of Orthopathy.* Mokelumne Hill, CA: Health Research; 1979.

36. Weir K. The roots of mental illness: How much of mental illness can the biology of the brain explain? *Monitor on Psychol.* 2012;43(6). http://www.apa.org/monitor/2012/06/roots.aspx

37. Dalton VS, Kolshus E, McLoughlin DM. Epigenetics and depression: return of the repressed. *J Affect Disord.* 2014;155:1-12.

38. Weaver ICG, Cervoni N, Champagne FA, et al. Epigenetic programming by maternal behavior. *Nat Neurosci.* 2004;7:847–854.

39. McGowan PO, Sasaki A, D'Alessio AC, et al. Epigenetic regulation of the glucocorticoid receptor in human brain associates with childhood abuse. *Nat Neurosci.* 2009;12:342-348.

40. Insel T. Director's Blog: The global cost of mental illness. The National Institute of Mental Health. Available at https://www.nimh.nih.gov/about/directors/thomas-insel/blog/2011/the-global-cost-of-mental-illness.shtml. Accessed November 5, 2017.

41. Bloom DE, Cafiero ET, Jané-Llopis E, et al. *The Global Economic Burden of Non-Communicable Diseases.* Geneva, Switzerland: World Economic Forum; 2011.

42. World Health Organization. Global burden of mental disorders and the need for a comprehensive, coordinated response from health and social sectors at the country level. World Health Organization; 2012. Available at http://apps.who.int/iris/bitstream/10665/78898/1/A65_10-en.pdf. Accessed November 6, 2017.

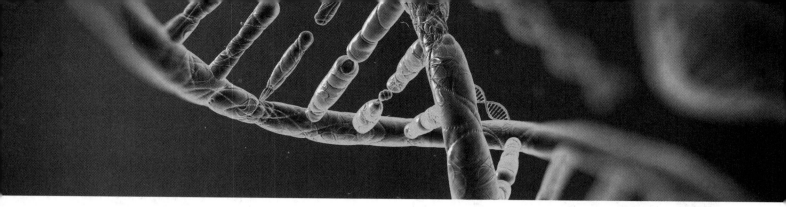

© vitstudio/Shutterstock

CHAPTER 13

Injury Etiology, Epidemiology, and Control

Loretta DiPietro and Mary Pat McKay

LEARNING OBJECTIVES

By the end of this chapter, the student will be able to:

- Identify uncontrolled energy as the agent in injury occurrence
- List and compare the major types of injuries
- Describe injury patterns among demographic subgroups in the United States and globally
- Explain the pathophysiology of different injury types
- Identify host and environmental factors that increase the risk of injury
- Discuss the factors affecting the public's understanding and acceptance of various risks
- Evaluate current strategies and policies for injury prevention and control

CHAPTER OUTLINE

▶ Introduction

Globally, injuries are the leading killer of young people between the ages of 4 and 34 years (National Center for Health Statistics, 2003).[1] In the United States, injuries are also the leading cause of death among persons aged 1–44 and the primary cause of lost years of productive life.[2] Approximately 68% of the 160,000 injury fatalities per year are unintentional, and of these, about 42,000 fatalities are from motor vehicle crashes. Injuries account for about one-third of all emergency department visits annually in the United States (approximately 35 million/year). The total cost of injuries, including acute and rehabilitative medical care, lost wages, and lost productivity approaches $406 billion/year—about 4% of the U.S. gross national

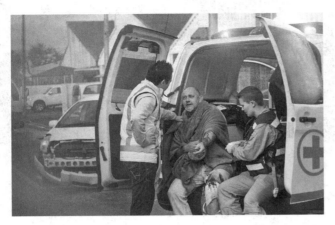
© Caiaimage/Trevor Adeline/Getty

product.[3] The **disability-adjusted life year (DALY)** is a measure of overall disease burden, expressed as the number of years lost due to ill health, injury, disability or early death. It was developed in the 1990s as a way of comparing the overall health and life expectancy of different countries. This metric combines morbidity and mortality to define the burden of injury beyond that of premature death to include equivalent years of healthy life lost by virtue of being sick or injured. The impact of both intentional and nonintentional injuries led the Centers for Disease Control and Prevention (CDC) to create a series of Healthy People 2020 objectives to reduce motor-vehicle crash-related deaths, increase the use of seat belts, and reduce firearm injuries, among others (see **TABLE 13-1**).

Injuries are generally defined as "intentional" or "unintentional." Examples of **intentional injuries** are assault, domestic violence, war, attempted homicide, or self-harm, whereas with **unintentional injuries** the event is not pre-calculated or planned (e.g., a slip on ice, a fall down stairs). It is important to consider that the majority of injuries are not "accidents." Indeed, most injuries are predictable and preventable. Similar to types of illness, injuries tend to cluster around specific risk factors and therefore are amenable to routine public health interventions. For instance, conflict resolution, limiting access to firearms, and treatment for substance addiction/mental illness have proven to be effective preventive measures for intentional injury. Similarly, seat belts/air bags, lowering the height of playground equipment, and protective helmets have been key to lowering the severity or fatality from unintentional crashes and falls.

▶ Mechanisms of Injury

The underlying agent in all types of injury is *uncontrolled energy* that is greater than what the tissues can absorb. There are several types of energy that cause injuries: (1) mechanical, such as falls, crashes, or gunshot; (2) chemical, e.g., poisoning; (3) thermal, e.g., burns from fire or steam, or frostbite; and (4) electrical, e.g., lightning strikes, electrocution. There are also injuries that are caused by the absence of oxygen (drowning, suffocation). The majority of

TABLE 13-1	Selected Year 2020 Objectives for Injury and Violence Prevention (IVP)
IVP 2.2	Reduce hospitalizations for nonfatal traumatic brain injuries to 77.0 hospitalizations per 100,000 population from a baseline of 85.6 hospitalizations per 100,000 population in 2007 (10% reduction goal).
IVP 11	Reduce unintentional injury death to 36.4 deaths per 100,000 population from a baseline of 40.4 deaths per 100,000 population in 2007 (10% improvement goal).
IVP 13.1	Reduce motor vehicle crash-related deaths to 12.4 deaths per 100,000 population from a baseline of 13.8 motor vehicle traffic-related deaths per 100,000 population.
IVP 15	Increase use of safety belts among drivers and right-front seat passengers to 92% from a baseline of 84% in 2009.
IVP 28	Reduce the number of residential fire deaths to 0.86 deaths per 100,000 population from a baseline of 0.92 deaths per 100,000 population in 2007.
IVP 31	Reduce nonfatal firearm-related injuries to 18.6 injuries per 100,000 population from a baseline of 20.7 injuries per 100,000 in 2007.
IVP 36	Reduce bullying among adolescents to 17.9% among students in grades 9–12 from a baseline of 19.9% in 2009.
IVP 41	Reduce nonfatal intentional self-harm injuries to 112.4 injuries per 100,000 population from a baseline of 124.9% in 2009.

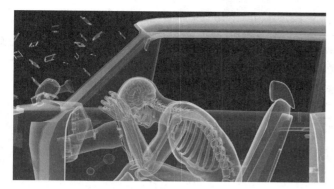
© angelhell/iStock/Getty Images Plus

injuries worldwide are the result of uncontrolled mechanical or **kinetic energy**.

The different types of tissue in the body have varying abilities to absorb and dissipate energy without injury, until a critical threshold is reached. Pain initially occurs just as the critical threshold is reached and provides the person the opportunity to act in order to limit resulting damage. Different kinds of tissue have diverse types of pain and pressure sensors, and therefore will respond uniquely to specific types of energy. For example, the skin has sensors that relay pain in response to significant pressure, stretch, or temperature. The role of protective equipment such as a seat belt, a gym mat, or a helmet is to distribute mechanical energy across a greater surface area in order to prevent the critical threshold from being reached.

▶ Epidemiology of Injury

As stated previously, most injuries are predictable and preventable and cluster around myriad risk factors. Similar to most illness, we can describe injury epidemiology in terms of agent, host, and environment (**FIGURE 13-1**). We have already discussed the agent of injury as uncontrolled energy of different types. Additionally, there are several host factors that may increase one's susceptibility of sustaining an injury and environmental factors that increase the contact between the agent and the host.

Host Factors

Age itself is a strong predictor of both intentional and unintentional injuries. This is especially so for injuries resulting from falls, due to either developmental issues in very young children or to functional and mobility limitations in older adults. Among infants younger than age 1, the most severe injuries from falls are the result of an adult leaving the infant unattended on a high surface. Newly walking toddlers are most at risk for serious falls down stairways. Yet, there is more public emphasis on infant falls than on fall-related safety in older people, even though injuries from these falls constitute a significant healthcare burden.[2] The most common cause of death among infants and small children is suffocation or drowning.[3] The most common cause of unintentional injury and death from injury among adults 65 and older is falling.[4]

Among school-age children (5–12 years), playground injuries were of significant concern 20–30 years ago; however, regulations limiting the height of playground equipment to under 5 feet, as well as changes in playground surfaces (away from asphalt toward rubber) have markedly reduced the severity of

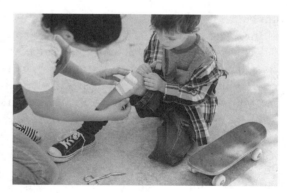
© Newman Studio/iStock/Getty Images Plus

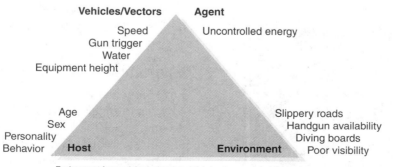

Vehicles/Vectors **Agent**
Speed Uncontrolled energy
Gun trigger
Water
Equipment height

Age Slippery roads
Sex Handgun availability
Personality Diving boards
Behavior **Host** **Environment** Poor visibility

Environment factors (physical and social) bring the agent and the host in contact with each other. Vehicles and Vectors carry or distribute the agent to the host.

FIGURE 13-1 Model of Disease Transmission Applied to Injury Risk

injuries from falls in this age group. In contrast, athletic injuries are now becoming a concern at younger ages, as competition in youth sports begins at earlier ages—when some children may not be adequately developed with regard to strength and agility compared with their peers. This is especially concerning with head injuries that result in concussions. At the same time, sport specialization at young ages has led to a greater reporting of overuse and knee injuries among adolescents.

Among Americans aged 5–24 years, the greatest risk for severe or fatal injury continues to be from motor vehicle crashes, and this is especially so with new (15–24 years) drivers (CDC, 2013).[3] Older age also increases the risk of injury and death from motor vehicles, due to sensory impairments in vision and hearing, along with declining cognitive function and reaction time. Unintentional poisoning is the leading cause of injury death in persons aged 25–64, with unintentional falls attributing the greatest injury-related fatalities in people over age 65 years. Only in one population subgroup, African-American men aged 15–44 years, does intentional injury (homicide) cause more fatalities than all types of unintentional injuries, including motor vehicle crashes.[3]

Sex (or gender) also is a strong determinant of injury occurrence. From an early age, boys are more likely to die from injuries than are girls. This disparity becomes almost exponential in adolescence and continues throughout the life span. The rate of nonfatal injuries is also higher in boys and young men compared with women; however, this trend reverses in older age, when the rate becomes higher in women ≥ 65 years compared with older men. At older ages, men die from injuries more frequently than women, but women sustain more injuries. The reasons for these sex differences in injury occurrence are not clear. Greater risk-taking behavior in boys and young men compared with their female counterparts has been implicated as a factor in their excess risk of injury; however, this has yet to be demonstrated conclusively.

Personality and behavior are also related to injury risk, as those who engage in riskier behaviors are more likely to become injured (regardless of gender). Examples of risk-taking behaviors include driving without a seat belt, cycling without a helmet, drinking and driving, and ignoring posted warning signs. Sensation- or thrill-seeking behavior takes risk taking to a higher level. Indeed, there are people who need constant thrill to feel "normal." Unfortunately, and similar to other addictions, one's tolerance for a given level of excitement will increase with time, thus requiring an even greater degree of risk-taking to achieve the same thrill level. Extreme sport enthusiasts and war correspondents who choose to continually put themselves at greater and greater risk are examples of such thrill-seekers.

No discussion about behavioral risk factors for injury would be complete without mentioning how alcohol ingestion significantly increases the risk of injury as well as the severity of a given injury. Alcohol is a **neurotoxin** and neurodepressant that causes measurable impairments in both physical and cognitive function. The initial effect of alcohol on the brain is a mild euphoria that is quickly followed by disinhibition. If the person continues drinking, the result is obvious discoordination and then unconsciousness. The effects of alcohol include an increased willingness to take risks (disinhibition) and a decreased ability to respond in a hazardous situation (discoordination, cognitive impairment). A blood alcohol concentration (BAC) as low as 0.05% can result in measurable functional impairments. Larger people will have a greater tolerance before impairments become noticeable due to a higher blood volume. The maximum legal cut-point for driving is a BAC of 0.08% (see **BOX 13-1**).

Alcohol use is implicated in about half of all drowning deaths and about 40% of motor vehicle fatalities (although this is down from 70% in 1966). Over 60% of trauma survivors who make it to the hospital are under the influence of alcohol. Excessive alcohol use is also strongly associated with intentional injuries, either as a perpetrator or as a victim.

Environmental Factors

Environmental factors are those that increase contact between the agent (uncontrolled energy) and the host. A winding, icy road and darkness will increase the risk of a motor vehicle crash for an inexperienced young driver; a throw rug placed at the top of stairs will increase the risk of a serious fall for an older person; an opened bottle of bleach will increase the risk of poisoning for a toddler; and the availability of a loaded

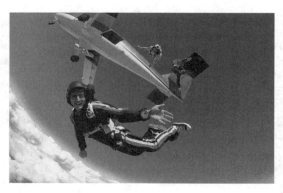

© Digital Vision/Thinkstock/Getty

BOX 13-1 Reducing Alcohol-Impaired Driving: Ignition Interlocks

Ignition interlocks are devices that can be installed in cars to prevent a driver who has a BAC above a specified level (usually 0.02–0.04%) from operating the car. The Community Preventive Services Task Force recommends the use of ignition interlocks for people convicted of driving under the influence (DUI) of alcohol based on strong evidence of their effectiveness in reducing re-arrest during the time that the interlocks are installed. Unfortunately, the public health impact of these devices is limited because only a small proportion of offenders actually install them. Installation of ignition interlocks could be mandated or offered as an alternative to suspending a driver's license (the amount of time they are installed typically matches the period for which the license would have been suspended). Public acceptance and sustained use of interlock devices could have a substantial impact on alcohol-related motor vehicle crashes.

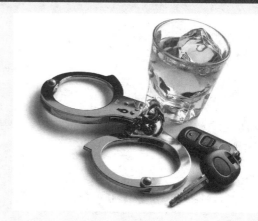

© DNY59/E+/Getty

The Task Force recommendation was based on results from two systematic reviews that considered a total of 15 studies:

- During the time that interlocks were in place, the proportion of re-arrests decreased by a median of 67% compared with comparison groups (13 studies).
- When interlocks were removed, re-arrests returned to a level similar to that of persons convicted of DUI who had not used such devices (11 studies).
- Drivers using interlocks had fewer alcohol-related motor vehicle crashes compared with those whose licenses had been suspended for a DUI (1 study).
- Overall, the prevalence of motor vehicle crashes among those with interlock devices was similar to that among the general driving population. On the other hand, those drivers using ignition interlocks had substantially more crashes than did those with suspended licenses—presumably because those with interlocks drove more than those with suspended licenses (2 studies).

Data from Elder RW, Voas R, Beirness D, et al.; Task Force on Community Preventive Services. Effectiveness of ignition interlocks for preventing alcohol-impaired driving and alcohol-related crashes: a community guide systematic review. *Am J Prev Med.* 2011;40(3):362-376.

handgun increases the risk of serious injury or death from a gunshot wound.

Perhaps the most successful interventions for injury prevention and control have been from modifications to the environmental factors. Jersey barriers alongside dangerous roads; childproof locks on bottles, cupboards, and toilet seats; barriers at the top and bottom of stairs and in electrical outlets; stop signs at dangerous intersections; and smoke detectors are all examples of simple strategies that have a large impact on reducing injury occurrence and severity. Rules, regulations, policies, and laws also have an impact on altering environmental conditions that increase injury risk; however, to be effective, these rules have to be adhered to by the public. Motorcycle helmets laws are extremely effective in reducing traumatic brain injuries from crashes; however, not all states in the United States have adopted these laws. In fact, only 19 states and the District of Columbia have a universal helmet law.[5] Similarly, gun laws that limit access to firearms are among the most contentious issues faced by public health and political officials (see **BOX 13-2**).

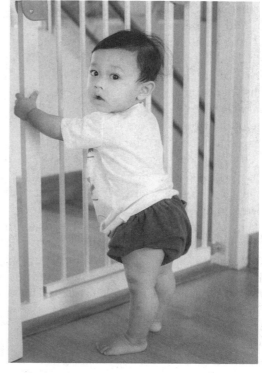

© Photo by MHIN/Shutterstock

▶ Pathophysiology of Injury

The type of tissue involved in a given injury event will determine the severity of the injury itself. Each tissue type in the body has different **viscoelastic properties** that affect its threshold for accommodating energy. The cornea of the eye suffers thermal injury more quickly than intact skin. Skin is relatively resistant to compression but will tear when stretched. The brain responds particularly poorly to compression because it has very low elasticity. Bone is very resistant to compression along its longitudinal (long) axis but is far less resistant to compression in cross section. Ligaments are capable of compression; however, excess stretching will tear them. In addition to properties inherent in the type of tissue, several host factors may alter the quality of certain tissue, making them more susceptible to injury. Age certainly is one such factor that affects the plasticity and resiliency of skin, bones, and blood vessels. Chronic conditions such as diabetes, osteoporosis, and cardiovascular disease also affect injury occurrence and severity because they negatively affect tissue integrity.

All types of injury (cuts, breaks, tears, and burns) heal in a set series of phases. First, there is bleeding at the site of the wound. In the case of open wounds due to cuts or lacerations, as the blood clots, the bleeding stops. Of course, open wounds caused by a sharp object like a knife or glass have less surrounding tissue damage than open wounds caused by blunt trauma (think line-drive to the face in baseball) or by rotating or "splash effect" trauma from a bullet. The greater the tissue damage, the more bleeding, thus possibly requiring stitches to repair the damaged tissue. Inflammation and swelling at the wound site happens next, and although this process is often quite painful, it is critical to healing.

During this initial phase of healing, the wound is quite fragile and susceptible to re-injury and to infection. After several days, **fibroblasts** organize in the wound and begin forming collagen, which connects the tissue and strengthens the site. Much of the strength of the area is repaired in the first two weeks, and the scab falls off at the end of that time. The wound continues to heal for several more months as the residual scar matures and the area is remodeled. As collagen is replaced, the thickness, stiffness, and redness of the scar diminishes. This final phase of healing is prolonged, and even minor wounds may take several years to reach their final appearance.

The healing of bone fractures occurs in a similar manner. There is an initial period of swelling, followed by slow healing, as **osteoblasts** produce collagen and other proteins and coat them with an adhesive so that calcium can stick to the collagen.

Interestingly, injuries that are most likely to be life-threatening, such as lacerations to vital organs, are less likely to be associated with permanent disability. Indeed, if someone survives a knife stab to the liver, future liver function will more than likely be normal. The same is not true, however, for a serious **traumatic brain injury (TBI)**. These injuries are life-threatening in the acute phase and often require an extensive period of recovery, with no expectation of return to pre-injury function. In the United States, an estimated 3.8 million sport-related TBIs occur annually, most of which are concussions.[6] Almost 15% of all high school sports-related injuries are concussions.[6] Significant spinal cord injuries almost always result in some permanent disability, with the extent of that disability dependent on where on the spinal cord the injury occurred. Unfortunately, there are few medical interventions that can dramatically change the long-term consequences of these serious injuries, thereby underscoring the need for preventing them in the first place.

The long-term psychologic sequelae of a serious injury are also important to discuss. **Post-traumatic stress disorder (PTSD)** is caused by an exaggerated and sustained fight-or-flight response following a traumatic event. PTSD relating to both intentional and unintentional injuries has created a substantial public health burden, as PTSD can affect the injured person and their families for years. Survivors of genocide, war, attempted homicide, and rape are especially affected (especially when significant disfigurement results). Why some people are more susceptible to PTSD than others who have experienced the same injury or level of trauma is not clear. PTSD has been linked to severe depression and anxiety, to alcohol and other substance abuse, and to family violence, and therefore, is in itself a risk factor for future intentional and/or self-inflicted injuries years after the initial event. Even if one does not meet the clinical criteria for PTSD, people may make certain alterations to their lifestyles in order to avoid further psychologic trauma (e.g., not driving again; avoiding stairwells).

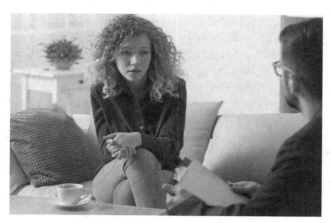

▶ Perception of Risk

The actual and the perceived risk of injury from a given exposure often are very different. Chauncey Starr first approached the question, "How safe is safe enough?" by a "revealed preference" approach.[7] This approach assumes that by trial and error, society arrives at some optimal balance between the risks and benefits associated with a given activity in order to arrive at patterns of acceptable risk-benefit trade-offs (i.e., the risk-mix). Starr suggested that: (1) acceptability of the risk associated with a given activity is approximately proportional to the third power of the benefits of that activity; and (2) given equal benefits, the public will accept risks from voluntary activities (such as skateboarding without a helmet) that are about 1,000 times greater than the actual risks from involuntary hazards (food additives).

Perceived risk is both quantifiable and predictable, and numerous psychometric studies have identified similarities and differences among different groups with regard to risk perceptions and attitudes. Indeed, the term "risk" has various meanings among different groups of people, and the psychologist Paul Slovic has identified several factors that define how the public perceives a given hazard. These perceptions are described here and summarized in **TABLE 13-2**.[8]

- *Dread* – When the consequence of an event is perceived to be horrific (a plane crash), the assessment of risk will be higher than it actually is.
- *Choice* – Having a choice about participating in a given activity often results in a perception of risk that is lower than it actually is (such as cigarette smoking). Thus, people will accept a higher level of risk if they feel that it is their choice to do so.
- *Control* – Most people need to have a sense of control over a situation and often perceive that they have more control than they actually do (such as control of a car on an icy surface or having a handgun in the house). This *control illusion* leads us to perceive risks as being less than they actually are.
- *Youth* – Risks that affect children often seem greater than those that affect adults. The potential consequences with regard to years of disability or years of productive life lost cause people to aim for a zero-risk environment for their children, while accepting the same level of risk (or even higher) for themselves.
- *Familiarity* – Knowledge and expertise with a certain activity or environment may cause us to perceive the associated risks as lower than what they actually are. For example, walking alone at night through urban streets seems less risky when it is one's own neighborhood, compared with when it is an unknown neighborhood.

TABLE 13-2 Factors Affecting Risk Perception	
Factor	**Perception**
How *serious* are the effects?	■ How serious is the potential harm in terms of monetary loss, loss of time, and stress? ■ Are the effects potentially catastrophic? Can one error lead to death, permanent disability, or financial ruin? ■ Are the effects reversible?
How *long-term* are the effects?	■ How immediate are the potential effects? ■ Are the effects reversible?
How *feared* are the effects?	■ Are the effects unusual or outside of normal experience? ■ Do views differ among demographic subgroups for demographic or other reasons?
How much *choice* and *control* do I have?	■ Who decides about whether or not to assume the risk? ■ Who is in charge and how trustworthy are they?

Modified from Slovic P. Perception of risk. *Science*. 1987;236:280-285.

- *Publicity* – If a risk has a lot of public attention (such as terrorist events), the risk is likely to be assessed as being more significant than it actually is.
- *Proximity* – One is more likely to assess the risk of a given situation to be greater if it is to be assumed by oneself or by his or her family, compared with if that risk is to be assumed by unknown people living in another city or in another country.
- *Risk-benefit trade-off* – If there are opportunities as well as risks mixed up together and a choice could lead to benefits, the risk may be considered lower than it actually is.
- *Trust* – Where the risk involved the actions of others, our perception of the risk involved will be significantly affected by the extent to which we trust the other party (e.g., airline pilots, surgeons, police officers).
- *Immediate vs. delayed consequences* – Behaviors such as smoking, drinking alcohol, and excessive sun exposure may be perceived as less risky than they actually are because the damage is not assumed for many years.
- *Reversibility* – Risks associated with outcomes that can be reversed or easily fixed (a broken bone from playing soccer) are perceived to be lower than those associated with irreversible outcomes (permanent brain trauma as a result of repeated concussions from playing football).

▶ Injury Control

Injury control is the broad term applied to both the prevention and treatment of injuries. Injury control comprises three levels of public health intervention: primary prevention (preventing the event from happening in the first place); secondary prevention (preventing the complications from an injury); and tertiary prevention (rehabilitation from injury and the prevention of re-injury). In 1968, William Haddon created a framework to help public health practitioners to organize the opportunities for intervention.[9] **Haddon's Matrix** divides time into pre-, during-, and post-event phases and also considers human, **vector/vehicle**, and environmental factors within each phase. Although **TABLE 13-3** illustrates the components of the matrix applied to motor vehicle injury control, this matrix can be applied to other types of injuries as well.

Within each cell of Table 13-3, there is an opportunity for intervention. The types of intervention include *education* (public service messages about why seat belts save lives), *engineering* solutions (car design, air bags, guardrails), *economic* incentives (fines for speeding or failure to use seat belts), *enforcement* (jail time for driving while intoxicated), and *empowerment* (changing social norms). These are known as the "Five Es" of injury control; a combination of all five elements is the most effective at lowering risk. For example, education campaigns alone during the 1970s (costing millions of dollars) resulted in only 14% of the American public wearing their seat belts by 1984. When states began to pass seatbelt legislation, along with fines between $10 and $25 for not wearing one (economic and enforcement), belt use began to increase. States that have strengthened their seatbelt laws (i.e., bigger fines) have observed further increases in their use, such that compliance in the United States is now over 80%. Advancements in automobile and road design

TABLE 13-3 Haddon's Matrix for Motor Vehicle Crashes			
	Human	**Vector/Vehicle**	**Physical/Social Environment**
Pre-Event	Intoxication Safety belt use Speed Alertness/sleepiness Experience	Tire pressure Brake functioning I beams Crumple zones	Speed cameras Weather Social culture Willingness to allow others to drive drunk
During Event	Frailty Age Size	Speed of impact Air bags Size Stiffness of surfaces Stability control	Flammability Guardrails Stiffness of fixed objects Barriers Embankments
Post-Event	Body mass index Age Comorbid conditions	Degree of crush Fuel system integrity	EMS response Trauma center availability Rehab programs

Data from Haddon W Jr. The changing approach to the epidemiology, prevention, and amelioration of trauma: the translation to approaches etiologically rather than descriptively based. *Am J Public Health Nation Health*. 1968;58:1431-1438.

over the past several decades (engineering) have also been highly effective at preventing crashes and reducing the severity of injury resulting from a crash.

Much of injury control has to do with changing human behavior; however, this is often difficult to accomplish as cultural habits are difficult to change and many people do not appreciate other people making decisions on their behalf. Public health intervention strategies can be defined as "active" or "passive." **Active strategies for injury control** require individuals to make a decision about their behavior—that is, they decide to put on a motorcycle helmet because they appreciate the protective qualities of the helmet or because they simply want to follow the law. Due to the recent research on sports-related TBIs, the CDC implemented a HEADS UP to Youth Sports public health campaign—an active public health strategy. The initiative is aimed at coaches, parents, and youth athletes to recognize, seek treatment for, and prevent concussions.[10] **Passive strategies for injury control** do not require individuals to make a decision on their own behalf because the protective mechanism is already in place. These strategies tend be more effective because they bypass human choice. The greatest advancements in motor vehicle safety have been due to passive strategies, such as air bags, passive restraints, anti-lock brakes, car design, road design, and protective barriers. Other passive strategies that have lowered injury occurrence and severity include better protective gear for contact sports like football and ice hockey, lowering the height of playground equipment, removing diving boards from swimming pools, and providing absorbent landing surfaces for playgrounds and gym floors.

Injuries are among the most common health problems for people all over the world. All injuries (intentional and unintentional) are the result of uncontrolled energy being applied to the tissues of the body above their tolerance thresholds. There are specific risk factors for specific types of injuries, and the type of injury can be predicted if the type, amount, and location of force applied are understood. Injuries can be predicted, prevented, and controlled using the same public health concepts as for any other disease.

CASE REPORT

Combat-Related Injuries

Jane is a 42-year-old military surgical nurse who served three tours in Iraq and Afghanistan between 2003 and 2011. Throughout her service, Jane had attended to the numerous and horrific consequences of improvised explosive devices. During her last tour, Jane survived a suicide bomb blast that killed three of her fellow nurses as they were sitting at a marketplace. Jane suffered a TBI from the blast and also lost her right arm and the sight in her left eye. Since returning home to the United States, Jane has reoccurring nightmares with vivid recollections of the blast. Because of the nature and extent of her injuries, Jane could no longer work in surgery. She lost interest in her friends and in once-enjoyable activities. Jane began to avoid crowded spaces and began drinking daily. In the past year, thoughts of suicide began to overwhelm her.

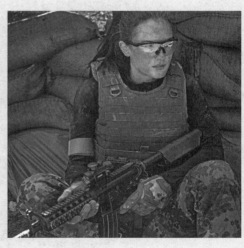
© Lorado/E+/Getty

1. What type of energy caused Jane's injuries?
2. Describe the pathophysiology of her different injuries with regard to the susceptibility of the various tissue types involved.
3. Based on Jane's behavioral symptoms, what psychiatric diagnosis would you give her?
4. What public health strategies could best address Jane's current physical, psychiatric, and social conditions?

Key Terms

Active strategies for injury control
Disability-adjusted life year (DALY)
Fibroblasts
Haddon's Matrix

Intentional injuries
Kinetic energy
Neurotoxin
Osteoblasts
Passive strategies for injury control

Post-traumatic stress disorder (PTSD)
Traumatic brain injury (TBI)
Unintentional injuries
Vector/Vehicle
Viscoelastic properties

Discussion Questions

1. The majority of the world's 1.7 million fatalities from motor vehicle crashes occur in developing countries, where public health efforts to control their impact must compete for scarce resources with HIV/AIDS, malaria, and other communicable diseases, as well as with food scarcity. Together, there are more fatalities from injuries (> 6 million total) than any of these competing issues. What would it take to get injuries onto the global public health radar and generate effective outreach programs?

2. All states require physicians, nurses, police officers, teachers, and others in authority to report any concern about child abuse and let the local social work system investigate the issue. Some legislators believe that there should be a similar requirement for reporting intimate partner violence. What are some of the potential consequences of such legislation?

3. Create a Haddon's Matrix for the issue of concussions in youth sports.

4. Given the prominence of chronic traumatic encephalopathy in the news, and its relation to violence, self-harm, and neurodegeneration, state your opinion about current "return-to-play" strategies in: (a) youth sports; (b) high school sports; (c) college sports; and (d) professional sports. Who should be in charge of enforcing these policies?

5. Create a passive strategy for the control of injuries due to handguns.

6. At the quarry outside of a local town are posted signs stating "NO SWIMMING"; yet in the last 3 years, there have been two deaths and three serious spinal cord injuries due to swimming and diving there. Why is this a public health concern? If you were the local health commissioner, how would you respond? Create a plan for injury control.

References

1. National Center for Health Statistics. *Ten leading causes of death by age group, United States, 2015* [chart]. Available at https://www.cdc.gov/injury/images/lc-charts/leading_causes_of_death_age_group_2015_1050w740h.gif. Accessed November 5, 2017.

2. Gelbard R, Inaba K, Okoye OT, et al. Falls in the elderly: a modern look at an old problem. *Am J Surg.* 2014;208(2):249-253.

3. Centers for Disease Control, National Center for Injury Prevention and Control. *WISQARS Ten leading causes of injury death by age group, United States 2013.* Available at https://www.cdc.gov/injury/images/lc-charts/leading_causes_of_injury_deaths_unintentional_injury_2015_1050w760h.gif. Accessed June 12, 2017.

4. Centers for Disease Control and Prevention. Press release: Falls are the leading cause of injury and death in older Americans. Thursday, September 22, 2016. Available at https://www.cdc.gov/media/releases/2016/p0922-older-adult-falls.html. Accessed November 5, 2017.

5. Insurance Institute for Highway Safety/Highway Loss Data Institute. Motorcycle Helmet Use. Available at http://www.iihs.org/iihs/topics/laws/helmetuse/mapmotorcyclehelmets. Posted June 2017. Updated November 2017. Accessed November 5, 2017.

6. Stein CJ, Meehan WP III. Concussion in youth sports. In: Micheli L, Stein C, O'Brien M, d'Hemecourt P, eds. *Spinal Injuries and Conditions in Young Athletes.* New York, NY: Springer; 2014: 47-54.

7. Starr C. Social benefit versus technological risk. *Science.* 1969;165:1232-1238.

8. Slovic P. Perception of risk. *Science.* 1987;236:280-285.

9. Haddon W Jr. The changing approach to the epidemiology, prevention, and amelioration of trauma: the translation to approaches etiologically rather than descriptively based. *Am J Public Health Nation Health.* 1968;58:1431-1438.

10. Centers for Disease Control and Prevention. HEADS UP to Youth Sports. Available at https://www.cdc.gov/headsup/youthsports/index.html. Updated February 1, 2017. Accessed June 12, 2017.

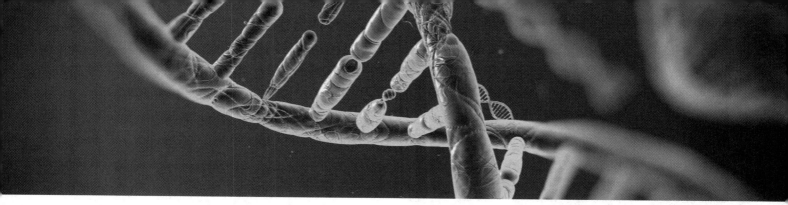

CHAPTER 14

The Natural History of Infectious Diseases

Victor K. Barbiero

LEARNING OBJECTIVES

By the end of this chapter, the student will be able to:

- Identify common infectious disease terms and definitions
- Describe the biologic interactions of organisms with each other and the environment
- Explore modes of disease transmission, the development of resistance, and breakpoint transmission
- Explain biologic equilibriums, the germ theory, and basic concepts of population biology, natural selection, and survival strategies, as they relate to the health of populations

CHAPTER OUTLINE

▶ Introduction

Over half of the world's population is plagued daily by an unforgiving battery of infectious diseases. These diseases limit physical and intellectual growth and impede economic progress for many of world's nations. In fact, infectious diseases affect over half of the world's population and account for about 36.5% of the disease burden worldwide, human immunodeficiency virus (HIV)/acquired immune deficiency syndrome (AIDS) kills about 1.1 million people annually, tuberculosis kills another

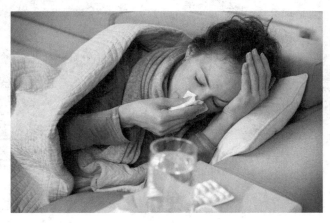

© Subbotina Anna/Shutterstock

1.5 million, respiratory disease kills about 1.4 million, diarrhea kills about 750,000, and malaria kills about 650,000. This chapter introduces the reader to the biologic processes that govern the survival and spread of pathogens. The reader will understand how complex interactions of the host–parasite (vector) relationship regulate disease transmission, how specific survival strategies enable pathogens to survive and develop resistance, and how understanding these processes can lead to more effective prevention and control interventions. Readers will gain a practical appreciation of the challenges and issues faced today in the control and elimination/eradication of diseases that have existed for millennia.

This chapter endeavors to put infectious diseases in their proper perspective. The nature of the host–parasite or vector–environment relationship is as natural and complex as life itself. If you consider infectious disease transmission, case management, prevention, and control holistically, you will gain a sound and useful appreciation of disease processes; and, more important, how the impacts of infectious diseases can be mitigated in the future.

▶ Natural History of Infectious Diseases

It is critically important for the student of infectious disease epidemiology to be familiar with Robert Koch's 1890 postulates (*The Henle-Koch Postulates*),[1] which are as follows:

- A germ causing a disease must be discoverable in all cases of the disease.
- The germ must grow in a pure culture.
- The germs in the culture must cause the disease in a susceptible host.
- The germs must be recoverable and transmit the disease to another susceptible host.

Koch first applied these postulates to his study of anthrax. After this, he moved on to human diseases like bacterial septicemia and tuberculosis. Koch's postulates are key to our understanding of infectious disease epidemiology. They enable us to define a pathogen in terms of initial infection, morbidity and mortality, means of replication, time of onset, and transmission from one host to another. These elements are the building blocks of infectious disease epidemiology and control. If we are able to understand how much mortality and morbidity a pathogen causes, how the pathogen replicates, how much time it takes to produce symptoms, how the pathogen is transmitted, and what is required for efficient transmission, we can better identify interventions to interrupt transmission and limit spread. For example, polio presents symptoms in only 0.5% (1/200) of those infected. Thus, Koch's postulates require the student of infectious disease epidemiology to consider the difference between a **case** and **infection** when considering the postulates, and more importantly, when monitoring surveillance efforts for control, elimination, and/or eradication.

Biologic Equilibriums

FIGURE 14-1 illustrates the concept of "biologic equilibrium." Just like water finds its own level, so too do organisms seek "equilibrium." This concept is vital to our understanding of the biology and natural history of infectious disease because it implies that organisms will usually adjust and adapt to their environment and strike a *viable* balance in the host–pathogen relationship. Evolutionarily speaking, this makes perfect sense and argues for the survival and spread of disease-causing organisms and their hosts,

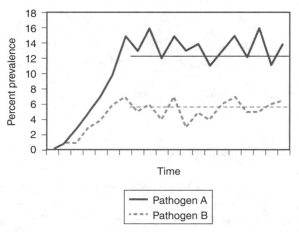

FIGURE 14-1 Biologic Equilibriums

Data from Barbiero VK. Adapted from Global Health and Development Course, GWU 2011 (Original Slide). 2015.

as well as all other organisms. Think about the common cold, or malaria, or HIV/AIDS, or even the influenza virus. These organisms adapt to their hosts not by killing 100% of those they infect, but by taking either a long time to kill their host and adapting to complex routes of transmission and/or attenuating (lowering their virulence) to better survive within their host.

The key to understanding biologic equilibriums is to predict at what point the pathogen will "level off" in the system. This is a difficult thing to do and varies with pathogens, hosts, the environment, seasons, and other elements such as behavior and culture. Even though pandemics occur, 100% of a host population is not infected or exposed; witness the Black Death (the plague caused by the bacterium *Yersinia pestis*) in the 14th century, the great swine flu pandemic of 1918 (in which the **case fatality rate** was approximately 3%), and even the present HIV/AIDS pandemic. Biologic balance is the basis for disease transmission and a key determinant of public health. It makes no teleologic sense for a pathogen to infect and kill 100% of its hosts because it will be unable to reproduce. Hosts (in this case humans) and pathogens strive for a viable balance anchored in **attenuation** and immunity—an equilibrium where the pathogen is "tolerated" within the biologic system and causes a minimal amount of morbidity and mortality. Witness the common cold; once this balance is achieved, both pathogens and hosts can survive and reproduce, and the disease is no longer considered a major public health problem. However, when an existing equilibrium is disturbed, the result can be severe outbreaks and even pandemics such as the 2014–2015 Ebola outbreak.

Natural Selection and Adaptation

Darwin's tenets of natural selection and adaption are anchored in an organism's ability to change, and with that change, survive. Approximately 60–80% of human pathogens arise from animal systems.[2] A relatively new human virus like Ebola, adapted to an animal life cycle, kills humans quickly, but transmits slowly. Although outbreaks will continue to occur, it is doubtful Ebola will become a pandemic (i.e., spreading across an entire country or the world). HIV also broke into the human cycle but has characteristics different from Ebola. It can be transmitted by body fluids when a person is initially infected and quite well. It then becomes less transmissible as the host's immune system decreases viral load. Then after a period of 5–7 years, it may recur, attack the

immune system more vigorously, and indirectly kill the host. Both Ebola and HIV are still evolving in the human system, and over time each will likely become less virulent in order to survive. Other viruses such as rhinoviruses, adenoviruses, and coronaviruses, among many others, cause the common cold. However, these viruses have been around humans for millennia and are better adapted to their human host. They infect millions, thus surviving and spreading, but kill few; thus, they effectively achieve a balance in the host–parasite–environment cycle.

For students of infectious disease epidemiology and ecology, the term evolutionary medicine (or Darwinian medicine) is gaining traction. Simply stated, *evolutionary medicine* refers to the application of evolutionary theory to health and disease. It focuses on how evolution and the adaptive and survival forces therein shape the distribution and prevalence of disease susceptibility and resistance, and the general health of populations.

Smart and Dumb Pathogens

Pathogens might be considered "smart" or "dumb." For the purposes of this discussion, a smart pathogen adapts to its host, causes little or no disease, and perhaps helps the host in some way. Thus, ultimately, "smart" pathogens could be categorized as **commensals** or **mutuals**, rather than **parasites**. **TABLE 14-1** presents a short list of "smart" and "dumb" pathogens based on the morbidity and mortality they cause. Understanding how pathogens reproduce and how they establish biologic equilibriums is a fundamental public health concept that governs endemicity, outbreaks, epidemics, and pandemics.

▶ Population Dynamics

"The power of population is indefinitely greater than the power in the earth to produce subsistence for man."
—Thomas Malthus, 1798

Thomas Malthus and Malthusian Projections

In 1798, Thomas Robert Malthus, then a curate in Surrey, England, published *An Essay on the Principle of Population*. His publication warned that high population growth would ultimately be checked by famine and disease. Malthus maintained populations would rise and fall in relation to the resources available and consumption of those resources by the

TABLE 14-1 Smart and Dumb Pathogens[a]

Pathogen	Smart/Dumb For Humans	Why...?
Bubonic Plague	Dumb	CFR = approximately 60–100%, kills large percentage, burns out in human population, in rats and fleas relatively smart.
Ebola	Dumb	CFR = approximately 41–85%, kills large percentage and kills quickly; will burn out in human population, then retreat to sylvan host and survive.
MRSA (Bloodstream)	Dumb	CFR = approximately 21%; high death rate, can be controlled when treated, newly emerged, will likely attenuate with continued human infection.
MERS	Dumb	CFR = 19%; like MRSA, high death rate, can be controlled when treated, newly emerged, will likely attenuate with continued human infection.
SARS	Dumb	CFR = approximately 15%; like MRSA and MERS, high death rate, can be controlled when treated, newly emerged, will likely attenuate with continued human infection.
HIV/AIDS	Smart	CFR = approximately 80–90%, but highest infectivity in first 3 weeks; then viral load drops, transmission drops, virus survives in host (HIV infection), in later stage virus recrudesces and impairs immune system leading to secondary/opportunistic infections (AIDS); average untreated survival approximately 5–10 years (depending on subtype); AIDS survival 6–19 months.
Smallpox	Smart	CFR = approximately 30%; even with high CFR, smallpox survived well in human populations, epidemics occurred, but natural, lifelong immunity in humans curtailed extended pandemics, no sylvan host.
Polio	Smart	CFR = approximately 2–5%; cases occur in approximately 5% (1/200) infections, thus co-existence in human population for millennia, natural, lifelong immunity conveyed to those exposed.
Measles	Smart	CFR = approximately 1–3%, low CFR, adapted to humans, natural, lifelong immunity conveyed to all exposed.
Malaria	Smart	CFR = approximately 0.47%; kills approximately 1/2,000 of those infected, elegant host–parasite–vector relationship, seasonal, 4 major species, 3 less virulent, approximately 30 million years of evolution contributes to survival of *Plasmodia*. *P. knowlesi* can infect humans but primarily infects wild monkey populations.
Anthrax	Smart	CFR = 10–50%; primarily a zoonosis, in humans high CFR, treatable with antibiotics, originated as a biologic warfare agent, thus ecologic balance disturbed, limited natural transmission in humans.
Hepatitis A	Smart	CFR = approximately 2%, low CFR, symptoms occur, but does not kill.
Influenza A	Smart	CFR = < 0.1%; outbreaks by distinct antigenic variants via antigenic shift, but doesn't kill, creates large amounts of morbidity, easily transmitted.
Hookworm	Smart	CFR negligible; few deaths, but high morbidity, survives in human environment; has zoonotic cousins *Ancylostoma caninum* and *Ancylostoma ceylanicum*.
Common Cold	Smart	CFR negligible, caused by a constellation of viruses, infects many but causes low morbidity, relatively easily transmitted.

Abbreviations: AIDS, acquired immune deficiency syndrome; CFR, case fatality rate; HIV, human immunodeficiency virus; MERS, Middle Eastern respiratory syndrome; MRSA, methicillin resistant *Staphylococcus aureus;* SARS, severe acute respiratory syndrome

[a] This characterization is for illustrative purposes only.

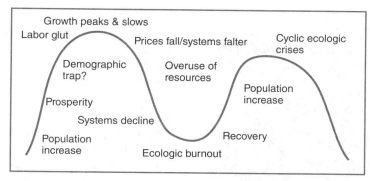

FIGURE 14-2 Malthusian Predictions

Data from Barbiero VK. Malthusian Projections. 2007. Adapted from Malthus RJ. *An Essay on the Principle of Population.* London, UK: Library of Economics and Liberty: 1798.

population (not unlike host–parasite relationships). He viewed a triad of fertility, food consumption, and mortality that would dictate the projection cycle and promote a balanced, albeit harsh, equilibrium model. Malthus's cycle projected high population growth and consumption, followed by a crash in the populations and "ecologic burnout," followed by a period of recovery, sustained growth, and an eventual (and inevitable) crash; that is, cyclical ecologic crises (**FIGURE 14-2**).

Although we have thus far avoided a population crash, famine and disease remain a part of life on earth, and human progress has the potential to disturb fragile biologic and ecologic equilibriums that may cause devastating impacts on population distribution, food production, disease transmission and distribution, and the survival of millions of people.

Demographic and Epidemiologic Transitions

The demographic transition characteristically has four stages (**FIGURE 14-3**).[3,4] Stage one, *the preindustrial stage*, presents high birth and high death rates, which provide for slow, stable growth. Stage two, *the transitional stage*, witnesses declining death rates with continuing high birth rates and accelerated growth. This accelerated growth is known as *the demographic momentum*, because as deaths decrease, the surviving birth cohorts will reach reproductive age and have children, often at a high fertility rate for at least one or two generations. Stage three, *the industrial stage*, forecasts declining birth and death rates due to better survival, and a slowing demographic momentum. Stage four, *the post-industrial stage*, maintains low death rates with fluctuating birth rates and a stable population.

There are profound health and development implications of the demographic transition. First, the

demographic momentum implies significant population growth, even though fertility may decline. Second, population age structures will begin to change, and more people will be in older segments of the population. Third, chronic diseases will emerge as the major cause of morbidity and mortality.

The shift from infectious disease outbreaks and famine to chronic and degenerative diseases is referred to as the **epidemiologic transition**. In 1971, Omran eloquently defined three phases of the epidemiologic transition: *the age of pestilence and famine; the age of receding pandemics*, and *the age of degenerative and manmade diseases.*[5] Thus, Omran posited that infectious disease pandemics would give way to manmade chronic and degenerative diseases as primary causes of morbidity and mortality. The World Health Organization (WHO) reports chronic diseases cause almost 70% of worldwide deaths.[6] Furthermore, with the increase of chronic diseases,

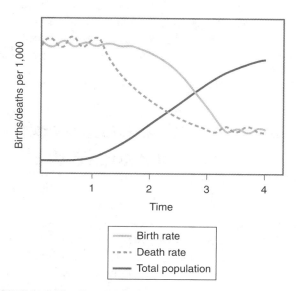

FIGURE 14-3 The Demographic Transition

Reproduced from United Nations Population Fund. Demography on the World Stage: The Demographic Transition. Available at http://papp.iussp.org/sessions/papp101_s01/PAPP101_s01_090_010.html. Published 2015. Accessed November 6, 2017.

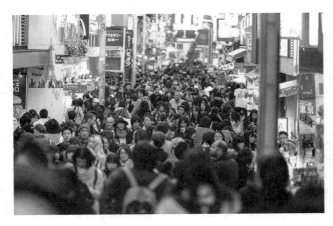

© Pola Damonte via Getty Images/Moment/Getty

low- and middle-income countries face a double burden of disease because both infectious and chronic diseases will continue to cause significant morbidity and mortality for the foreseeable future.

It is important to understand that demographic and epidemiologic shifts give rise to important changes in host–pathogen relationships and disease dynamics across the planet. Healthcare needs will likewise change, and a greater need for chronic disease management will emerge. Given high rates of urban growth, planners, politicians, and public health experts have much to consider. Sound management of the demographic transition will require an in-depth assessment of future health (and other) costs for a growing and aging population. In the short and medium terms, governments will have to derive an effective and operational balance to address the infectious disease burdens of the poor, and the growing proportion of chronic diseases affecting older populations, both rich and poor, in both rural and urban areas. Leaders must consider practical policies and programs to stabilize population growth, and cope with the inevitable repercussions of these two transitions.

▶ Disease Transmission: Modes of Transmission and Control

Infectious disease transmission is neither haphazard nor cursory, but rather a product of evolutionary biology and highly specific adaptations. For these reasons, the **eradication**, **elimination**, and even the control of infectious diseases represent formidable challenges for prevention, treatment, and cure. Thus, opportunities to control, eliminate, or eradicate diseases must be carefully considered by planners in terms of financing, opportunity costs, and the time frame or horizon of success.

Sound disease control applies proven tools to weaken the chain of transmission and reduce incidence so the disease is no longer a public health problem. **BOX 14-1** depicts seven major modes of infectious disease transmission and eight general control interventions. Food- and waterborne diseases are directly linked to contamination via the fecal–oral route, generally poor personal hygiene and sanitation, and the lack of potable water. HIV and hepatitis B are primarily sexually transmitted, but both are also transmitted by transfusions and unsafe injections. Vector-borne diseases like malaria, Zika, and West Nile virus, which are carried by mosquitos, and onchocerciasis (river blindness), transmitted by a parasitic freshwater worm, are anchored in a specialized host–vector–pathogen relationship. Aerosol-transmitted germs like *Mycobacterium tuberculosis* depend on close proximity between the host and pathogen because transmission occurs via droplet inhalation. Nontraumatic contact with animals via skin or traumatic contact via bites and scratches also can transmit pathogens such as *Bacillus anthracis* (anthrax) and rabies virus.

Controlling infectious diseases by prevention is more cost-effective than treatment. Vaccination is one of the most efficient means of reducing morbidity and mortality. However, the integrity of health delivery systems, albeit improving, often limits delivery, as we see with measles deaths, which totaled about 146,000 in 2013.[7] Mass chemotherapy can be applied when feasible, for example in controlling onchocerciasis, intestinal worms, and lymphatic filariasis. However, drugs must be inexpensive, stable, and effective if administered only once or twice a year. Massive chemotherapy programs can be implemented, but costs, supplies, and sustained support must be considered. Drug conservation, patient adherence, and drug availability are required to allay resistance and ensure effectiveness over time.

Vector control represents a time-tried endeavor, but rarely stands alone, and is applied as part of an integrated approach that includes appropriate

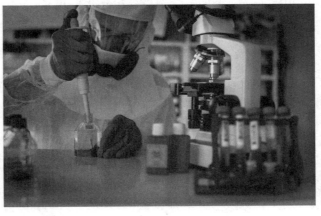

© luchschen/Shutterstock

BOX 14-1 Modes of Infectious Disease Transmission and Methods of Control

Modes of Infectious Disease Transmission

- **Foodborne** – ingestion: *Salmonella, E. coli, Entamoeba histolitica*, hepatitis A
- **Waterborne** – ingestion: cholera, rotavirus
- **Bloodborne/Sexual** – hepatitis B and C, HIV
- **Vector-borne** – malaria, onchocerciasis, West Nile virus, filariasis, schistosomiasis, etc.
- **Inhalation** – tuberculosis, influenza, meningitis
- **Nontraumatic contact** – anthrax
- **Traumatic contact** – bites, scratches: rabies, cat scratch disease (*Bartonella*)

Methods of Infectious Disease Control

- **Vaccination** – smallpox, polio, measles, pneumonia, rotavirus, pediatric tuberculosis, diphtheria, pertussis, tetanus, hepatitis B, human papilloma virus, yellow fever, meningitis, influenza
- **Mass Chemotherapy** – onchocerciasis, hookworm, lymphatic filariasis
- **Vector Control** – malaria, dengue, yellow fever, onchocerciasis, West Nile virus
- **Improved Water, Sanitation, Hygiene** – diarrhea, all fecal–oral route diseases
- **Improved Care Seeking, Disease Recognition** – maternal health, neonatal health, diarrheal disease, acute respiratory disease, malaria, etc.
- **Case Management (Treatment) and Improved Caregiving** – diarrheal disease, acute respiratory illness, malaria, etc.
- **Case Containment, Recognition, Policy Enforcement** – avian influenza, meningitis, cholera, Ebola, etc.
- **Behavioral Change** – HIV, sexually transmitted infections, all other diseases.

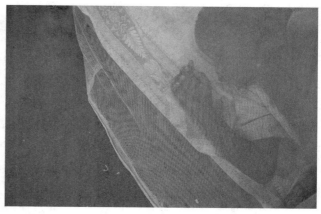
© punghi/Shutterstock

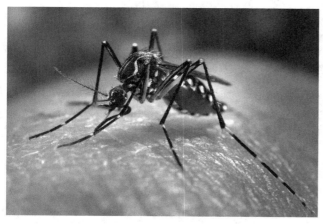
James Gathany/CDC/Prof. Frank Hadley Collins, Dir., Cntr. for Global Health and Infectious Diseases, Univ. of Notre Dame

treatment and personal protection. Water supply, sanitation, and personal/community hygiene can reduce the incidence and severity of diarrheal diseases, but costs and maintenance condition their success.

Educating families (especially mothers) about early disease recognition, care seeking, and rudimentary case management with affordable home treatments is a difficult but necessary element of sound disease-control practice. Disease recognition early in an infection can save millions of children who often arrive at health facilities moribund and almost beyond help. Outbreak containment often poses challenging obstacles, as witnessed by the 2014–2015 Ebola outbreak. Strict policy and containment strategies are required to stem outbreaks before they spread too far. Lastly, behavior change to reduce disease transmission at the individual, family, and community levels represents a cross-cutting issue for control. It is important to nurture healthy behavioral norms, anchored in prevention, disease recognition, care seeking, and treatment. The example of insecticide-treated nets (ITNs) represents a successful intervention achieved through access, affordability, sustained investment, and most importantly, inculcating a behavioral norm to use ITNs to prevent malaria. If positive normative behavior is achieved, more effective disease control interventions will be realized.

▶ Survival Strategies: r- and K-Strategist Populations

For our purposes, **r-strategists** and **K-strategists** connote reproductive patterns that organisms use to survive. If you are an organism that lives in a harsh environment where life and death come and go with changes in the environment you live in, such as weather, tides, temperature, food availability, or inside a host organism, one strategy would be to increase production of offspring in order to give more progeny a chance of survival even under unpredictable and

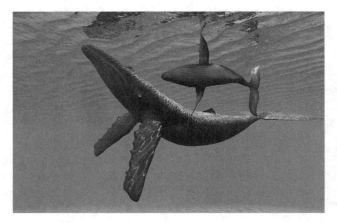

© Catmando/Shutterstock

unforgiving conditions. Strategically, you would produce a lot of "cheap" offspring requiring little energy and parental investment. They would mature quickly and consequently produce many offspring themselves. The chances of your simple species surviving through adaptation will increase, as well as through the absolute numbers of progeny produced. If you lose 95% of your offspring, 5% still remain and they will likely be better adapted to the vagaries of their environment. Similarly, their offspring with continue to adapt and survive better than their parents, grandparents, and great-grandparents. Most invertebrates (viruses, bacteria, worms, insects, and plants) follow this high reproductive strategy, and they are successful. They are found around the globe in stable environments, as well some of the harshest environments on the planet. These are the *r-strategists*.

K-strategists have usually adapted to a more stable environment, where sudden, unpredictable changes are less likely. Often, K-strategists approach the *carrying capacity (K)* of their environment. K-strategists (e.g., whales) often live relatively longer lives than r-strategists (e.g., fish), are larger, and have a higher percentage of their offspring survive.[8]

It is important to understand that the reproductive strategies exhibited by r- and K-strategists are equally effective in terms of survival. It is also important to note that there can be some overlap among the characteristics of r- and K-strategists. For example, Tsetse flies produce only 7 eggs in their lifetime and geckos produce only 1 or 2 eggs, qualifying as K-strategists for progeny, but r-strategists for other characteristics. The take-home message is that organisms have various reproductive strategies governed by their environment and physiology. They adapt to their environment to survive, be it the African savannah, a barrier reef in the Caribbean, the mountains of Colorado, or the blood, organs, or organelles of other organisms. Be they r-strategists or K-strategists, both are eminently successful (**FIGURE 14-4**).

▶ Breakpoint Transmission

Perhaps one of the most fundamental concepts in infectious disease epidemiology and control is the concept of **breakpoint transmission**, introduced by Professor George McDonald in 1965. Breakpoint transmission is simply defined as "the point at which a parasite population is at such a low level that it cannot sustain itself in the environment." **FIGURE 14-5** illustrates the concept of breakpoint transmission using smallpox, polio, and malaria as examples.

Smallpox was able to be eradicated because it was highly recognizable, and because over 90% of susceptible individuals were immunized, the virus could not spread to additional susceptible hosts. "**Herd immunity**" was established and sequestered viral

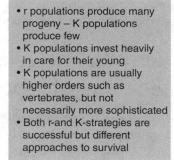

- r populations produce many progeny – K populations produce few
- K populations invest heavily in care for their young
- K populations are usually higher orders such as vertebrates, but not necessarily more sophisticated
- Both r-and K-strategies are successful but different approaches to survival

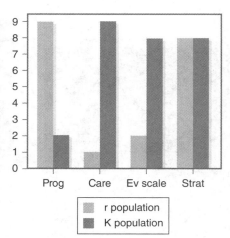

FIGURE 14-4 r and K Populations

Data from Barbiero VK. Illustrative Graph: GWU SPHHS. 2003.

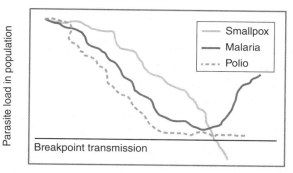

FIGURE 14-5 Breakpoint Transmission

Data from Barbiero VK. Illustrative Graph: Breakpoint Transmission. GWU SPHHS, PH 180 Course. 2003. Adapted from Macdonald G. The dynamics of helminth infections, with special reference to schistosomes. *Trans R Soc Trop Med Hyg.* 1965;59(45):489-506.

spread until it eventually died out. Polio, the second candidate for eradication, is on the brink of its own breakpoint, but not quite there yet. Continued massive immunization campaigns are required in places like Pakistan and Afghanistan to bolster herd immunity and limit viral spread to susceptible persons.

The malaria elimination program in Sri Lanka in the early 1960s presents an important alternative lesson for eradication programs. The program was an indoor residual spray campaign using dichloro-diphenyl-trichoroethane (DDT) aimed at eliminating the mosquito vector (*Anopheles culicifa-cies*) and thus permanently interrupt transmission. It was a **vertical program**, run in parallel to the existing health system with separate budgets, personnel, equipment, and supplies. The program also enjoyed deep and broad external technical U.S. and programmatic assistance from WHO, the Centers for Disease Control and Prevention, and international donors. Sri Lanka's malaria elimination program achieved great success; it reduced annual malaria incidence from over 700,000 cases annually to less than 17 reported cases in 1963.

Experts thought the "breakpoint" had been achieved and stopped their elimination efforts. They were wrong. Malaria returned to Sri Lanka with a vengeance, exploding to over 535,000 cases by 1969 and the subsequent abandonment of elimination efforts in Sri Lanka, and eventually worldwide, due to lack of support and insecticide resistance to DDT.[9] This example teaches us that interrupting transmission of a pathogen and complete elimination of a parasite from a geographic area is no simple task.

▶ Drug Resistance

Over the past decades, the WHO noted that "antimicrobial resistance has been detected in all parts of the world; it is one of the greatest challenges to global public health today, and the problem is increasing."[10] Major infectious diseases such as tuberculosis, pneumonia, methicillin-resistant *Staphylococcus aureus* (MRSA), Middle East respiratory syndrome (MERS), and malaria are resistant to some of the most powerful drugs available. It is important to understand that drug resistance inevitably will occur if drugs are put into a health system. This is because the job of a pathogen is to survive, and survival, as Charles Darwin noted, means organisms adapt to their environment; they adapt to environmental and biologic pressures and strike an equilibrium. Similarly, pathogens will adapt to drug pressure over time.

FIGURE 14-6 illustrates how bacteria become drug resistant.[11] Because of random mutations, most bacterial populations will contain some individuals that are resistant to certain antibiotics (or other pressures). In the case of bacteria, when these antibiotics are introduced into a system, most of the susceptible bacteria will be killed, but the resistant forms

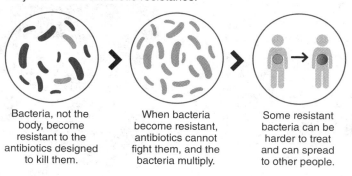

Antibiotic resistance occurs when bacteria no longer respond to the drugs designed to kill them. Anytime antibiotics are used, they can cause antibiotic resistance.

Bacteria, not the body, become resistant to the antibiotics designed to kill them. > When bacteria become resistant, antibiotics cannot fight them, and the bacteria multiply. > Some resistant bacteria can be harder to treat and can spread to other people.

FIGURE 14-6 How Bacterial Populations Become Drug Resistant

Reproduced from Centers for Disease Control and Prevention. What is antibiotic-resistant bacteria? Available at https://www.cdc.gov/antibiotic-use/community/pdfs/aaw/AU_What-is-antibiotic-resistant-Infographic_8_5x5_5_3_508.pdf. Accessed December 13, 2017.

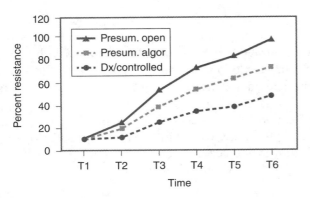

FIGURE 14-7 Resistance to Drugs

Data from Barbiero VK. Developed by Barbiero for Global Health & Development course 2005-2013. 2015.

will survive. With continued antibiotic pressure (i.e., treatments), the resistant bacteria are selected and eventually become the dominant form of the bacterial population. These are the bacteria that are transmitted, and thus resistance spreads throughout the host population.

FIGURE 14-7 illustrates two major points: first, drug resistance is inevitable; and second, we can delay, but not prevent, the emergence of drug resistance through better diagnosis and treatment. The graph indicates that in an open system, where people are treated presumptively, the slope of the resistance curve will be steep and higher rates of resistance will occur in a shorter time period. If more specific and sensitive algorithmic assessment tools are applied prior to treatment, then the emergence of resistance can be delayed for a longer period of time. The best-case scenario promotes accurate clinical and laboratory diagnosis of infection and subsequent appropriate treatment. However, even with the best efforts of diagnosis and treatment, resistance will eventually emerge because multiple survival factors come into play for the pathogen and host. These factors include the inherent ability of pathogens to mutate and adapt, adherence to the drug regimen by patients, the continuous availability of the drugs in the system, and the quality of the drugs available. In many resource-poor countries, these factors align to promote, rather than delay, drug resistance.

▶ Eradication versus Control: Smallpox Eradication

Remember the definitions of eradication, elimination, and control? It is essential that these strategies, and the differences between them, are considered when deciding how to reduce the prevalence and impact of a disease.

Clearly, important successes have been realized in areas such as smallpox and polio eradication, guinea worm elimination, and diarrheal disease control.[12] But, as discussed, biologic systems are resilient, adapted to, and balanced with, their environment. Only one human disease, smallpox, has been eradicated; we are close to polio and guinea worm eradication, but the job is not complete.

The variola virus causes smallpox; it is in the virus family poxviridae. *Variola major* produces the most common and severe form of the disease. Smallpox is thought to have existed for more than 12,000 years. During the 20th century, it is estimated that there were 300 million to 500 million deaths from smallpox worldwide, death rates for unvaccinated populations averaged 30%.[13-15] In the late 1960s, an estimated 10–15 million people were infected annually.[16]

On May 8, 1980, the World Health Assembly declared smallpox was eradicated. This was a monumental achievement for mankind. However, the success of smallpox eradication contrasted with the costly failures of other eradication campaigns, notably malaria eradication. Smallpox eradication was nothing short of an operational and administrative masterpiece that used a global, "vertical" campaign approach—one that was approved locally, but managed by outside experts. However, it was simultaneously integrated into existing health infrastructures and had to take advantage of available resources, including health personnel, teachers, community elders and members (including children), and religious leaders, among others. Technically, a number of key factors converged to make eradication possible (**BOX 14-2**).

From the outset, surveillance was a key to success—just as surveillance is key to successful polio eradication. However, unlike polio, smallpox is easily recognizable by local health workers and members of the community. Good communication and follow-up were essential but managed to work well, and the last case was identified in Somalia in 1977.

BOX 14-2 The "Eradication Potential" of Smallpox

- Highly effective vaccine conveying lifelong immunity
- Vaccine and natural immunity acquired
- Smallpox is a disease of moderate infectivity (not highly infectious)
- Cases are easily recognized
- The vaccine is thermally stable
- The vaccine was relatively easy to administer (bifurcated needle)
- People could get vaccinated at any time, young or old, thus an "open vaccine window"

Today, many speak of eradication and elimination of specific diseases, but eradicating a pathogen is no easy task. Before embarking on a global eradication strategy that may take decades to succeed, impede broader system-strengthening investments, and cost billions of dollars, public health professionals must consider the biologic basis of disease transmission, and the compelling need and ability of organisms to survive, adapt, and strike a biologic equilibrium with their hosts. Thus, control, elimination, and eradication decisions require careful consideration of feasibility, costs, human resource requirements, the status of the health delivery system, opportunity costs, and the amount of time and effort required to eradicate an organism from our planet.

In the future, controlling many diseases through strengthened systems and community engagement may be a better strategy than a singular effort of elimination or eradication. In 1998, Dr. Donald A. Henderson, former Head of the Global Smallpox Eradication Program, eloquently commented on the future of disease eradication.[17] He wrote:

In looking to the future, however, I believe it is critical that we should not be blinded to a range of new public health program paradigms by staring too fixedly at the blinding beacon of a few eradication dreams.[17(p21)]

In sum, it is important to remember that transmission breakpoints do exist; however, to achieve eradication, pathogens must cross the point of no return; that is, not enough opportunities to viably reproduce. Also, biologic equilibriums do exist, but the balance can be upset by a variety of external and internal forces. Drug resistance can be delayed, but resistance will emerge if drugs are put into the system—it is only a matter of time. Modes of transmission will vary with pathogens, and therefore, it is important to understand them and to respect them all. Finally, eradication is a noble endeavor; however, it is no simple task. Public health strategies demand an in-depth consideration of a broad array of potential opportunity costs and consequences. In many cases, effective disease control, rather than eradication, may be the more appropriate goal.

Key Terms

Attenuation	Elimination	K-strategists
Breakpoint transmission	Epidemiologic transition	Mutuals
Case	Eradication	Parasites
Case fatality rate	Herd immunity	R-strategists
Commensals	Infection	Vertical program

Discussion Questions

1. How does the biologic equilibrium relate to public health, disease transmission, and disease elimination? List three or four characteristics and comment on how these characteristics may impede or facilitate disease control.
2. What are some of the key issues in the development of disease resistance? How can we better limit disease resistance?
3. Describe/define breakpoint transmission and its relevance to disease control, elimination, and eradication. Present a discussion of a real-world disease to support your explanation.
4. Draw graphs that illustrate the development of drug resistance. Provide brief comments on your impressions of drug use and the potential for resistance.
5. Discuss the pros and cons of an eradication policy. What are the opportunity costs associated with eradication?
6. Define control, elimination of infection, elimination of disease, and eradication. Provide general comment (your opinion) on pursuing these investments.
7. Describe r- versus K-strategist organisms; provide two examples of each and relate the strategy to survival and possible susceptibility to disease.

References

1. Evans AS. Causation and disease: The Henle-Koch postulates revisited. *Yale J Biol Med*. 1976;49(2):175-195.
2. Morens DM, Fauci AS. Emerging infectious diseases: threats to human health and global stability. *PLoS Pathog*. 2013;9(7):1-3.
3. United Nations Population Fund. Demography on the World Stage: The Demographic Transition. Available at http://papp .iussp.org/sessions/papp101_s01/PAPP101_s01_090_010 .html. Published 2015. Accessed November 6, 2017.

4. Montgomery K. The Demographic Transition. Available at http://pages.uwc.edu/keith.montgomery/Demotrans/demtran.htm. Posted 2000. Accessed November 6, 2017.

5. Omran AR. The epidemiologic transition; a theory of the epidemiology of population change. *Millbank Mem Fund Q.* 1971;49:509-538.

6. World Health Organization. Top 10 Causes of Death. WHO Media Center. Available at http://www.who.int/mediacentre/factsheets/fs310/en/index2.html. Updated January 2017. Accessed November 6, 2017.

7. World Health Organization. Measles. WHO Factsheet #286. http://www.who.int/mediacentre/factsheets/fs286/en/. Updated October 2017. Accessed November 6, 2017.

8. University of Miami Biology Department. r and K selection. Available at http://www.bio.miami.edu/tom/courses/bil160/bil160goods/16_rKselection.html. Posted 2015. Accessed November 6, 2017.

9. Gramiccia G, Beales G. The recent history of malaria control and eradication. In: Wernsdorfer WH, McGregor I, eds. *Malaria: Principles and Practice of Malariology.* London, UK: Churchill Livingstone; 1989:1366-1367.

10. World Health Organization. Worldwide Country Situation Analysis - Summary: Response to Antimicrobial Resistance. Geneva, Switzerland: WHO; 2015. Available at http://www.who.int/antimicrobial-resistance/publications/situationanalysis/en/. Accessed November 6, 2017.

11. Centers for Disease Control and Prevention. What is antibiotic-resitant bacteria? Available at https://www.cdc.gov/antibiotic-use/community/pdfs/aaw/AU_What-is-antibiotic-resistant-Infographic_8_5x5_5_3_508.pdf. Accessed December 13, 2017.

12. Levine R. *Millions Saved: Proven Successes in Global Health.* Washington, DC: Center for Global Development; 2004.

13. Davis CP, Stöppler MC. Smallpox. Available at http://www.medicinenet.com/smallpox/article.htm. Posted 2015. Accessed November 6, 2017.

14. Centers for Disease Control & Prevention. Smallpox. Available at https://www.cdc.gov/smallpox/index.html. Updated July 12, 2017. Accessed November 6, 2017.

15. Heymann D. Smallpox. In: *Control of Communicable Disease Manual.* 20th ed. Washington, DC: American Public Health Association.

16. World Health Organization. Emergency preparedness, response: smallpox. Available at http://www.who.int/csr/disease/smallpox/en/. Accessed November 6, 2017.

17. Henderson DA. Eradication: lessons from the past. *Bull World Health Org.* 1998;76(suppl 2):17-21. Available at http://europepmc.org/articles/PMC2305698. Accessed November 6, 2017.

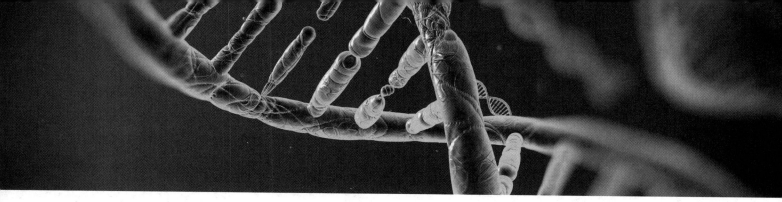

CHAPTER 15

Malaria

Victor K. Barbiero

LEARNING OBJECTIVES

By the end of this chapter, the student will be able to:

- Describe the biology of malaria transmission and the clinical manifestations of malaria disease and infection
- Explain the epidemiology and ecology of malaria relative to transmission and infection
- Identify the vector biology of malaria at the global level
- Describe the diagnosis and treatment of malaria, the pharmokenetic properties of drugs, issues of drug resistance, and the potential for vaccines
- Explore malaria prevention and control and technical challenges therein

CHAPTER OUTLINE

▸ Introduction

Malaria is an age-old tropical disease that occurs in many parts of the world. In the 1800s, malaria was endemic in Washington, DC, where the swamps of Foggy Bottom (one mile from the White House) served as breeding sites for the mosquito vectors of malaria. Malaria parasites attack our red blood cells (RBCs), using the cells as a vessel to multiply and infect other blood cells. The symptoms of malaria are many and include headache, fever, chills, nausea, diarrhea, joint and muscle pain, spleen enlargement, kidney failure, and brain damage. Severe malaria can kill an individual in days; uncomplicated malaria causes illness that can be confused with many other infections. An important diagnostic feature of malaria is an intermittently spiking fever occurring every 48 or 72 hours, depending on the species of malaria—but fever intervals can vary, thus requiring accurate diagnosis of the parasite in the blood. Treatment will clear the infection if appropriate and timely. An estimated 3.4 billion people

Symptoms of Malaria

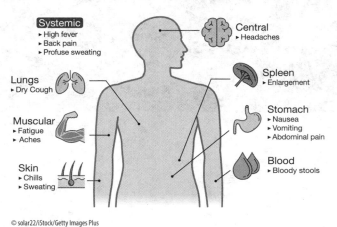

Systemic
▸ High fever
▸ Back pain
▸ Profuse sweating

Central
▸ Headaches

Lungs
▸ Dry Cough

Spleen
▸ Enlargement

Muscular
▸ Fatigue
▸ Aches

Stomach
▸ Nausea
▸ Vomiting
▸ Abdominal pain

Skin
▸ Chills
▸ Sweating

Blood
▸ Bloody stools

© solar22/iStock/Getty Images Plus

are at risk to malaria, and 1.2 billion are at high risk. Malaria infects over 200 million people annually and kills over 600,000; approximately 90% of the deaths are in sub-Saharan Africa.

History

Malaria, caused by a nucleated protozoan parasite in the genus *Plasmodium*, has affected humankind for millions of years. The earliest accounts of malaria come from China in 2700 BC, and references to the disease have been found on Egyptian hieroglyphics.[1] The mosquito vector, members of the genus *Anopheles,* likely emerged in Africa 30 million years ago and from there spread worldwide. In the early 17th century, South American Indians used the bark of the cinchona tree (a substance rich in quinine, a potent antimalarial) to treat fevers. Malaria derives its name from the Italian "*mal aria*" or "bad air." Alphonse Laveran discovered malaria in the blood of an Algerian patient in 1880.[1] In 1897, Ronald Ross, a British military doctor stationed in India, discovered that the mosquito transmitted malaria and later won the Nobel Prize for Medicine in 1902.

The global distribution of malaria is a tragic consequence of a resilient parasite–host–vector

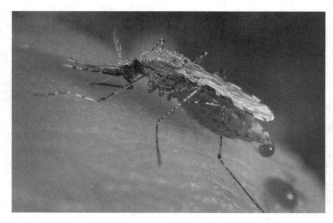

James Gathany/CDC

relationship and the inadequacy of healthcare systems in many developing countries. However, great progress has been made, and between 2010 and 2015, malaria mortality fell 29% globally and 31% in sub-Saharan Africa alone; the decline in the Western Pacific Region was even more dramatic, at 58% during the same period.[2] Weak systems, human behavior, difficult diagnosis, and natural and manmade emergencies, including conflicts, make malaria control a very challenging endeavor. With collective global efforts such as the World Health Organization's (WHO's) Roll Back Malaria (RBM) Program, The Global Fund for AIDS, TB, and Malaria, the U.S. government's President's Malaria Initiative, and investments by private foundations such as the Bill & Melinda Gates Foundation, the burden of malaria can continue to decline, but a sustained global commitment is imperative.

Malaria Endemicity

Malaria as a disease differs geographically and biologically (**FIGURE 15-1**). In Africa, home to the most efficient vector, *Anopheles gambiae*, and the likely birthplace of malaria parasites as well, a fine-tuned adaptation between man, parasite, vector, and the environment has evolved, making malaria a formidable and enduring public health problem. Geographic variability, human behaviors, and transmission potentials vary within and among regions, and thus the dimensions of malaria as a public health problem also vary. Over 200 million cases occur each year, with 80% of those cases in Africa. Globally, over 3 billion people are at risk. An estimated 429,000 deaths occur annually (with a range of 235,000–639,000).[2] African children under 5 years of age are most vulnerable to malaria and comprise approximately 75% of worldwide deaths. A mere 20% of malaria cases worldwide come to the attention of the healthcare system, with 80% of care sought in the private sector (traditional healers, shops, and pharmacies). Total annual direct costs are estimated to be USD $12 billion.[3] Malaria remains a leading cause of school and work absences. It can impede a child's ability to learn and may consume up to 30% of a household's disposable income for the poorest of the poor. Thus, malaria has a double-edged sword effect because it is both a disease of poverty and a cause of poverty.

▸ Epidemiology of Malaria

Types and Distribution of Malaria Parasites

Five species of *Plasmodium* cause malaria in humans: *P. vivax, P. falciparum, P. malariae, P. knowlesi,* and

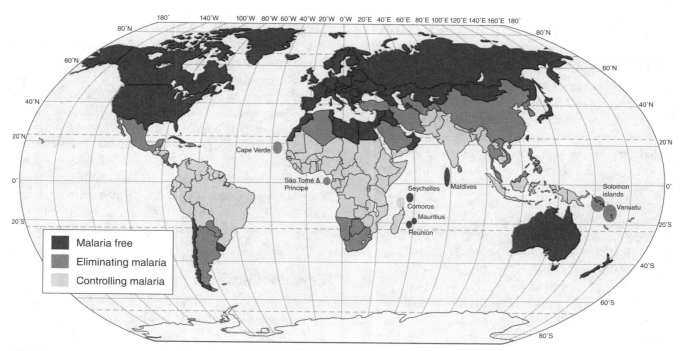

FIGURE 15-1 The Endemicity of Malaria

Data from Centers for Disease Control and Prevention. Malaria: where malaria occurs. Available at https://www.cdc.gov/malaria/about/distribution.html. Updated March 17, 2017. Accessed December 15, 2017.

P. ovale (see **TABLE 15-1**). *P. vivax* and *P. falciparum* are the most common, and *P. falciparum* is the most virulent. *P. vivax* is more abundant globally, accounting for most of the malaria in Asia and Latin America. *P. falciparum* is found mostly in the tropics, causes most of the acquired malaria in Africa, and causes most of the malaria mortality worldwide. In total, 95% of all malaria infections are either due to *P. vivax* or *P. falciparum*. *P. knowlesi* primarily infects macaques, which may then transmit malaria to humans.

There is great geographic variability in the parasite, vectors, transmission, mortality, and morbidity of malaria. *P. vivax*, although widespread, does not cause a great deal of mortality. If left untreated, the infection can last 2–3 months, with more than 50% of patients experiencing a relapse. *P. ovale* is similar to *P. vivax*, but it produces a milder form of malaria. Often, *P. ovale* infection resolves without treatment. Both *P. vivax* and *P. ovale* infections produce fevers on a 48-hour cycle, associated with bursting of blood cells by mature schizonts. This 48-hour periodicity is referred to as *tertian malaria*. *P. malariae* displays a 72-hour cycle and is referred to as *quartan malaria*. *P. falciparum* may occur on a 48-hour cycle but is usually irregular. *P. falciparum* routinely causes anemia and can adhere to the endothelium of capillaries and postcapillary venules, which leads to obstruction of microcirculation, pulmonary edema, and tissue anoxia (i.e., it blocks the passage of blood). In the brain, this causes cerebral malaria; in the kidneys, it can cause necrosis and renal failure.

TABLE 15-1 Five Species of *Plasmodium* That Cause Malaria in Humans	
Species	**Characteristics**
P. vivax	Most abundant globally; spread by *Anopheles* mosquito
P. falciparum	Most virulent; mostly found in the tropics; causes most malaria mortality; spread by *Anopheles* mosquito
P. malariae	Associated with nephrotic syndrome; spread by *Anopheles* mosquito; wide range of prepatent period (16–59 days)
P. knowlesi	Infects macaques; distributed primarily in Malaysia (Borneo in particular)
P. ovale	Causes tertian malaria; spread by *Anopheles* mosquito; prepatent period of 12–20 days; primarily distributed in sub-Saharan Africa

▶ Malaria Life Cycle and Vectors

The Life Cycle of Malaria

Malaria is transmitted when the female *Anopheles* mosquito takes a human "blood meal." The mosquito requires heme, an iron-containing compound found in hemoglobin, to develop her eggs. Because the female mosquito is needed for human *Plasmodium* to sexually reproduce, the *Anopheles* is the *definitive* or *final* host for human *Plasmodium*. Humans are *intermediate hosts*, meaning they are required for the asexual development of the parasite. Malaria can also be transmitted by blood transfusion from an individual with an active infection, or congenitally from an infected mother to her baby. Both transfusion and transplacental transmission are relatively rare.

The life cycle of malaria is stunningly elegant. It is a complex host–parasite relationship that has enabled human malaria to survive and thrive for millennia (**FIGURE 15-2**). The life cycle comprises three stages: the *exoerythrocytic cycle*, the *erythrocytic cycle*, and the *sporogonic cycle*.

Exoerythrocytic Cycle

When an infected female *Anopheles* mosquito takes a blood meal, she injects uninucleate **sporozoites** from her salivary glands into the bloodstream. The sporozoites migrate to liver parenchymal cells in approximately 30 minutes. In the liver cells, the sporozoites develop into spherical, multinucleate, liver-stage **schizonts**, which contain 2,000–40,000 **merozoites**. In *P. vivax* and *P. ovale* infections, the liver-stage schizonts may be delayed for 1–2 years.[4] The quiescent liver-stage schizont is called a **hypnozoite** and can cause a relapse. The liver stage of the parasite's development is called **exoerythrocytic schizogony** or the exoerythrocytic cycle.

Erythrocytic Cycle

After 5 to 21 days (or 1–2 years), depending on the species of *Plasmodium*, mature schizonts rupture and the merozoites emerge into the bloodstream; each merozoite can infect an RBC. The single merozoites undergo asexual reproduction forming **trophozoites**. Once mature, the parasitized cell is

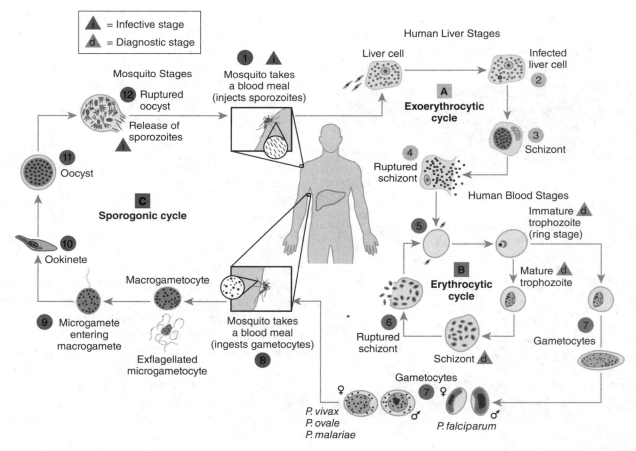

FIGURE 15-2 The Life Cycle of Malaria

Reproduced from Centers for Disease Control and Prevention. Malaria: about malaria: biology. Available at https://www.cdc.gov/malaria/about/biology/index.html. Updated March 1, 2016. Accessed December 15, 2017.

referred to as an erythrocytic schizont, which contains 8–36 merozoites. When the mature schizont ruptures, the merozoites are released to infect other blood cells. During this process, some parasites differentiate into sexual erythrocytic stages called **gametocytes**. The time required for **erythrocytic schizogony**, which releases the successive generations of merozoites, varies with the species of *Plasmodium*, thus causing the classic periodicity of malarial fevers already mentioned.

Sporogonic Cycle

The gametocytes are infective to the female *Anopheles* mosquito and when ingested develop into male and female gametes (**microgametes** and **macrogametes**, respectively). In the stomach of the mosquito, the gametes undergo fertilization and form a zygote, which differentiates into an elongated **ookinete**. The ookinete invades the gut wall of the mosquito and forms an **oocyst**. Over a 2- to 3-week maturation period, the oocyst matures and ruptures, releasing sporozoites that make their way to the salivary glands of the mosquito. At the next blood meal, the sporozoites are inoculated into the bloodstream of a human and the cycle begins again. It is important to note that a female *Anopheles* mosquito must live 2–3 weeks after taking an infective blood meal in order to transmit malaria. This has important implications for malaria prevention and control.

Vectors of Malaria

By definition, a vector is an organism that is required by another organism to complete its life cycle or simply carry the organism to its intermediate or final host; furthermore, a vector can be either the final or intermediate host of an organism. The evolutionary biology of the host–parasite relationship for human malaria has given rise to a myriad of *Anopheles* vectors that span the globe and are elegantly adapted to micro- and macroclimates and habitats around the world (with the exception of Antarctica). There are about 3,500 species of mosquitos and approximately 430 *Anopheles* species; only 30 or 40 transmit malaria.[5] *Anopheles* mosquitos can feed on humans (**anthropophilic**), animals (**zoophilic**), or both. They characteristically fly 1–3 kilometers and feed at dusk or dawn (crepuscular) or at night (nocturnal). Some *Anopheles* feed indoors and some feed outdoors (exophagic); and some rest indoors (endophilic) and some rest outdoors (exophilic). Feeding and resting behaviors are important to understand in order to implement the most effective control interventions. For example, if an *Anopheles* species is primarily endophilic and endophagic, bed nets may be a very effective control intervention.

Anopheles vectors are found in nonendemic areas as well as areas where malaria has been eliminated such as the United States. Thus, the potential for indigenous malaria transmission remains if the parasite is imported. Major vectors in Africa are *An. gambiae*, *An. funestus*, and *An. arabiensis*; in North Africa, *An. pharoensis* dominates. *An. culicifacies*, *An. fluviatilis*, *An. dirus*, *An. minimus*, and *An. punctulatus* are major transmitters in sub-Saharan Africa and East Asia and the Pacific regions (**FIGURE 15-3**). Like all mosquitos, *Anopheles* have four stages of their life cycle: egg, larva, pupa, and adult. Females lay 50 to 200 eggs that float on standing water.[5] They can live in freshwater or saltwater marshes, rice fields, mangrove swamps, ditches, streams, temporary rain pools, forests, sunlit pools, and even tree holes. Thus, control is quite challenging. Larvae hatch within 2–3 days (2–3 weeks in colder climates) and breathe through spiracles, small holes in their abdomen. They feed on algae, bacteria, and other microorganisms. The larva molts into a pupa, and after a few days, the adult mosquito emerges. The entire process can take as little as 5 days but usually takes 10–14 days in tropical conditions. Adult mosquitos mate within a few days. The males form large swarms and the females fly into the swarms to mate. The female seeks a blood meal and the eggs develop in 2–3 days. She lays the eggs and then seeks another blood meal. Females can live for 1–3 weeks. This successive feeding–egg-laying cycle enables the development of the *Plasmodium* in the mosquito and facilitates the transmission of malaria parasites.

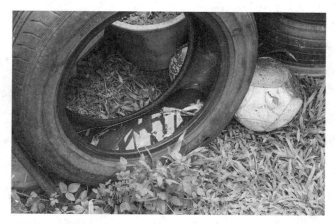

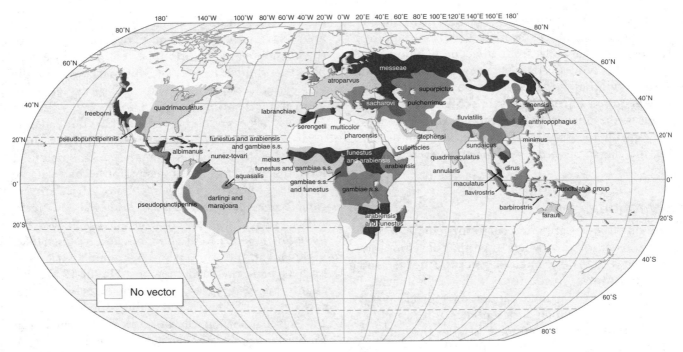

FIGURE 15-3 Malaria Vectors Worldwide

Reproduced from Kiszewski A, Mellinger A, Spielman A, Malaney P, Sachs SE, Sachs J. A global index representing the stability of malaria transmission. *Am J Trop Med Hyg*. 2004;70(5):486-498.

▶ Clinical Malaria

Pathophysiology of Malaria

No pathology is associated with sporozoites, the liver stage of the parasite, the initial merozoites released from the liver, or gametocytes. When erythrocytic schizogony occurs, the malaria parasite feeds on hemoglobin and other proteins within the RBC, causing various and progressive degrees of anemia. It replicates and creates a toxin called **hemozoin** and other toxic compounds. When the erythrocytic schizonts mature, they rupture the cell, releasing these compounds, which likely trigger an immune response. Macrophages and other cells are released, which trigger the production of cytokines such as **tumor necrosis factor** and other soluble cellular factors. These cytokines are likely responsible for the fever in malaria patients. These products of the immune response are likely responsible for the cyclical fevers and chills, sweats, and other symptoms associated with malaria. As mentioned, in cases of *falciparum* malaria, infected RBCs adhere to the walls of the capillaries and venules and obstruct blood flow and oxygen, causing tissue damage. The severity of disease appears to be associated with the degree of **parasitemia** (percent RBCs infected).

Genetic Factors That Influence Infection and Mortality

There are a number of inherent and acquired factors that influence the susceptibility and severity of malaria infection. It now seems clear that persons who carry the **sickle cell trait** are relatively protected against severe disease and death caused by *Plasmodium falciparum* malaria.[6] Although individuals with sickle cell anemia are easily infected, the *P. falciparum* parasite develops poorly, thus causing less illness. People who do not have **Duffy blood group** antigen receptors on their erythrocytes have RBCs that are refractory to infection by *P. vivax* merozoites. Most of the people in West Africa and much of East Africa do not have this receptor (that is, they have the Duffy-negative phenotype) and they are thus more protected from *P. vivax* infection.[7] **Glucose 6-phosphate dehydrogenase (G6PD) deficiency** and some other hemoglobinopathies such as hemoglobin E and thalassemias are more prevalent in malaria-endemic areas and are thought to provide protection from malarial disease.[8] However, these associations are less compelling.

Immunity to Malaria

People residing in malaria-endemic regions acquire immunity to malaria through natural exposure to malaria parasites (acquired immunity). This results only after continued exposure from multiple infections with malaria parasites over time. Humans can acquire immunity to any species of *Plasmodium*. Acquired immunity does not necessarily prevent infection but provides protection against the severe effects of malaria. Thus, after several years of continued exposure, people develop an immunity that limits high-density parasitemia but does not offer sterile protection. Furthermore, acquired immunity can wane and disappear if the individual is not exposed to parasites for an extended period of time. Acquired immunity is both antibody-based and cellular-based, targeting all stages of the parasite. Antibodies can be made to sporozoites, liver stage, blood stage, and sexual stages of the parasite. Antibodies target the parasites and infected cells, marking them for the body's killer cells. Natural killer lymphocytes and neutrophils attack malaria parasites. Macrophages engulf the antibody-targeted parasites and parasitized RBCs and kill them. Antibody-mediated acquired immunity can be transferred from mother to the fetus across the placenta, providing the newborn with some degree of protection. However, this passively transferred immunity wanes within 6 to 9 months, leaving the child vulnerable to infection.[9] Because of a child's immature immune system, children are particularly at risk, as evidenced by the high number of deaths in children less than 5 years old caused by severe malaria.

Clinical Syndromes

Clinical malaria is a spectrum of morbidity and mortality. Malaria can be mild or severe, complicated or uncomplicated, acute or chronic. Severe malaria is almost exclusively caused by *P. falciparum*. It is particularly severe in children under 5 years of age, pregnant women, and nonimmune populations, although both men and women of all ages can be infected and incur severe disease. The nonspecific nature of malaria symptoms makes it difficult to diagnose. Malaria symptoms, particularly fevers, can mirror symptoms from other diseases such as diarrheal disease and other viral and bacterial infections. Thus, malaria can be definitively diagnosed only by laboratory testing, namely microscopy or rapid diagnostic tests, which are discussed later in this chapter. Clinical manifestations may vary with the intensity of transmission and the inoculation rate of parasites into the exposed host. In Africa, where *P. falciparum* is most prevalent, almost all of the severe malaria is in children under 5 years of age. Outside of Africa, where *P. vivax* is most prevalent, all ages are at risk of severe disease

and death. All populations at risk of malaria can be reinfected, because there is no sterile immunity, but the severity of disease may decrease due to a degree of acquired immunity.

FIGURE 15-4 depicts the acute and chronic aspects of malaria infection. Acute disease normally occurs in non-immune populations and begins with a nonsevere fever. Due to the lack of acquired immunity, infected individuals can rapidly progress to severe disease. *P. falciparum* infections can rapidly migrate to the brain, causing cerebral malaria and death. Chronic disease occurs worldwide and causes a great deal of morbidity and mortality. Because individuals can be reinfected in endemic areas, chronic anemia can also develop, even though the individual may be asymptomatic. Chronic infections cause chronic anemia, which in turn leads to developmental disorders and can cause death if left untreated in populations who are anemic and often nutritionally stressed. *P. vivax* and *P. ovale* can cause a **relapse** because the parasite can emerge from dormant liver-stage schizonts. *P. falciparum* and *P. malariae* can **recrudesce** when clinical symptoms abate, but the infection is not entirely cleared from the system; the merozoites multiply, infecting large numbers of RBCs and causing illness (**BOX 15-1**).

Malaria during pregnancy is a unique problem and is particularly dangerous to the mother, fetus, and newborn. Every year approximately 32 million pregnancies occur in areas the WHO considers to be stable malaria transmission areas. The burden of malaria in pregnancy occurs mainly in sub-Saharan Africa, where an estimated 35 million pregnant women live in endemic areas.[10] Among African mothers, 3–15% suffer severe anemia, accounting for 10,000 malaria-related, anemia

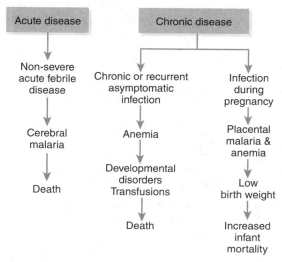

FIGURE 15-4 Acute and Chronic Malaria Infection

- Depending on the species of *Plasmodium* involved, relapse and recrudescence may occur and vary in their effects.
- **Relapsing malaria** means *Plasmodium* can re-emerge from liver stages after the blood stage merozoites have disappeared; this occurs because certain *Plasmodium* form quiescent liver stages called hypnozoites in addition to the erythrocytic stage.
- These hypnozoites can become activated after the initial infection has been cleared.
- *P. vivax* and *P. ovale* cause relapsing malaria because both give rise to hypnozoites in the liver.
- *P. vivax* may relapse from a few weeks up to 5 years and *P. ovale* for 1 to 1.5 years.
- **Recrudescent malaria** occurs when the erythrocytic stages re-emerge after the infection no longer causes symptoms; the infection recrudesces and the patient becomes symptomatic.
- *P. falciparum* and *P. malariae* can recrudesce but do not form hypnozoites, so they do not cause relapses.
- *P. falciparum* can break out for up to 12 months, but *P. malariae* can cause clinical malarial attacks 2 decades after the original infection.

deaths per year. Globally, malaria causes about 30% of low birth weight in newborns and up to 200,000 infant deaths per year.[11] Pregnant women, particularly primagravids, appear to be more susceptible to malaria and are at a higher risk of developing severe and fatal disease.[12] Malaria can seriously weaken the mother, causing hyper-parasitemia and consequent severe anemia, fever, hypoglycemia, and sepsis, all of which impact her ability to carry and deliver the fetus. In the most severe cases, malaria can cause hemorrhaging, killing both the mother and fetus. Malaria parasites can also cross the placenta and infect the fetus, which occurs most often in *P. falciparum* infections. When the fetus is infected, malaria may cause intrauterine growth retardation, preterm delivery, abortions, or stillbirths. A congenital infection in the newborn can cause low birth weight, prematurity, severe malaria, and death.

Cerebral Malaria

As you remember, cerebral malaria is caused by *P. falciparum* because it has the ability to adhere to the walls of capillaries and postcapillary venules. Cerebral malaria is defined as any mental abnormality in a person with malaria. The case fatality rate is 15–25% for children in Africa.[13] Persons at greatest risk include children, older persons, pregnant women, nonimmune persons, and those with a chronic illness. The histopathologic hallmark of cerebral malaria is engorgement of cerebral capillaries and venules with parasitized and nonparasitized RBCs and hypoglycemia. Current understanding of the pathogenesis of cerebral malaria implicates parasitized RBC sequestration in the brain, leading to localized ischemia, hypoxia, and the release of nitric oxide and cytokines, notably tumor necrosis factor, in these areas of sequestration.

▶ Malaria Diagnosis, Treatment, and Vaccines

Malaria Diagnosis (Microscopy, PCR, RDTs)

The definitive diagnosis of malaria requires identification of the parasite in the blood by thick and thin blood smears (**FIGURE 15-5**). The former will identify the presence of the parasite and the latter will identify the species of the parasite; both will help in more effective treatment and case management. For example, if the ring forms or banana-shaped gametocyte are identified, the diagnostician can conclude the infection is *P. falciparum* and treat accordingly. Slide preparation and microscopy require meticulous effort and adherence to methodology; thus, effective diagnosis is a difficult challenge in the field where reagents, personnel, and quality control are often lacking. To address this challenge, new techniques have been developed to make diagnosis easier and improve determining the presence and identification of the parasite.

Malaria can be definitively diagnosed by a biochemical technique called a **polymerase chain reaction (PCR) assay**. The PCRs amplify deoxyribonucleic acid fragments, thus specifically identifying the presence and species of the parasite. Although PCR assays can be used to diagnose the individual, they are too expensive and complicated for general surveillance and clinical diagnosis. A **rapid diagnostic test (RDT)** is an alternative way to quickly detect specific malaria antigens (proteins) in the blood and confirm the presence and species of malaria parasites. The RDTs are often called "dipstick tests" because a drop of blood is collected on a test strip infused with specific reagents. After 15 minutes, the presence of specific bands on the strip indicate if the patient is infected and by what species. In resource-poor settings, RDTs are a reasonable alternative to microscopy for surveillance and clinical diagnosis. But RDTs do have limitations. In remote, tropical areas, high temperatures can affect the quality of the test and reduce shelf life, thus requiring routine resupply. Even though easier than microscopy, diagnosis requires trained personnel and supervisors for accuracy, especially in remote villages. Because malaria can be fatal very quickly, RDTs must be highly sensitive.

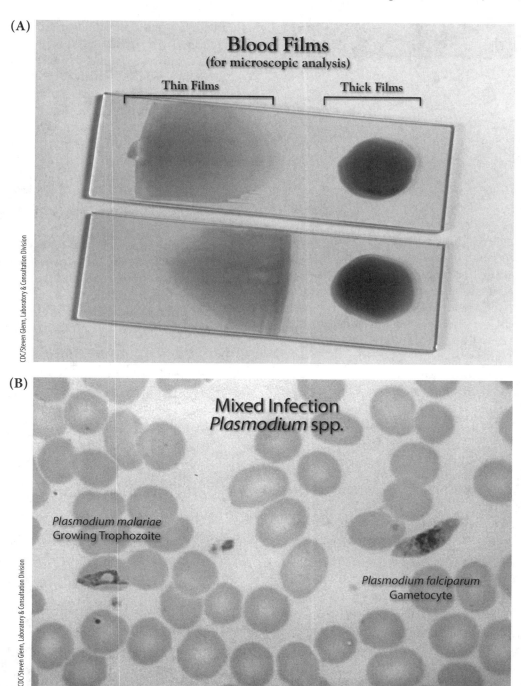

(A)

Blood Films
(for microscopic analysis)

Thin Films   Thick Films

CDC/Steven Glenn, Laboratory & Consultation Division

(B)

Mixed Infection
Plasmodium spp.

Plasmodium malariae
Growing Trophozoite

Plasmodium falciparum
Gametocyte

CDC/Steven Glenn, Laboratory & Consultation Division

FIGURE 15-5 (A) Thin and thick blood smears. The former will identify the presence of the parasite and (B) the latter will identify the species of the parasite.

Lastly, positive tests should be followed by prompt and appropriate treatment, and negative tests should be verified by microscopy. Thus, RDTs are not perfect but can help promote better diagnosis and treatment in remote and underserved areas.

Treatment of Malaria

Accurate and appropriate treatment of malaria is essential in order to reduce malaria mortality and morbidity. Antimalarials have been available for hundreds, if not thousands, of years. Quinine, originally derived from the bark of the cinchona tree, remains an effective antimalarial today. Other drugs such as cholorquine, mefloquine, and sulfadoxine-pyrimethamine (SP) (Fansidar) have been widely used but face growing levels of drug resistance that render them less effective across the globe (**BOX 15-2**). Artemisinin, a relatively new drug for malaria (called qinghaosu in Chinese), was discovered in China where it is traditionally used as medicine for malaria and skin diseases. It comes from the shrub *Artemisia annua*.

- Chloroquine
- Mefloquine
- Quinine
- Sulfadoxine
- Quinine sulfate
- Primaquine
- Artemisinin Combination Therapy (ACTs) (Coartem)

Artemisinin is widely recommended for use in combination with other antimalarials to treat malaria and delay resistance. This is referred to as ACTs, artemisinin-based combination therapies. These ACTs are the gold standard for treatment of uncomplicated malaria, and combination therapy can help delay resistance. Coartem, the trade name for artemether and lumefantrine, is highly effective and was added to the WHO's essential drug list to treat severe and uncomplicated malaria in endemic areas. However, if ACTs are used indiscriminately, resistance will eventually develop to the combination therapies as well. For severe and/or cerebral malaria, intravenous or intramuscular treatment is recommended with quinine or injectable artemisinins. It is important to note treatment must be accompanied by supportive care, including hydration, monitoring of glucose and electrolytes, and transfusion (if severe anemia exists). Treatment for pregnant women involves a prophylactic dose of ACTs during the quickening stage (18–24 weeks gestation) and on through delivery to reduce malaria deaths and congenital transmission.

Drug-Resistant Malaria

As Darwin wrote in the late 1800s, survival depends on who is the "fittest" in a given ecosystem. Genetic mutations drive evolution, enable adaptation, and promote survival. All organisms strive to adapt, reproduce, and survive, including parasites. Developing resistance to drugs is an appropriate survival strategy for parasites, as is developing less virulence in order to allow the hosts to survive so they can be available for future generations of the pathogen. All organisms will adapt if challenged by external forces, be they climate, food availability, or drug toxins. *Plasmodium* species have developed drug resistance to every drug developed to treat and cure the infection. (Similarly, mosquitos develop resistance to insecticides to survive.)

The path to resistance is relatively simple and anchored in natural selection. Drug levels can fluctuate over time based on drug availability, tolerance of the drug by the patient, and the patient's adherence to drug regimens. Some parasites will survive the lower concentrations, and some will develop resistance

naturally by mutation. Mutations in the genes of *Plasmodium* occur spontaneously but are relatively uncommon. However, some of these mutations are associated with reduced sensitivity to an antimalarial drug. In either case, the surviving parasites are "naturally selected" to reproduce, yielding a higher population of resistant forms. If a mosquito bites the infected patient, it can transmit these resistant parasites. These forms eventually become the dominant form, thus giving rise to **resistant malaria**. The realities of drug resistance are depicted in the profiles of resistance to *Plasmodium* species presented in **FIGURE 15-6** and **BOX 15-3**.

Combination therapy is designed to avoid or delay drug resistance. Combination therapy can prevent selective mutations and consequent drug resistance by the simultaneous use of *two or more antimalarial drugs* with different modes of action. Using two or more antimalarials at the same time

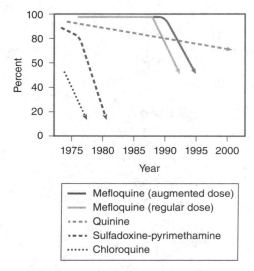

FIGURE 15-6 Resistance to Antimalarials

- Errors in drug prescription and/or administration
- Problems with drug absorption (vomiting and/or diarrhea)
- Fall in drug concentration after passing blood peak level
- Constant mutation
- Abundance of drug in the system
- Migration/displacement/war
- Poor drug adherence by patient
- Poor drug quality – knockoffs/ counterfeits
- Poorly regulated private sector
- Sharing, selling, hoarding conserving by patients and sellers

reduces the probability of parasite resistance to both drugs. For example, suppose we have two drugs, drug A and drug B. Assume the probability of a resistant mutation to drug A is 1 in 10^4 and the probability of a resistant mutation to drug B is 1 in 10^6. Then, the probability of a mutation resistance to both A and B $= 10^4 \times 10^6 = 10^{10}$. Thus, combination therapy will effectively reduce the probability of widespread drug resistance. Drug resistance can also be allayed by accurate diagnosis, treatment, and follow-up by care providers, monitoring drug supply and quality, reducing costs, and simple packaging to promote adherence by the patient. However, natural selection is a powerful force, and scientists are already detecting drug resistance to Coartem.

Malaria Vaccines

It has been said that an effective vaccine for malaria has been 5 years away for the last 25 years. Although promising vaccines exist, to date, no satisfactory vaccines are available to prevent or cure malaria. However, great progress has been made and researchers are looking for a vaccine on three major fronts (**FIGURE 15-7**). The sporozoite vaccine is an **infection-blocking vaccine**. It is aimed at attacking the sporozoite, thus blocking the plasmodium before it gets to the liver. The second is a preventive and curative vaccine. This **blood-stage vaccine** aims at the merozoite stage, blocking merozoite replication, and thus retarding infection and disease. This vaccine is the most promising to date, but dose requirements and efficacy compromise the vaccine's widespread use. The third vaccine aims at the gametocyte and is a **transmission-blocking vaccine**, attacking and killing gametocytes so they cannot infect the mosquito. Most vaccine research efforts understandably focus on *P. falciparum*.

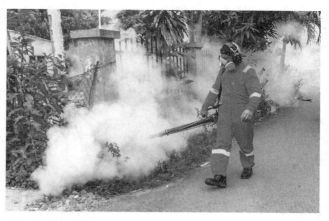
© Yusnizam Yusof/Shutterstock

▶ Malaria Interventions and Control

Malaria Control Policies

Malaria prevention and control are feasible and practical if sound and sustained political and financial commitment is available. Key interventions include antimalarial treatment, personal protection, and vector control. WHO's RBM Program was created to identify appropriate technical interventions and mobilize resources for prevention and control. The program focused on **integrated malaria control**, comprised of three linked interventions: (1) appropriate and effective treatment; (2) personal protection via insecticide-treated bed nets; and, when appropriate, (3) vector control through indoor residual spraying and source reduction (limiting mosquito breeding sites). Integrated malaria control is being implemented in many countries and has received attention and traction at the highest levels of governments worldwide. The RBM secretariat was disbanded in 2015 and that same year the WHO proposed a Global Technical Strategy for Malaria 2016–2030—a blueprint for countries to reverse and eliminate the spread of malaria.

Malaria Control

There is worldwide agreement on the key interventions required to "roll back" malaria. For Africa, the Abuja Declaration of 2001 provided three objectives: (1) 60% of children should receive prompt and effective treatment; (2) 60% of pregnant women should have access to and receive **intermittent preventive treatment for pregnant women (IPTp)**; and (3) 60% of children and pregnant women will possess and sleep under an **insecticide-treated bed net (ITN)**. ITNs are impregnated with a biologically safe insecticide bonded to the net and are being widely distributed

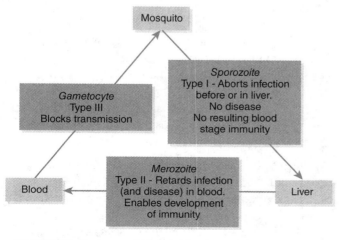

FIGURE 15-7 Features of Malaria Vaccines

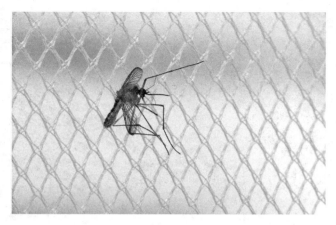

© Milkovasa/Shutterstock

by governments, nonprofits, and the private sector through social marketing campaigns to promote expanded demand and use by mothers and children.

Prompt and effective treatment depends on recognition of the fever, and accurate diagnosis (over 40% of malaria diagnoses are not malaria). Furthermore, appropriate drugs must be available and affordable, and lastly, patients must comply with and adhere to the specific regimen. The private and public sector must ensure counterfeit drugs are not available.

IPTp is prophylaxis for pregnant women; the drug of choice is SP. IPTp begins at about 20 weeks, during the "quickening stage" (the moment the mother feels the baby move), and continues through birth. A minimum of two doses is recommended, but four doses are preferable (one per month). The WHO estimates 32 million women could benefit from IPTp. In order to ensure IPTp effectiveness, pregnant women should attend antenatal clinics (ANCs) within the first trimester and have four visits over their pregnancy. Women should obtain a bed net early in their pregnancy at the ANC. Providers should advise women of the risks to themselves and their babies. An effective partnership with the reproductive health elements of the system is important in order to reinforce malaria prevention for the mother and baby. WHO also recommends intermittent preventive treatment with SP in the first year of life (IPTi). "IPTi reduces clinical malaria, anemia, and severe malaria for infants. Treatment is given three times during the first year of life at approximately 10 weeks, 14 weeks, and 9 months of age, corresponding to the routine vaccination schedule of the Expanded Program on Immunization."[14]

Long-lasting ITNs (LLITNs) represent an effective intervention to prevent malaria; however, they must be used properly and maintained (i.e., holes must be sewn or patched). Mosquitos often bite at dusk or early evening, and children and women may not be in bed yet; thus, they may be exposed. LLITN social marketing (subsidized) programs are widespread and encourage

use. Costs range from $5 to $10 per net and they remain effective for 5–7 years. LLITNs can reduce all-cause child mortality by almost 20% if used effectively. National campaigns improve distribution in endemic areas and raise awareness about malaria prevention and control.

Vector control, through **indoor residual spraying (IRS)**, a somewhat costly and invasive effort, is applied in specific situations where epidemic malaria transmission occurs and logistic-system integrity enables effective application and cleanup. The insecticide is sprayed on house walls and can remain active for up to 6 months. Mosquitos often rest inside on walls before or after blood meals and become exposed to the insecticide. The insecticide kills the mosquito before it takes another blood meal. Another method of vector control is larviciding with biodegradable larvicides. Lastly, source reduction at the community level relies on effective communication and commitment by local leaders, but also on the identification of breeding sites and the availability of appropriate larvicides and/or tools to drain potential breeding sites. (Source reduction is particularly difficult in Africa because the vector, *Anopheles gambiae*, is ubiquitous and breeds in all types of standing water, including puddles made by cow hooves.)

Each intervention holds great promise, as does a malaria vaccine. However, a great deal remains to be done before these goals are realized. Vigilance, commitment, and continued support for appropriate interventions and service delivery are required to successfully control malaria. **FIGURE 15-8** presents how these interventions can be integrated in communities to reduce malaria mortality and morbidity.

▶ Challenges to Effective Malaria Control

Malaria remains one of the most deadly vector-borne diseases on earth. Although great strides have been made in reducing malaria mortality and morbidity, much remains to be done. In Africa, almost every fever is considered malaria, and this makes accurate treatment difficult. Many African countries and rural parts of India have been unsuccessful in using many of the new tools or interventions due to the following:[15-17]

- Weak health systems
- Limited access to health services by large rural populations
- Lack of community knowledge of malaria transmission and symptoms
- Reliance on traditional healers for treatment of fevers

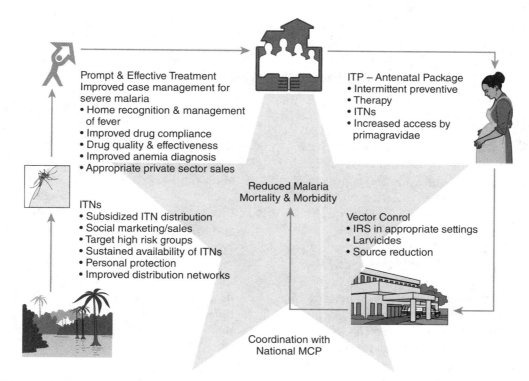

FIGURE 15-8 Malaria Control Interventions

- Lack of skilled providers and poor health provider performance
- Health worker confusion about IPTp-SP guidelines
- Patient skepticism of health risks of receiving SP during pregnancy
- Inaccurate diagnosis
- Inadequate availability of antimalarials, bed nets, and other commodities
- Inconsistent use of ITNs even when available
- Unregulated markets for drugs, inadequate logistics and supply lines
- Less-than-perfect patient adherence to drug regimens
- Educational materials that rely on dominant language literacy

Barriers to sustained LLITN use and IRS application center on costs and logistics for governments, communities, and individuals. Lastly, knowledge and beliefs about the available interventions and recognition of the severity of malaria disease hamper efforts to reduce morbidity and mortality. *It is important to understand that tools and interventions are only as good as their application.*

In summary, the burden of malaria in the personal and social contexts is huge. It is a cause of poverty and a result of poverty, a development issue as well as a public health issue. Controlling malaria will take continued resources and commitments by governments and donors alike. Integrated approaches are essential; there are no magic bullets. Strengthened health systems and infrastructure will improve access to drugs and improve the management of severe malaria. Conserving drugs through accurate diagnosis and treatment is imperative. We are winning the war against malaria, but continued efforts are required to limit malaria morbidity and mortality so that it is no longer a major public health problem.

Key Terms

Anthropophilic
Blood-stage vaccine
Duffy blood group
Erythrocytic schizogony
Exoerythrocytic schizogony
Gametocytes
Glucose 6-phosphate-
    dehydrogenase (G6PD)
    deficiency

Hemozoin
Hypnozoite
Indoor residual spraying (IRS)
Infection-blocking vaccine
Insecticide-treated bed net (ITN)
Integrated malaria control
Intermittent preventive treatment
    for pregnant women (IPTp)
Macrogametes

Merozoites
Microgametes
Oocyst
Ookinete
Parasitemia
Polymerase chain reaction (PCR)
    assay
Rapid diagnostic test (RDT)
Recrudesce

Recrudescent malaria	Schizonts	Trophozoites
Relapse	Sickle cell trait	Tumor necrosis factor
Relapsing malaria	Sporozoites	Zoophilic
Resistant malaria	Transmission-blocking vaccine	

Discussion Questions

1. There exists a debate on the benefits and costs of disease eradication vs. disease control. For malaria, what do you think is the best approach? For this question, define eradication and control, and other relevant terms, state your opinion, and justify your position.

2. What are the major challenges to reducing malaria mortality and morbidity in Africa? How should these challenges be addressed?

3. Define integrated control in your own words. What element of integrated control is the most challenging? Why? What are the challenges facing the development of an effective malaria vaccine?

4. Where are the best opportunities to integrate malaria control in the general public health system? What needs to be done to effectively integrate malaria control in the system?

5. If you were the Minister of Health in Tanzania, and you had a budget of $100 million for all health activities, how much would you spend on malaria, and how would you spend it?

6. Pick a malaria-endemic country in Africa and describe the epidemiology of malaria. Also, describe the present efforts to control malaria in that country including government and donor support.

References

1. Centers for Disease Control and Prevention. The history of malaria, an ancient disease. Available at https://www.cdc.gov/malaria/about/history/. Accessed June 19, 2017.

2. World Health Organization. Malaria. Fact sheet: world malaria report 2016. Available at http://www.who.int/malaria/media/world-malaria-report-2016/en/. Updated December 13, 2016. Accessed June 19, 2017.

3. Centers for Disease Control and Prevention. Impact of malaria. Available at https://www.cdc.gov/malaria/malaria_worldwide/impact.html. Updated April 15, 2016. Accessed June 19, 2017.

4. Paget T. Protozoa. In: Denyer SP, Hodges NA, Gorman SP, Gilmore BF, eds. *Hugo and Russell's Pharmaceutical Microbiology*. 8th ed. Indianapolis, IN: Wiley-Blackwell; 2011.

5. Centers for Disease Control and Prevention. *Anopheles* mosquitoes. Available at https://www.cdc.gov/malaria/about/biology/mosquitoes/. Updated October 21, 2015. Accessed June 19, 2017.

6. Centers for Disease Control and Prevention. Protective effect of sickle cell trait against malaria-associated mortality and morbidity. Available at https://www.cdc.gov/malaria/about/biology/sickle_cell.html. Updated February 8, 2010. Accessed June 19, 2017.

7. Langhi DM, Bordin JO. Duffy blood group and malaria. *Hematology*. 2006;11(5):389-398.

8. Waicman H, Galacteros F. [Glucose 6-phosphate dehydrogenase deficiency: a protection against malaria and a risk for hemolytic accidents]. *Comptes Rend Biol*. 2004; 327(8):711-720.

9. Dobbs KR, Dent AE. Plasmodium malaria and antimalarial antibodies in the first year of life. *Parasitology*. 2016;143(2): 129-138.

10. Chico RM, Dellicour S, Roman E, et al. Global Call to Action: maximize the public health impact of intermittent preventive treatment of malaria in pregnancy in Sub-Saharan Africa. *Malaria J*. 2015;14:207. doi: 10.1186/s12936-015-0728.

11. United Nations Children's Fund. Fact Sheet: Malaria kills 1,200 children a day: UNICEF. Available at https://www.unicef.org/media/media_81674.html. Updated April 23, 2015. Accessed June 20, 2017.

12. van Eijk AM, Hill J, Noor AM, Snow RW, ter Kuile FO. Prevalence of malaria infection in pregnant women compared with children for tracking malaria transmission in sub-Saharan Africa: a systematic review and meta-analysis. *Lancet*. 2015;3(10): e617-e628.

13. Seydel KB, Kampondeni SD, Valim C, et al. Brain swelling and death in children with cerebral malaria. *N Engl J Med*. 2015;372(12):1126-1137. doi: 10.1056/NEJMoa1400116.

14. World Health Organization. Malaria. Available at http://www.who.int/immunization/programmes_systems/interventions/malaria/en/. 2017. Accessed December 18, 2017.

15. Maslove DM, Mnyusiwalla A, Mills EJ, McGowan J, Attara A, Wilson K. Barriers to the effective treatment and prevention of malaria in Africa: A systematic review of qualitative studies. *BMC Int Health Hum Rights*. 2009;9:26. doi: 10.1186/1472-698X-9-26.

16. Sundararajan R, Kalkonde Y, Gokhale C, Greenough PG, Bang A. Barriers to malaria control among marginalized communities: a qualitative study. *PLoS One*. 2013;8(12):e81966. doi: 10.1371/journal.pone.0081966.

17. Mubyazi GM, Bloch P. Psychosocial, behavioural and health system barriers to delivery and uptake of intermittent preventive treatment of malaria in pregnancy in Tanzania – viewpoints of service providers in Mkuranga and Mufindi districts. *BMC Health Serv Res*. 2014;14:15. doi: 10.1186/1472-6963-14-15.

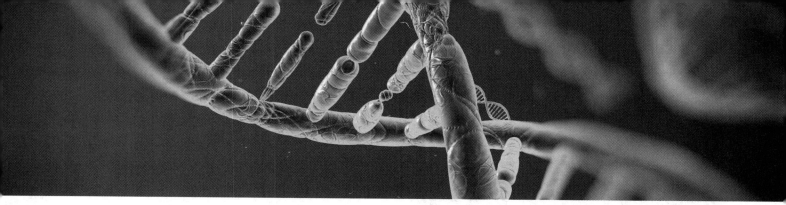

© vitstudio/Shutterstock

CHAPTER 16

Tuberculosis

Victor K. Barbiero

LEARNING OBJECTIVES

By the end of this chapter, the student will be able to:

- Describe the epidemiology and etiology of tuberculosis
- Explain the diagnosis and treatment of tuberculosis and multi-drug resistant tuberculosis
- Compare optimal interventions for tuberculosis control
- Summarize the comorbidities associated with tuberculosis and the HIV–TB interface
- Define the key terms required to discuss tuberculosis as a public health problem

▶ Introduction

Tuberculosis (TB) is the most prevalent disease on earth; over 2 billion people are infected with TB. It kills approximately 1.5 million people annually—about 4,100 people per day.[1,2] The bacteria *Mycobacterium tuberculosis* causes TB; it most often infects the lungs (about 80%) but can affect other parts of the body, such as the bones, kidneys, and central nervous system.

TB is both curable and preventable. A vaccine for TB called the Bacille Calmette–Guerin (BCG) vaccine was developed in 1921. It is recommended as a childhood vaccine in high-prevalence countries to prevent tuberculosis meningitis and **miliary tuberculosis** (widespread, multi-organ TB infection) in children, but BCG does not protect against adult TB.

TB infects over 30 million people annually and approximately 9 million become ill. For human immunodeficiency virus (HIV) negative people, the

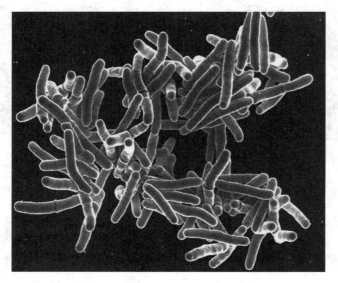

National Institute of Allergy and Infectious Diseases (NIAID)/CDC

lifetime risk of falling ill with TB is about 10%. TB is a leading cause of death in people aged 15–44 (the most productive age group) and kills an estimated 500,000 women annually. TB infects about 550,000 children annually and kills approximately 80,000 HIV-negative children. However, TB is a major opportunistic infection and killer of HIV-positive people, causing about 25% of all HIV-related deaths (i.e., of the 1.1 million annual deaths from HIV, approximately 275,000 deaths are attributable to TB coinfection).

Over 95% of TB cases and deaths occur in low- and middle-income countries (LMICs); South and East Asia have the highest number of TB cases, but Africa has the highest incidence of TB with an estimated case

ratio of 280/100,000. About 80% of reported TB cases occur in 22 countries.

Active tuberculosis (i.e., TB disease) is characterized by cough, fever, severe night sweats, and weight loss, but symptoms may be mild for many months. "People with active TB can infect 10–15 other people through close contact over the course of a year."[1] If left untreated, about one-third of those infected will die, one-third will self-cure, and one-third will remain infectious.[3,4] However, persons with compromised immune systems, such as people living with HIV, with undernutrition or diabetes, or people who use tobacco, and those who are being treated with immunosuppressive drugs, have a much higher risk of falling ill.

TB kills approximately 1.5 million people annually, 360,000 of whom are HIV-positive. About 480,000 **multidrug-resistant tuberculosis (MDR-TB)** cases occurred in 2013, which was about 3.5% of the total cases. TB accounts for about 34 million disability-adjusted life years annually. TB coinfection with HIV fuels TB transmission and makes case management more complicated. Twenty-two high-burden countries account for 80% of TB cases. Africa has the highest estimated incidence with 280 cases per 100,000 population, but the most populous countries of Asia, like India, China, Indonesia, and Pakistan, comprise more than half (56%) of the new cases annually (**FIGURE 16-1**). A TB patient loses 3 to 4 months per year due to illness and an estimated 20–30% of annual household income. In South Africa, probably because of the TB–HIV interface, lost earnings are estimated at up to 16% of the nation's gross domestic product.

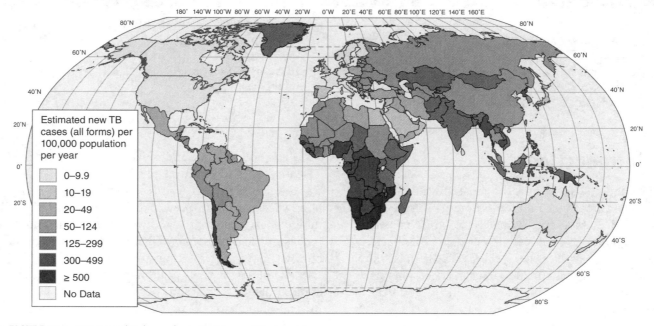

FIGURE 16-1 Estimated Tuberculosis Incidence Worldwide

Reproduced from World Health Organization. *Global Tuberculosis Report 2014*. Geneva, Switzerland: World Health Organization; 2014. Available at http://apps.who.int/iris/bitstream/10665 /137094/1/9789241564809_eng.pdf?ua=1. Accessed November 13, 2017.

About 60% of cases and deaths occur in men, probably due to higher reporting, but also possibly because of greater exposure and perhaps susceptibility. Even so, TB causes more deaths among women than all other causes (i.e., approximately 510,000 TB female deaths annually vs. approximately 280,000 annual maternal deaths). In addition, an estimated 80,000 children died from TB in 2013. About 1.2 million (12%) of the total 10.4 million TB cases reported in 2015 were among HIV-positive people, and approximately 360,000 HIV deaths (24%) were attributable to TB.[5] Africa accounts for about 80% of HIV-positive TB cases and TB-associated HIV deaths. MDR-TB represents a serious issue for TB control. In 2013, about 3.5% of new cases and about 20.5% of previously treated TB cases were MDR-TB; half of those cases were in India and China. Of the 480,000 MDR-TB cases in 2013, about 9.0% (43,000) were extensively drug resistant. Only an estimated 97,000 MDR-TB patients were started on treatment in 2013, with a global treatment success rate of 48%. About 0.9% (43,200) developed **extensively drug-resistant tuberculosis (XDR-TB)**. Worldwide, even with disturbing rates of MDR-TB and XDR-TB, the TB death rate dropped 45% between 1990 and 2013.

▶ Transmission and Natural History of Tuberculosis

TB is spread through the air from one person to another; thus, crowded conditions such as buses, markets, taxis, movie theaters, elevators, and other close-quarter environments are ideal places where the TB bacillus can spread. The bacteria are put into the air when a person with active TB in the lungs or throat coughs or sneezes, speaks, sighs, or otherwise exhales the bacteria into the air (**FIGURE 16-2**). The spray may include millions of droplets containing TB bacilli nuclei, which can remain suspended in the air for hours.[6] People nearby can breathe in these airborne nuclei and become infected. The longer a person is exposed to droplet TB nuclei (for

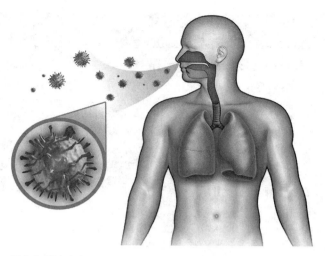

© Andrea Danti/ShutterStock

example, on a crowded bus), the more likely an infection will develop. Although susceptibility to infection may depend on an individual's immunity or the specific strain of bacteria, TB remains a highly infectious pathogen. TB cannot spread by shaking hands, sharing food or drink, bed linens, kissing, or so forth; viable bacilli must be placed into the air from an infected individual and inhaled by a susceptible individual.

It is important to understand the difference between active TB and TB infection. When a person inhales the TB carrier's droplets into the lower airways, the body's alveolar macrophages are attracted and contain the bacteria in the phagocyte's cytosolic vesicles.[7] At this point, the body's immune cells can eliminate the bacteria. However, if the TB bacteria are not killed at the initial site of infection, they can replicate in the lung and cause active TB. This is referred to as **primary tuberculosis**, which occurs in 5–10% of those infected. For most people, the immune system will contain and control the infection; the person will be infected but show no symptoms. This is called **latent TB infection**; that is, the organism is present, but dormant, and the person cannot infect others. The bacteria are walled off in lumps of scar tissue called **tubercles**. At this point, the bacteria can remain dormant for decades or a lifetime, or, it can eventually be eliminated. However, in 5–10% of latent infections, TB bacteria also can become **reactivated**, and the person becomes sick and can transmit the disease to others. This usually occurs because of a weakening immune system (**BOX 16-1**).

The lifetime risk of developing active TB for a non-HIV-positive person is 10%. If a person is HIV positive, or immunocompromised from other conditions, the risk of developing active TB is 10% *annually*. For this reason, the TB–HIV interface is a very important public health issue in terms of TB transmission and TB–HIV morbidity and mortality.

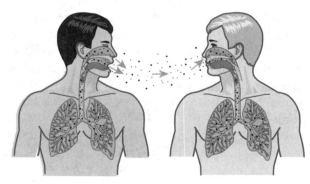

FIGURE 16-2 How Tuberculosis Spreads

BOX 16-1 Tuberculosis Profile

TB Infection vs. Disease

- ■ **TB infection** – The organism is present, but dormant; cannot infect others
- ■ **TB disease (active TB)** – A person is sick and can transmit disease to others if present in the lungs
- ■ **10% Lifetime Risk** – Chance of developing active TB disease in a HIV-negative or otherwise immunocompetent individual
- ■ **10% Annual Risk** – Chance of developing TB disease if coinfected with HIV/or immunocompromised from another cause (cancer, chemotherapy, undernutrition, poorly controlled diabetes)

TB Transmission

- ■ TB is spread through the air via droplets
- ■ TB enters the human body through the lungs
- ■ TB can affect any organ system: lungs, bone, kidney, central nervous system
- ■ 80% of TB cases are pulmonary
- ■ Typical active disease presentation: persistent cough > 3 weeks duration, bloody sputum, decreased appetite, weight loss, general weakness, night sweats
- ■ A person with active pulmonary TB can infect 10–15 other people per year

---

▶ Diagnosis of Tuberculosis

Active **pulmonary TB** is characterized by a persistent cough for more than three weeks, decreased appetite, general weakness, chest pain, blood in the sputum, weight loss, chills, fever, and profuse night sweats. However, not all persistent coughs are TB, especially in LMICs, where a myriad of agents can cause respiratory disease. Due to the risk of contagion to others, timely and accurate diagnosis and treatment are essential.

Sputum smear microscopy, originally developed by Robert Koch in the 1880s, remains the cheapest method for detecting pulmonary TB. The identification of an active infection through a sputum-spear microscopy is a high priority for TB control and treatment. A patient with a positive sputum smear can infect 10–15 people annually. Definitive diagnosis depends on the examination of at least three smears taken at intervals, with at least two smears being tuberculin positive. If microscopy is inconclusive, the patient may be prescribed antibiotics, and if symptoms persist, the patient may be referred for a chest x-ray, which can detect tubercles from the initial infection. However, this is a clinical diagnosis and requires expert skill by the care provider; furthermore, no chest x-ray pattern is absolutely typical. X-ray results may be due to TB or caused by another respiratory condition. Approximately 10–15% of positive-smear patients may not be diagnosed with TB from an x-ray. Lastly, up to 40% of x-ray-diagnosed TB cases are false positives (not TB). Thus, diagnosis is not definitive based on chest x-rays.

In the former Soviet Union, chest x-rays were commonly used to diagnosis and treat pulmonary

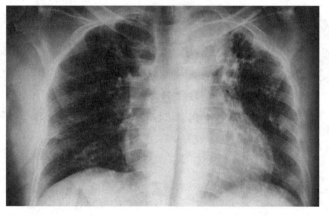

© Puwadol Jaturawutthichai/Shutterstock

TB, probably causing a great deal of misdiagnosis and perhaps giving rise to the spread of MDR-TB. Alternative diagnostics to sputum-smear microscopy and x-rays exist. Sputum culture in liquid and solid media are sensitive and specific; however, these require time (2–8 weeks for a negative classification), sound laboratory technique, and timely follow-up.

A third option for TB diagnosis is the Xpert MTB/RIF test. This self-contained, rapid diagnostic test is based on DNA extraction and molecular nucleic amplification. The Xpert MTB/RIF test is similar in sensitivity to culture and can simultaneously detect drug resistance to rifampicin. It requires specific equipment and at least 1–2 days training for a skilled technician. The World Health Organization (WHO) approved the Xpert MTB/RIF test in 2010. Test results can be obtained in just 90 minutes.[8] However, the equipment and reagents are expensive, but costs will hopefully decline in the future.

▸ Treatment of Tuberculosis

For the most part, TB is a treatable and curable disease. Between 2000 and 2013, the WHO estimates there was a 45% decline in TB mortality and 37 million lives were saved through TB diagnosis and treatment. The control of TB depends on timely and effective diagnosis, and complete treatment of active TB with appropriate drugs. *Implementing a poor TB program is worse than no TB program at all*, because a poor TB program can give rise to MDR-TB and XDR-TB.

The treatment strategy for TB is called **directly observed therapy, short-course (DOTS)**. The DOTS strategy is a clinical intervention and a community-based public health approach to treatment. It focuses on the direct observation of drug adherence by the patient by a relative, a community member, or a health worker, throughout the course of treatment. The strategy is more than an intervention; it is a management strategy anchored in the health system. The WHO DOTS strategy depends on five essential, practical components. These are:

- Sustained political commitment to a national TB program
- Adequate access to quality-assured sputum smears and microscopy
- Regular, uninterrupted supply of quality-assured anti-TB drugs
- Standardized regimens of short-course chemotherapy under direct observation by conscientious observers from the community
- Sound monitoring, reporting, and evaluation for program implementation, supervision, and effectiveness (i.e., clinical drug failures, assessment of success rates, and drug availability and adherence)

New cases of TB are placed on a standard Category I DOTS regimen. DOTS consists of a 6-month regimen of four **first-line drugs**: isoniazid (INH), rifampin (RIF), pyrazinamide, and ethambutol for the first 2 months (8 weeks, 56 doses), and then continuing INH and RIF for the following 4 months either daily (126 doses) or intermittently (36 doses) (2 times per week).[9,10] DOTS is just what it means: a relatively short course of directly observed therapy. Typically, approximately one-third of patients are not adherent, and it is impossible to predict which patients will take the drugs for 6 months and which patients will not. Patients who have failed or interrupted the Category I regimen, or who have relapsed after receiving the full treatment and being considered cured, will be placed on a Category II regimen. This regimen is an 8-month, repeat regimen of Category I drugs, plus an injectable antibiotic for the first 2 months.

As the WHO DOTS strategy aptly states, in order for DOTS to be effectively implemented and sustained, politicians must recognize TB as a public health problem of national proportions and dedicate resources for personnel, training, diagnosis, and medicine. Furthermore, the private sector and public at large need to perceive TB as a threat to their personal well-being and businesses. Yet, in the United States, DOTS is not supported by all health insurance programs. Once an active case is identified, appropriate drugs are required in adequate supply for 6 months. Adherence with the complete DOTS regimen is required for effective therapy; thus, direct observation ensures adherence and appropriate treatment for the entire course. As noted, healthcare workers, nongovernment organization (NGO) staff, community volunteers, religious leaders, and other community members provide observation and usually deliver the medicines to the patient. However, interference with patient autonomy is of ethical concern. Systematic monitoring and accountability are needed to pinpoint problems and learn from successes.

Good drug management for TB treatment (and all other diseases) requires genuine and effective cooperation among the public sector, private sector, and other partners. At the international level, multinational suppliers, procurement agencies, and international donors help ensure an adequate supply of appropriate drugs. Local manufacturers may also play a role in the government supply and distribution system. TB treatment is anchored in sound procurement, adequate stocks, effective and equitable drug distribution, ensuring patient adherence to the full drug regimen (DOTS), flexible selection of effective drugs based on available stocks, current resistance profiles, patient tolerance of the drugs, drug costs, and oversight at the regional, district, and community levels. Lastly, the entire logistics and management system must be framed in a sound policy framework that enjoys sustained commitment from the highest levels of central, regional, and district government (**FIGURE 16-3**).

If regimens are incomplete for any reason, MDR-TB can develop, which is difficult or impossible to cure. China successfully controlled TB through national commitment, a rapid rollout of DOTS, and an organized program anchored in accurate diagnosis and complete observed therapy.[11] Accurate diagnosis of smear-positive individuals is essential to conserve drugs, limit the spread of the bacteria, mitigate drug resistance, and reduce morbidity and mortality. In Russia, the former Soviet Union, and other countries, MDR-TB is a growing concern and will require attention, deep government commitment, adequate supplies of second- and third-line drugs, and sound management by governments, NGOs, and the private sector in those countries.

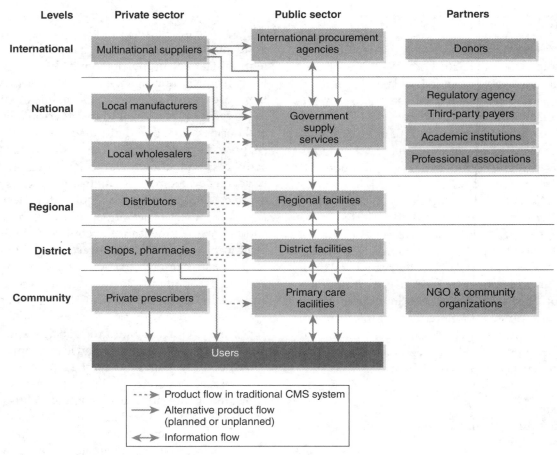

FIGURE 16-3 Drug Management in the Real World

Data from Bloom A. Tuberculosis: Finally Joining This Century. PowerPoint presentation delivered March 5, 2013; George Washington University Global Health and Development Course; PH 3133.

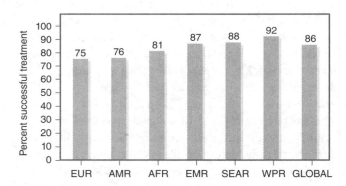

FIGURE 16-4 Treatment Success for New and Relapse Cases Globally and for the Six WHO Regions, 2012

Reproduced from World Health Organization. *Global Tuberculosis Report 2014*. Geneva, Switzerland: World Health Organization; 2014. Available at http://apps.who.int/iris /bitstream/10665/137094/1/9789241564809_eng.pdf?ua=1. Accessed November 13, 2017.

Globally, the treatment of TB has been a success. Successful treatment in most WHO regions approaches or is greater than 80%, with a global average of 86% (**FIGURE 16-4**).[12] The WHO estimates that 5.3 million (61%) of the approximately 10.4 million new cases of TB were treated in 2015. Importantly, the size of the 2012 global cohort of TB cases treated rose from 1 million in 1995 to 5.3 million, reflecting

the success of the global TB effort. Lower treatment rates in the Americas and European regions are likely due to a higher number of patients who were not evaluated, and higher rates of failed treatments or lost patients, or the death of a patient (**BOX 16-2**).

▶ Tuberculosis Drug Resistance

Resistance by the tuberculin bacilli comes in two forms: MDR-TB and XDR-TB; both, for the purposes of our discussion, are manmade.[6,11,12] Although random mutations occur frequently, TB resistance is generally a function of poor drug management and misuse (**BOX 16-3**). TB treatment (and most disease therapy) is not perfect and TB treatment is no exception. Monotherapy vs. combination therapy coupled with imperfect adherence, low-quality drugs, and presumptive therapy all contribute to selective resistance by the pathogen. Today, every TB strain has some form of resistance; albeit those are not widespread, but the potential to spread widely clearly exists. MDR-TB is defined as a TB bacterium that is resistant to at least INH and RIF, the anchors of TB therapy at present. This MDR-TB is curable but requires

---

BOX 16-2 Definition of Treatment Outcomes Used in 2015 Global TB Data Collection

- **Cured** – Bacteriologically confirmed pulmonary TB patient who was smear- and culture-negative in the last treatment and on one previous occasion
- **Completed Treatment** – A TB patient who completed treatment without evidence of failure, but with no record of sputum or culture negativity
- **Died** – A TB patient who died from any cause during treatment
- **Failed** – A TB patient whose sputum smear or culture is positive at month 5 or later during treatment
- **Lost to Follow-up** – A TB patient who did not start treatment or whose treatment was interrupted for two consecutive months or more
- **Not Evaluated** – A TB patient for whom no treatment outcome is assigned; this includes cases "transferred out" to another treatment unit as well as cases for whom the treatment outcome is unknown to the reporting unit
- **Successfully Treated** – A TB patient who was cured or who completed treatment with evidence of sputum or culture negativity
- **Cohort** – A group of patients in whom TB has been diagnosed, and who were registered for treatment during a specific time period

Reproduced from World Health Organization. *Global Tuberculosis Report 2015*. Geneva, Switzerland: World Health Organization; 2015. Available at http://www.who.int/tb/publications/global _report/gtbr15_main_text.pdf. Accessed February 20, 2018.

BOX 16-3 Drug-Resistant Tuberculosis

TB Drug Mismanagement and Misuse

- Poor adherence by patients
- Provision of wrong medicine, wrong dose, wrong length of time for taking drugs
- Inadequate and/or interrupted supply of required drugs
- Poor quality drugs (counterfeits, knockoffs)

Patient Aspects That Give Rise to Resistant TB

- Patients do not take their drugs regularly
- Patients do not take all of their drugs
- Patients develop TB again after being treated in the past
- Patients come from areas where drug-resistant TB is common
- Patients have spent time with someone known to have MDR- or XDR-TB

Data from Centers for Disease Control and Prevention. Drug-resistant TB. Available at http://www.cdc.gov/tb/topic/drtb/default.htm. Reviewed January 17, 2017. Accessed November 13, 2017.

---

second-line drugs (and sometimes third-line drugs) that are more expensive and require extended regimens of 2 years or more. Two newer drugs—bedaquiline and delamanid—show promise in the treatment of MDR-TB. The XDR-TB is resistant to INH and RIF, but also to any fluoroquinolone and at least one of the three second-line antibiotics (amikacin, kanamycin, or capreomycin). The XDR-TB is resistant to the most potent TB antibiotics and is much more difficult to cure (in fact, often it is considered virtually untreatable). XDR-TB is particularly dangerous for people with HIV infection or other conditions that suppress the immune system. These individuals are much more likely to develop TB disease once infected, and also have the potential to spread the XDR-TB strain to other individuals.

Clearly, the most effective way to prevent and mitigate the impact of TB drug resistance is effective therapy anchored in impeccable drug compliance. Doses should not be missed, and therapy should never be discontinued prior to completion, even when the patients' symptoms have disappeared. If patients are not tolerating the drugs well, they should inform their care providers. Avoiding exposure to TB-resistant patients is also important but even more difficult in many ways than high compliance. Five prevention-to-cure priority actions are required for the management and mitigation of MDR-TB (**BOX 16-4**).

▶ HIV–TB Interface and Comorbidities

There is a widespread correlation of coinfection between TB and HIV. A direct relationship exists between HIV prevalence and TB incidence. HIV-positive individuals infected with TB are 30 times

1. High-quality treatment of drug-susceptible TB to prevent MDR-TB
2. Expansion of rapid testing for, and consequent detection of, MDR-TB
3. Immediate access to quality care for MDR-TB patients
4. Infection control
5. Increased political commitment (including adequate funding for current and expanded interventions and research to develop new diagnostics, drugs, and treatment regimens)

Data from Laya BF, Sto. Domingo MCL, Javier XM, Sanchez M. The burden of drug resistant tuberculosis. *TB Corner*. 2015;1(1):1-5.

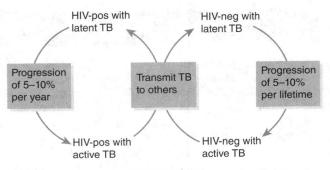

FIGURE 16-5 Impact of HIV–TB Co-Infection

Data from Bloom A. Tuberculosis: Finally Joining This Century. PowerPoint presentation delivered March 5, 2013; George Washington University Global Health and Development Course; PH 3133.

more likely to develop TB disease. TB is the leading cause of death in HIV-positive individuals. HIV–TB coinfection not only contributes to the progression of TB disease morbidity and consequent mortality, but also facilitates the transmission of TB from HIV-positive/TB-positive individuals to both HIV-positive and HIV-negative individuals. Coinfection may also increase the reactivation of latent TB infection and increase the rate of recurrent TB, either by reactivation or reinfection (**FIGURE 16-5**).[9,13]

The expanded implementation of DOTS alone will not control TB in countries with high prevalence of HIV; more aggressive, joint TB–HIV interventions are required. TB control can be a major contributor to HIV treatment and control and vice versa. In 2012, the WHO instituted a global TB–HIV Policy. The Policy has three major elements: establish mechanisms to deliver integrated TB–HIV services; reduce the burden of TB in persons living with HIV; and reduce the burden of HIV in patients with presumptive and diagnosed TB. This integrated approach relies on coordination of planning and service delivery, HIV and TB testing and treatment, reducing the burden of TB in HIV-positive people, and reducing the HIV burden in TB patients (**BOX 16-5**).[14]

BOX 16-5 WHO TB/HIV Policy 2012

A. Establish and strengthen the mechanisms for delivering integrated TB and HIV services

A.1. Set up and strengthen a coordinating body for collaborative TB/HIV activities functional at all levels
A.2. Determine HIV prevalence among TB patients and TB prevalence among people living with HIV
A.3. Carry out joint TB/HIV planning to integrate the delivery of TB and HIV services
A.4. Monitor and evaluate collaborative TB/HIV activities

B. Reduce the burden of TB in people living with HIV and initiate early antiretroviral therapy (the Three I's for HIV/TB)

B.1. Intensify TB case-finding and ensure high quality antituberculosis treatment
B.2. Initiate TB prevention with Isoniazid preventive therapy and early antiretroviral therapy
B.3. Ensure control of TB Infection in healthcare facilities and congregate settings

C. Reduce the burden of HIV in patients with presumptive and diagnosed TB

C.1. Provide HIV testing and counselling to patients with presumptive and diagnosed TB
C.2. Provide HIV prevention interventions for patients with presumptive and diagnosed TB
C.3. Provide co-trimoxazole preventive therapy for TB patients living with HIV
C.4. Ensure HIV prevention interventions, treatment and care for TB patients living with HIV
C.5. Provide antiretroviral therapy for TB patients living with HIV

Reproduced from World Health Organization. *WHO Policy on Collaborative TB-HIV Activities: Guidelines for National Programmes and Other Stakeholders*. Geneva, Switzerland: World Health Organization; 2012. Available at http://apps.who.int/iris/bitstream/10665/44789/1/9789241503006_eng.pdf?ua=1&ua=1. Accessed November 13, 2017.

Furthermore, the WHO also recommends the "Three I's" to prevent and manage TB–HIV coinfection: intensified case finding (to ensure all HIV-positive individuals are tested for TB and the converse: isoniazid preventive therapy (provision of preventive therapy to HIV-positive individuals to help prevent TB infection); and infection control for TB (in healthcare settings to prevent TB spread).[15,16]

TB and HIV are also linked because DOTS can prolong the life of people living with AIDS, and TB control programs can be vehicles for identifying HIV-positive patients, thus making case identification, TB and HIV treatment, and active case management more efficient and effective. Furthermore, DOTS represents an important model for HIV treatment, a regimen that also requires strict adherence to be effective and to reduce antiretroviral drug resistance. However, treatment of a coinfected individual does present some difficulties due to atypical presentations of TB infection (e.g., **extrapulmonary tuberculosis**) and complex interactions between TB drugs and antiretrovirals. Thus, trained healthcare providers are needed and additional investment is required to manage potential side effects and drug interactions, and the milieu of social, clinical, and epidemiologic issues associated with TB–HIV coinfection.

▶ Interventions and Control of Tuberculosis

Globally, TB control is progressing well. The WHO estimates that TB mortality fell by about 45% between 1990 and 2013. Prevalence fell by an estimated 41% during the same period, but more cases are reported due to growing populations and the HIV–TB interface.[12] An estimated 37 million lives have been saved.

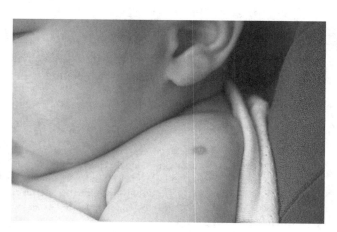

© Kwangmoozaa/Shutterstock

Of the 6.1 million cases reported in 2013, 5.7 million were new infections and 0.4 million were already on treatment. The remaining 3.0 million cases were either unreported or not diagnosed, highlighting the challenges of TB control.

The BCG vaccine is the only licensed TB vaccine in the world. It is a live, attenuated vaccine administered to infants globally, and to neonates soon after birth in TB-endemic areas.

Approximately 120 million people are immunized via the BCG vaccine annually, and over 4 billion people have been immunized since it was developed. It is most efficacious against miliary and meningeal TB in infants and children, but less so against pulmonary TB in adults and adolescents. Because of its limitations, there is concern that without additional or more effective vaccines, the WHO's new Stop TB target to virtually eliminate TB—meaning less than one active TB case per 1 million people annually—by 2050 will not be met.[17]

About 87% of the world's countries are implementing DOTS and an estimated 77% of populations in those countries are "covered." The WHO estimates DOTS treatment success is reported at about 86% in smear-positive patients for all new TB cases. However, much remains to be done, and scaling up access to treatment to ensure full coverage with full compliance, quality drugs, and sustained drug management remains a challenge for the future. Additionally, implementing preventive therapy regimens in high-burden areas is a strategy not yet fully explored. Presently, more than 50 companies are involved with the development of new TB diagnostics, and there are 10 new or repurposed anti-TB drugs in late-phase clinical development.

In 2014, the World Health Assembly approved an End TB Strategy. The overall goal of the strategy is to end the TB epidemic with a 90% reduction in TB deaths and a 90% reduction in new TB cases by 2035.[5] The control of TB is a realistic goal; we have effective drug combinations, a practical drug-delivery stratagem to ensure compliance in DOTS, and a platform bolstered by the HIV–TB interface that can facilitate the identification of HIV-positive and HIV-negative TB cases. As with all control interventions, vigilance, government commitment, system strengthening, fiscal and human resources, appropriate diagnostics and care, better reporting, and improved care-seeking behavior by TB-infected individuals will be required to achieve the objectives of the End TB Strategy and free billions from the worldwide burden of TB.

🔍 *CASE REPORT*

Potential Public Health Nightmare

In 2007, a 31-year-old lawyer named Andrew Speaker caused headline news when he travelled abroad while knowingly infected with TB. During a series of medical visits, a chest x-ray and sputum culture had indicated infection with TB, although Speaker was asymptomatic. His sputum sample was sent for culture, but before the results were available, Speaker and his fiancée left on a previously planned trip to Europe for their wedding and honeymoon. According to government accounts, health officials met with Speaker and urged him not to travel but did not specifically forbid him from doing so. According to Speaker, the language used was unclear, so he did not acknowledge the severity of the warning.

Andrew Speaker and his fiancée flew to Paris on May 12. In late May, the Centers for Disease Control and Prevention (CDC) reportedly contacted Speaker and advised him not to travel home on a commercial airliner because updated test results showed that he had XDR-TB and that a TB clinic in Denver, CO was waiting for his arrival for treatment. The Department of Health and Human Services put Speaker on a no-fly list, but he was already en route from Prague to Montreal. There, he rented a car and crossed the border into the United States. He was flown by air ambulance to the National Jewish Hospital in Denver, where he was put in isolation and started on treatment. Speaker insists that he was repeatedly told he was not contagious.

1. Should Andrew Speaker have been banned from travel to Europe?
2. What steps should the CDC have taken in this case?
3. What was Speaker's responsibility to others?

Key Terms

Active tuberculosis
Directly observed therapy, short-course (DOTS)
Extensively drug-resistant tuberculosis (XDR-TB)
Extrapulmonary tuberculosis

First-line drugs
Latent TB infection
Miliary tuberculosis
Multidrug-resistant tuberculosis (MDR-TB)
Primary tuberculosis

Pulmonary TB
Reactivated
Second-line drugs
Tubercles

Discussion Questions

1. What is the difference between latent and active TB?
2. Describe the natural history and pathophysiology of TB infection. What governs the emergence or reactivation of TB?
3. What are the best ways to diagnose TB? What is the least effective way?
4. Name three ways that MDR-TB can emerge and spread.
5. Why is TB incidence higher in Africa than in Southeast Asia even though Southeast Asia has more TB infections and cases?
6. What are the treatment regimens for Category 1 and 2 TB infections and for the treatment/management of MDR-TB?
7. Describe DOTS. What are the advantages and challenges of the DOTS strategy?
8. Describe the TB–HIV interface. What are the key issues regarding TB and HIV? What strategies exist to mitigate the negative consequences of the TB–HIV interface?
9. What are the five elements of the WHO platform to mitigate the spread of MDR-TB? What challenges are associated with each element?

References

1. World Health Organization. Tuberculosis Fact Sheet – Media Center Fact Sheet #104. Available at http://www.who.int/mediacentre/factsheets/fs104/en/. Published 2015. Updated October 7, 2017. Accessed November 13, 2017.
2. Bloom A. Tuberculosis: Finally Joining This Century. PowerPoint presentation delivered March 5, 2013; George Washington University Global Health and Development Course; PH 3133.
3. World Health Organization. *Global Tuberculosis Report 2014*. Geneva, Switzerland: World Health Organization; 2014. Available at http://apps.who.int/iris/bitstream/10665/137094/1/9789241564809_eng.pdf?ua=1. Accessed November 13, 2017.
4. Centers for Disease Control and Prevention. Tuberculosis Web Page. Available at http://www.cdc.gov/tb/. Reviewed May 6, 2017. Accessed July 7, 2017.

5. World Health Organization. *Global Tuberculosis Report 2016.* Geneva, Switzerland: World Health Organization; 2016. Available at http://apps.who.int/medicinedocs/documents /s23098en/s23098en.pdf. Accessed November 13, 2017.

6. Amor YB. Tuberculosis: the deadly comeback of an old infectious disease. In: Battle CU, ed. *Essentials of Public Health Biology – A Guide for the Study of Pathophysiology.* Sudbury, MA: Jones and Bartlett Publishers; 2009: 311-320.

7. Levine R. Tuberculosis in China – Case 3. In: Center for Global Development, *Millions Saved*; 2000. Available at https://www.cgdev.org/doc/millions/MS_case_3.pdf. Accessed November 13, 2017.

8. Albert H, Nathavitharana RR, Isaccs C, Pai M, Denkinger CM, Boehme CC. Development, roll-out and impact of Xpert MTB/RIF for tuberculosis: what lessons have we learnt and how can we do better? *Eur Respir J.* 2016;48:516-525.

9. Centers for Disease Control and Prevention. Treatment for TB disease. Available at http://www.cdc.gov/tb/topic /treatment/tbdisease.htm. Updated August 11, 2016. Accessed November 13, 2017.

10. Coberly JS, Chaisson RE. Tuberculosis. In: Nelson KE, Williams CM, Grahm NMH, eds. *Infectious Disease Epidemiology: Theory and Practice.* Aspen Publishers, Inc.: Gaithersburg, MD; 2001:411-438.

11. Centers for Disease Control and Prevention. Drug-resistant TB. Available at http://www.cdc.gov/tb/topic/drtb/default.htm. Reviewed January 17, 2017. Accessed November 13, 2017.

12. World Health Organization. *Global Tuberculosis Report 2017.* Geneva, Switzerland: World Health Organization; 2017. Available at http://www.who.int/tb/publications /global_report/en/. Accessed November 13, 2017.

13. Maher D, Harries A, Getahun H. Tuberculosis and HIV interaction in sub-Saharan Africa: impact on patients an programmes: implications for policies. *Trop Med Int Health.* 2005;10:734-742. Available at http://onlinelibrary.wiley.com /doi/10.1111/j.1365-3156.2005.01456.x/epdf

14. World Health Organization. *WHO Policy on Collaborative TB–HIV Activities: Guidelines for National Programmes and Other Stakeholders.* Geneva, Switzerland: World Health Organization; 2012. Available at http://apps.who .int/iris/bitstream/10665/44789/1/9789241503006_eng .pdf?ua=1&ua=1. 2012. Accessed November 13, 2017.

15. World Health Organization. HIV – Scaling up the Three I's for TB/HIV. Available at http://www.who.int/hiv/topics /tb/3is/en/. Accessed November 13, 2017.

16. Skolnik R. *Global Health 101.* 3rd ed. Burlington, MA: Jones & Bartlett Learning; 2016:330-333.

17. Wejse C. Tuberculosis elimination in the post Millennium Development Goals era. *Int J Infect Dis.* 2015;32:152-155.

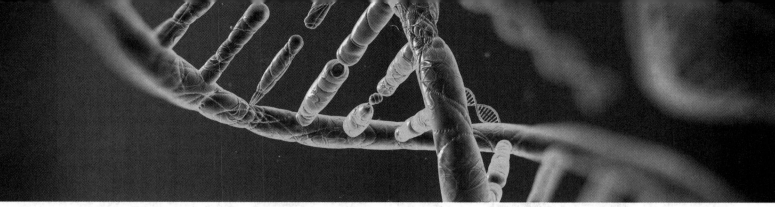

CHAPTER 17

HIV/AIDS

Victor K. Barbiero

LEARNING OBJECTIVES

By the end of this chapter, the student will be able to:

- Describe the epidemiology, natural history, and immunobiology of HIV/AIDS
- Describe the diagnosis and treatment of HIV/AIDS
- List the interventions for the prevention and control of HIV/AIDS
- Discuss the technical and operational challenges to achieving an AIDS-Free generation
- Describe global policy on HIV/AIDS prevention and control
- List the priorities of the major HIV/AIDS multi- and bilateral organizations, NGOs, FBOs, private foundations, and other organizations worldwide
- Define the key terms required to discuss HIV/AIDS as a public health problem

CHAPTER OUTLINE

▶ Introduction

The **human immunodeficiency virus (HIV)** and **acquired immune deficiency syndrome (AIDS)** can be justifiably considered the plague of the 21st century. AIDS was initially recognized publicly in the United States in 1981, and since that time, about 35 million people have died from HIV.[1] Rarely has a single pathogen caused greater consequence on the human condition than HIV/AIDS, and never has there been greater attention, political commitment, and devotion of resources to a global health problem (including smallpox and polio eradication). No cure exists, and although effective drugs are available and drug prices have declined,

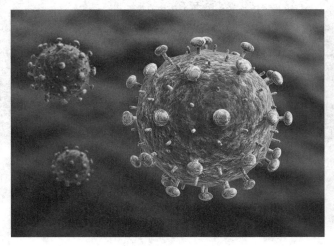

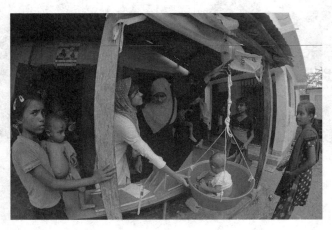

regimens remain toxic and require careful adherence and appropriate clinical oversight. Incidence is declining in some populations,[2] AIDS mortality is slowing, and prevalence is on the rise because of the increased distribution and use of lifesaving antiretroviral (ARV) drugs. It is unclear when an effective **vaccine** will be available, but great progress has been made on defining the natural history of HIV infection and clarifying the immunobiology that governs infection. Laboratory and field research continues to shed light on how the virus can be treated, prevented, and/or cured by drugs or vaccines.

▶ Global Statistics on HIV/AIDS

The World Health Organization (WHO) and the Joint United Nations Programme on HIV/AIDS (UNAIDS) estimate there are approximately 36.7 million people infected with HIV globally; of these, about 1.8 million are children under 15 years of age.[1,3] These figures are updated annually and semi-annually, but importantly, the number of people living with HIV infection is rising due to increased access to and use of treatment and, consequently, survival. With appropriate and timely treatment and care, an HIV-infected person's life expectancy can be similar to that of a non-HIV-positive individual. About 2.1 million new infections occurred in 2015,[3] compared to approximately 3.0 million in 2001 (a 33% decline), and about 1.2 million people died from AIDS-related infections, compared to approximately 1.8 million deaths in 2005.[4]

In 2016, approximately 18.2 million HIV-positive people were on ARV therapy.[3] An estimated 13.4 million children were orphaned because of AIDS, and approximately 150,000 children < 15 years were newly infected with HIV.[3] Awareness

about HIV transmission and prevention in young people has increased from approximately 25% in 2001 to approximately 35% in 2014, implying much work still needs to be done regarding awareness and consequent behavior change to mitigate infection. About 911.4 million men have been voluntarily circumcised since 2008 (as of 2015), and voluntary medical male circumcision (VMMC) remains a key preventive intervention for HIV.[5] In sub-Saharan Africa (SSA), 1.7 billion condoms were procured compared to 0.4 billion in 2001, a 425% increase. Life expectancy for people living with HIV has increased from approximately 36+ years in 2001 to approximately 55+ years in 2014. Investments in the global response for HIV/AIDS have increased from $4.9 billion in 2001 to $21.7 billion in 2015 (**FIGURE 17-1**).[6]

▶ The Epidemiology and Impacts of HIV/AIDS

The majority of people living with HIV/AIDS live in low- and middle-income countries (LMICs). Of the 37 million HIV infections globally, 25.5 million (69%) occur in SSA, and 5.1 million (14%) occur in Asia and the Pacific. However, the prevalence in Africa is about 4.8% and HIV prevalence in Asia is about 0.2%. Africa comprises approximately 73% of AIDS-related mortality (730,000 deaths per year) and accounts for about 827,000 million of the world's 1.8 million new infections (46%).[7] Although other regions have significant transmission and express different modes and drivers of transmission, the burden of HIV infection in Africa and resulting levels of morbidity and mortality require SSA to receive a large share of the global investment into HIV/AIDS (**FIGURE 17-2** and **TABLE 17-1**).

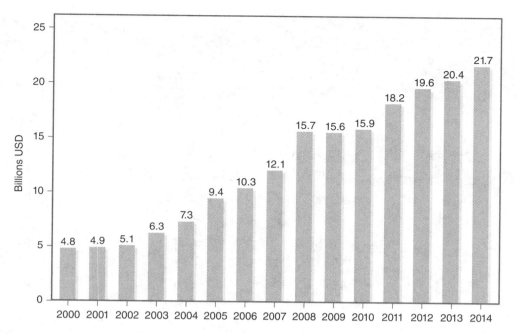

FIGURE 17-1 Global Resources for HIV Prevention and Control, 2000–2014

Data from UNAIDS. *How AIDS Changed Everything*. Available at http://www.unaids.org/sites/default/files/media_asset/20150714_FS_MDG6_Report_en.pdf. Published 2015.

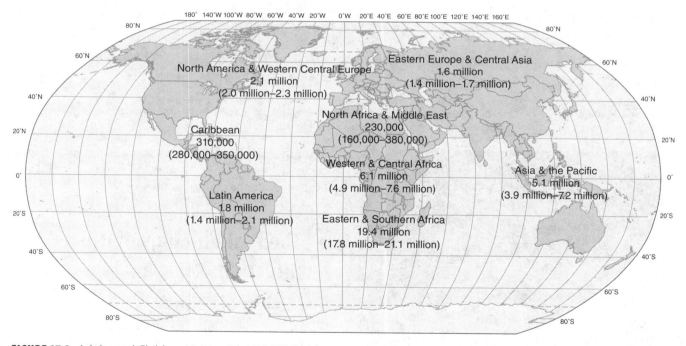

FIGURE 17-2 Adults and Children Living with HIV, 2016

Reproduced from UNAIDS. Core epidemiology slides. Available at http://www.unaids.org/sites/default/files/media_asset/UNAIDS_2017_core-epidemiology-slides_en.pdf. June 2017. Accessed January 4, 2018.

Approximately 17 million (47%) people living with HIV globally do not know they have the virus. HIV is the world's single most lethal infectious disease, yet most people today still do not have access to adequate and affordable prevention, care, and treatment. Although great progress has been made in understanding the immunobiology of infection and viable opportunities to block viral replication, a cure remains elusive. Effective first- and second-line drugs exist and enable infected individuals to live healthy lives and reduce the potential for HIV transmission to others. HIV not only impacts the individual, but

TABLE 17-1   Regional HIV and AIDS Statistics and Features, 2016

	Adults and Children Living with HIV	Adults and Children Newly Infected with HIV	Adult and Child Deaths Due to AIDS
Eastern & Southern Africa	**19.4 million** [17.8–21.1 million]	**790,000** [710,000–870,000]	**420,000** [350,000–510,000]
Western & Central Africa	**6.1 million** [4.9–7.6 million]	**37,000** [270,000–490,000]	**310,000** [220,000–400,000]
Middle East & North Africa	**230,000** [160,000–380,000]	**18,000** [11,000–39,000	**11,000** [7,700–19,000]
Asia & the Pacific	**5.1 million** [3.9–7.2 million]	**270,000** [190,000–370,000]	**170,000** [130,000–220,000]
Latin America	**1.8 million** [1.4–2.1 million]	**97,000** [79,000–120,000]	**36,000** [28,000–45,000]
Caribbean	**310,000** [280,000–350,000]	**18,000** [15,000–22,000]	**9,400** [7,300–12,000]
Eastern Europe & Central Asia	**1.6 million** [1.4–1.7 million]	**190,000** [160,000–220,000]	**40,000** [32,000–49,000]
Western & Central Europe and North America	**2.1 million** [2.0–2.3 million]	**73,000** [68,000–78,000]	**18,000** [15,000–20,000]
TOTAL	**36.7 million** [30.8–42.9 million]	**1.8 million** [1.6–2.1 million]	**1.0 million** [830,000–1.2 million]

Note: The ranges around the estimates in this table define the boundaries within which the actual numbers lie, based on the best available information.
Reproduced from UNAIDS. *UNAIDS Data 2017*. Available at http://www.unaids.org/en/resources/documents/2017/2017_data_book. Published 2017. Accessed January 31, 2018.

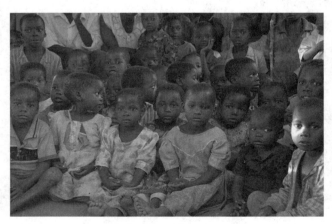

© africa924/Shutterstock

entire families and communities. It affects family cohesion, impacts the care and nurturing of children, and creates large numbers of AIDS orphans. Extended families must care for the ill and other family members, producing financial and emotional stress that permeates the community and can affect the prosperity of entire nations. Labor forces, the armed forces, police forces, the educational system,

agricultural productivity, governance, and national security have all been affected, especially in the high-prevalence countries of Africa.

▶ The Pathobiology of HIV Infection

The Biology of Viruses

Viruses are subcellular agents comprised of single or double strands of deoxyribonucleic acid (DNA) or **ribonucleic acid (RNA)**. They are unable to replicate outside their specific host's cells and are thus classified as **intracellular**, obligate organisms. Viruses are usually species-specific and have adapted pathways to survival for specific hosts. They "reproduce" by invading and commandeering host-cell reproductive machinery. They often destroy parts of or the host's entire cell on their path to replication. They usually target specific cells in a specific host, such as liver cells, respiratory cells or, like HIV, immune cells that regulate the host's immune system. Their specificity is called tropism, and this is governed by four factors: (1) suitable receptors on the host's cells that allow the virion to bind to the cell; (2) the ability of the host cell to support viral replication; (3) the ability of the virus to enter the host cell; and (4) whether the host cell's machinery supports viral viability in terms of infection, replication, and exit. For example, influenza infects respiratory tract cells and infectious droplets can be inhaled by another susceptible host. Enteric viruses infect the gut and are shed through feces and can contaminate water or food. HIV is a bloodborne virus that can infect immune cells and can be shed through body fluids such as blood and semen but cannot survive long outside a human host cell.

Viruses may be pathogenic, causing harm to the host, or nonpathogenic, meaning they infect the host's cells, but are limited in their spread and can be transmitted to another susceptible host before they cause illness or death. An organism's objective is to reproduce; if it kills its host too quickly or kills too many of its hosts, it will not survive.

Viral specificity relates to specific structures on a target–host cell that enable it to attach to that cell in a specific host. These structures are called **receptors**. If the virus finds its receptor, it can attach and enter the host cell and begin to replicate; if not, the virus will continue to "seek" an appropriate cell. If it fails to find an appropriate receptor, or its attachment is blocked in some manner, it will eventually cease to exist in that host.

Viruses have a small genome size compared to bacteria and humans. Although their genetic makeup is relatively simple, they are among the most successful "biologic entities" on the planet. However, viruses are elegant entities in any case. The viral genome contains genetic information that regulates its proteins and nucleic acids, and controls the machinery of the host cell to support intracellular viral replication. Some viruses are comprised only of nucleic acid and a protein coat for structure and protection called a **capsid**. The protein coat also permits attachment of the virion to the membrane of the host cell. In some cases, when the virus leaves the cell through **budding**, it can pick up parts of the cell's membrane, thereby giving the virus an envelope. Certain viruses like HIV may have spikes composed of glycoproteins that can assist in the union of the virus and host cell.

HIV is a member of the *Retroviridae* family and has a single-stranded RNA as its genome. It has a capsid structure and a lipid membrane/envelope and glycoprotein receptors (**FIGURE 17-3**).

Although simple in structure, viruses in general, and particularly HIV, are quite successful in terms of their evolutionary success. Generally, viruses have four

steps that enable them to infect their host: (1) implantation/attachment at the cell's portal of entry by finding specific receptors; (2) local replication within the cell; (3) infection by the virus to organs or organelles; and (4) spread/transmission of the virus to sites where it can enter the outside environment and find new hosts (**BOX 17-1**). Many viruses can exist within the cells of a host and infect other cells at low levels, thus not killing the host, but rather causing mild illness or no illness at all. Some viruses are extremely pathogenic, such as the Ebola virus, but their high pathogenicity will eventually sequester the virus geographically and cause the virus to die out. Most viruses co-exist with their hosts, causing mild illness. As discussed in a following section, HIV replicates quickly in an acute stage, but

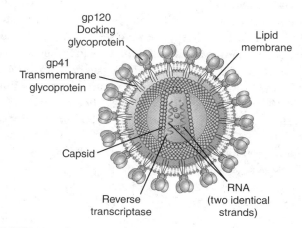

FIGURE 17-3 Structure of the HIV Virion

BOX 17-1 General Steps for Viral Infection in Humans and Other Hosts

- **Implantation** – To enter the host cell, viruses must bind to the cell via specific proteins that attach to specific receptors and enter the cell
- **Replication** – The virus incorporates itself into the nucleus of the cell and its genetic material is replicated using the host cell's own replication machinery
- **Infection** – A new virion is formed, and these exit the cell and infect other cells; thousands can form in one cell, and upon exiting, the host cell is destroyed, causing symptoms and disease, and other cells are infected
- **Spread/Transmission** – New virions can infect other cells and replicate, but also find a way to exit the host and find their way to new, susceptible hosts (HIV can exit the host through body fluids during sex, in the birth canal during labor, or by blood transfusion)

then the amount of virus in the plasma decreases and remains low in the asymptomatic stage. However, in time (approximately 7–10 years), the immune system wears down and eventually gives rise to AIDS, where opportunistic infections eventually kill the host.

▶ Immunity and HIV

Resistance to infectious agents is based on three major aspects of the body's immune system. The first is nonspecific resistance, which basically prevents an infectious agent from entering the body, or destroys it when the pathogen enters at certain points. Skin, tears, and stomach acid represent aspects of our nonspecific barriers against infection. However, these barriers pale in comparison to the nature and specificity of our immune system, which produces battalions of cells and chemicals to eliminate and fight infection. The immune system is complex and consists of many parts that form a cascade of events to kill or otherwise inactivate infectious agents. Textbooks are written on immunology, and a complete discussion of HIV immunology is beyond the scope of this chapter. However, a basic understanding of HIV immunity is important in order to understand how our bodies react to, suppress, and eventually succumb to HIV.

As we know from immunology, the immune system involves the actions of principally two types of white blood cells; namely, B lymphocytes and T lymphocytes (B cells and T cells, respectively). The B cells produce specific antibodies against specific pathogens and/or foreign substances called antigens. The interaction of antibodies and antigens is called humoral immunity or antibody-mediated immunity. Antibodies basically surround the antigen and target it for destruction by other components of the immune system or neutralize it so it cannot enter the cells it was targeting. The process of antibody-mediated immunity specific to HIV begins with the interaction of the virus with the cells of our immune system.

The T lymphocytes have specific proteins on their surface and have different functions, which enable them to produce various, but specific, chemicals to destroy foreign antigens, or signal the production of other chemicals that can destroy the antigen. This part of the immune response is called cell-mediated immunity. These chemical substances are also important to enable the immune system to detect foreign antigens that may enter the body. Once a B or T cell interacts with specific antigens, a small subset of these cells forms **memory cells**, while the others continue to mount a humoral or cellular response to combat the infection. The memory cells circulate in the body for long periods of time, keeping the specific information

on specific antigens. If the same antigen enters the body later, the memory cells will respond to the antigen and mount a rapid, protective, immune response. This rapid response is the foundation of immunity and keeps us from getting reinfected by the same pathogens, like polio, measles, and other infectious diseases. Vaccines can stimulate this immune process by placing dead or attenuated pathogenic agents, or immunogenic parts of agents into the body. The immune response is mounted, but more importantly, the body creates memory cells that convey long-term and sometimes lifetime immunity. It is hard to imagine a more elegant and effective means of protection from disease. However, infectious diseases often develop ways to circumvent the immune system and immune response and, in the case of HIV, infect the very cells that are sent to protect the individual.

Similar to other *Retroviridae*, HIV has a specific replication cycle and must face and elude the body's immune system. Like the immune system, the HIV life cycle is complex, yet simultaneously elegant. Ironically, one class of T lymphocytes contains the surface protein CD4, which facilitates HIV entry to the T cell. Thus, HIV is able to enter the T lymphocyte and destroy it while simultaneously producing billions upon billions of virions that infect and kill other T lymphocytes (**BOX 17-2** and **FIGURE 17-4**).

Unfortunately, the CD4 T lymphocyte is central to the normal functioning of the immune response,

---

BOX 17-2   General Steps for HIV Infection in Humans and Other Hosts

- HIV's major envelope glycoprotein (gp120) binds specifically to the CD4 protein on human white blood cells, the cells at the forefront of fighting infection. This first binding allows HIV to bind subsequently with other white blood cell protein receptors.
- After binding, HIV enters the cell and its single-stranded RNA is converted to double-stranded DNA by the viral enzyme **reverse transcriptase**.
- The new viral DNA makes its way from the cytoplasm to the nucleus, where it is inserted into the human DNA through another enzyme called **integrase**; now the viral DNA is part of the human DNA and each time the human DNA is replicated, so too is the viral DNA.
- New HIV proteins are made when new human proteins are made from the transcription of the human DNA (including the viral DNA).
- New HIV proteins join to form new HIV virions.
- These new virions leave the human cell through *budding*; they mature and become able to infect other T lymphocytes.

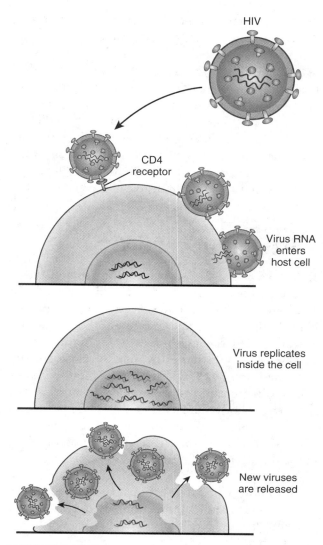

HIV

CD4
receptor

Virus RNA
enters
host cell

Virus replicates
inside the cell

New viruses
are released

FIGURE 17-4 HIV Entry into the Cell

and the destruction of large numbers of these cells over the course of HIV infection eventually causes an impaired immune response or immunodeficiency. This impairment allows other infectious agents, both new and previously recognized, to infect the body. These **opportunistic infections** enter the body, reproduce, spread, and eventually kill the individual. AIDS is the condition when the body's immune system can no longer function, and the individual's body cannot recognize, remember, or contain infectious agents, and thus succumbs to diseases that otherwise would not be lethal.

▶ The Natural History of HIV Infection

As we can appreciate, epidemiologically, HIV is an insidious pathogen. It attacks the human immune system but does not cause symptoms for 2–10 years.

HIV **viral load** peaks in the human bloodstream in about two to three weeks after infection; this is called the **acute phase of HIV infection**.[8-10] At this point, there are few signs or symptoms of infection other than flu-like symptoms, rash, or myalgia (muscle pain). However, the newly infected individual is probably most infectious at this time. The acute stage of infection lasts approximately 3–4 weeks, but seroconversion can take up to 2–3 months. Acute infection is characterized by persistently infected T cells, and the release of considerable amounts of the virus. At this point, the viral load typically will be very high and the CD4 count drops dramatically. After seroconversion, antibodies are produced, and the body limits the spread of the virus but does not eliminate the virus or eliminate viral replication. At this stage of infection, the infected individual still exhibits few symptoms; this stage is called **clinical latency (asymptomatic stage)**. The immune system is working well, albeit viral replication is still going on. The virus appears to be held in a quasi-steady state of infection, but after briefly recovering, the CD4 T cell count continues to decline over time. The asymptomatic stage can last a few years or a decade or more. In the later stage of infection (i.e., AIDS), CD4 counts are low (usually < 200 CD4 T cells/mm³), and the infected individual suffers from, and eventually succumbs to, opportunistic infections[9] (**TABLE 17-2**).

In high-income countries, the presence of HIV can be detected during the acute phase by identifying viral DNA via a polymerase chain reaction assay. However, at present, these tests are not widely available in LMICs and the rapid tests are antibody-based. In the acute phase of HIV infection, the virus cannot readily be detected because antibody levels are low or have not yet been made by the body. In this stage, the individual shows no symptoms but is the most highly infectious because of a high viral load in the blood. After the third week, antibodies rise to reduce the amount of circulating virus and a low level of "viral load" is maintained until later in life when the immune system wanes and the virus begins to replicate once more, giving rise to AIDS.

This model is worrisome because it implies that effective prevention is required during the acute phase of infection. Typically, only 50% of those in less-developed countries know their HIV status, and their perception of high-risk acts (multiple sex partners, needle sharing, etc.) is often weak. Given the high transmission potential of HIV in the acute phase, the virus can and does spread even though comprehensive prevention measures are in place, because these measures do not routinely focus on the relative risk of infection in the first weeks and months of infection.

TABLE 17-2 Opportunistic Infections in HIV/AIDS Cases

AIDS Opportunistic Infection

Candidiasis of bronchi, trachea, or lungs
Candidiasis, esophageal
Cervical cancer, invasive
Coccidioidomycosis, disseminated or extrapulmonary
Cryptococcosis, extrapulmonary
Cryptosporidiosis, chronic intestinal (duration > 1 mo)
Cytomegalovirus disease (other than liver, spleen, or nodes)
Cytomegalovirus retinitis (with vision loss)
Encephalopathy, HIV-related
Herpes simplex: chronic ulcer or ulcers (duration > 1 mo) or bronchitis, pneumonitis, or esophagitis
Histoplasmosis, disseminated or extrapulmonary
Isosporiasis, chronic intestinal (duration > 1 mo)
Kaposi sarcoma
Lymphoma, Burkitt (or equivalent term)
Lymphoma, immunoblastic (or equivalent term)
Lymphoma, primary, of the brain
Mycobacterium avium complex or *Mycobacterium kansasii* infection, disseminated or extrapulmonary
M. tuberculosis infection, any site (pulmonary or extrapulmonary)
Mycobacterium infection with other species or unidentified species, disseminated or extrapulmonary
Pneumocystis pneumonia
Pneumonia, recurrent
Progressive multifocal leukoencephalopathy
Salmonella septicemia, recurrent
Toxoplasmosis of the brain
Wasting syndrome due to HIV infection

Data from Centers for Disease Control and Prevention. Opportunistic Infections. Available at https://www.cdc.gov/hiv/basics/livingwithhiv/opportunisticinfections.html. Updated May 30, 2017.

Intervention programs need to promote deeper individual perceptions of risk coupled with knowledge of HIV status, secondary abstinence, monogamy, correct and consistent condom use, and risk-based testing and counseling soon after a perceived high-risk act takes place. Even with the success achieved over the last 15 years, a greater understanding of HIV transmission is still required today in order to mount sound prevention interventions at the appropriate time.

Curiously, there are certain individuals that can be infected with HIV, but the infection does not progress to full-blown AIDS. These individuals are called **long-term non-progressors**. These individuals comprise approximately 5% of the HIV-infected population. Non-progressors have detectable viral loads (although

low) but maintain normal CD4 counts.[11] Even if their CD4 count drops, it does not drop low enough to cause immunosuppression and make the individual susceptible to opportunistic infections or to have the individual classified as having AIDS. Long-term non-progressors can transition to progressive infections over time and develop AIDS. These individuals are being studied to try to find out why their body tolerates HIV infection, why their immune systems are less affected, and what mechanisms are responsible for limiting HIV infection and conveying a significant degree of protection.

▶ Transmission of HIV

HIV can be transmitted via blood, semen, vaginal fluids, breast milk, in utero, and during labor. HIV has to be transmitted directly though specific body fluids from one person to another. It cannot be transmitted through air or water, contact with the skin of an infected individual, or close contact other than sex (**BOX 17-3**). Thus, HIV is entirely preventable if precautions are applied to prevent the exchange of body fluids with an infected person to a noninfected person, or vertically from mother to child. Viral concentration in body fluids depends on the duration of HIV infection and the success of treatment. We know how HIV is transmitted, and we know how to avoid infection; the key is to appreciate the relative risk of infection and to take proper precautions to avoid infection. This seems a simple task, but today, with around 2 million new HIV

BOX 17-3 HIV Transmission Routes

HIV can be transmitted by:

- Semen
- Vaginal fluid
- Blood
- During pregnancy (in utero)
- During labor
- Breast milk

HIV cannot be transmitted by:

- Saliva
- Tears
- Sweat
- Vomit
- Urine
- Feces
- Water

infections occurring annually, transmission routes remain robust.

Sexual Transmission of HIV

HIV is present in semen, vaginal fluids, and cervical fluids. Semen contains a higher concentration of HIV than vaginal fluid. Viral concentration can change due to the duration of infection and/or treatment as well as during menstruation. Unprotected sex (whether heterosexual or homosexual) is considered a high-risk behavior for HIV transmission. Sexual activities that cause trauma and increase exposure to blood by infected semen or other body fluids represent the highest risk of infection. Receptive penile-anal intercourse is the highest risk because it causes microscopic tears in the rectum. Tears in the vaginal lining can also occur during penile-vaginal intercourse, but not as easily. This does not imply an infected woman does not pose a risk to her male partner; indeed, significant risk exists, but the risk is considered lower. Similarly, oral sex performed on an HIV-infected partner (male or female) is also risky, although of lower risk,[12] as HIV might enter microscopic tears in the mouth and cause transmission. Deep kissing theoretically may also effect transmission if the noninfected partner has microscopic tears in his or her mouth, but this is not considered a significant route of HIV infection.

Transmission of HIV by Blood

There are a number of ways that HIV can be transmitted by blood. In the past, blood transfusions posed an important risk due to poor applications of blood safety. However, over the last 10–15 years, blood safety has improved in many countries and although blood transfusion can be risky in some places, today it is a declining transmission issue. In fact, in Canada, blood donations are now accepted from men who have sex with men (MSM), provided their last sexual contact (with another man) was > 5 years prior.[13] Even in high-prevalence SSA countries, blood transfusions reportedly account for a low proportion of new HIV infections.[14] Still, in some countries, blood transfusions may remain risky because of less extensive blood donor selection, poor quality control concerning sterility of blood and equipment, and, generally poor blood-testing practices.

Perhaps the most important bloodborne transmission of HIV involves injecting chemical substances while sharing needles. Injecting drug users (IDUs) represent small but often very high-risk populations for HIV exposure and infection. IDUs in the United States represent a significant at-risk population, and this is especially concerning as across all U.S. demographic groups, injection drug use is on the rise.[15] IDUs also help drive HIV transmission in Russia and the former Soviet Union. Africa, South Asia, and East Asia have significant IDU populations as well. Needle exchange policies and programs can be effective but require sound management, support, and strict adherence by the users. **Harm reduction** must also be considered when attempting to reduce HIV transmission among IDUs; it may include methadone treatment, safe needle exchanges, and policies that reduce stigma associated with injecting drug use and IDUs in general. Harm reduction may be defined as: *a set of practical strategies and ideas aimed at reducing negative consequences associated with drug use; it is also a movement for social justice built on a belief in, and respect for, the rights of people who use drugs.*[16] Issues associated with harm-reduction strategies and policies are complex and often there is a lack of consensus among governments, politicians, technicians, communities, and IDU populations regarding the approval and implementation of such strategies. However, harm reduction can be an important tool in the holistic approach to reducing HIV transmission among IDUs, their partners, and their communities. Some data indicate that opioid agonist therapy, needle and syringe programs, and HIV testing and treatment for IDUs are the most effective and cost-effective public health interventions for IDUs, when implemented singly or in combination.[15]

Two other possibilities of HIV infection through blood involve piercing/tattooing and injection of steroids. In both of these situations, individuals may share needles/tools or the needles may not be cleaned properly prior to reuse.

Mother-to-Child Transmission

The WHO states, "In the absence of any interventions, transmission rates [from mother to child] range from 15 to 45%. This rate can be reduced to below 5% with effective interventions during the periods of pregnancy, labor, delivery, and breastfeeding."[17]

Mother-to-child transmission (MTCT; vertical transmission) is relatively rare in the United States and other high-income countries because most pregnant women in these countries seek and obtain high-quality prenatal care and are tested for HIV. If found to be infected, these women are given ARV therapy during the second and third trimesters, which lowers the possibility of infection to the fetus dramatically. Furthermore, performing a cesarean section rather than vaginal delivery lowers the percentage even more. Because breast milk has been shown to transmit HIV (as high as 15% infection rates), HIV-positive women in high-income countries can formula-feed their infants with minimal risk.

In low-income countries, especially in Africa where HIV average crude prevalence is 5% or more, options for prevention of MTCT are more limited. Cesareans are not often available, and formula can be contaminated with non-potable water. Thus, from a public health point of view, the benefits of breast-feeding outweigh the risks of not breastfeeding for the infant in low- and even in some middle-income countries, regardless of the HIV status of the mother. Further, not all women in low-income countries know or understand the periods of potential MTCT, nor do they have adequate knowledge of preventive MTCT strategies.[18] The global investments in ARV therapy now enable many women to access ARVs during their pregnancy to prevent MTCT. In 2015, 23% of pregnant HIV-positive women still did not have access to ARVs, leading to 150,000 children infected with HIV.[19]

▶ Diagnosis and Treatment of HIV Infection

HIV Testing and Diagnosis

Testing for HIV infection is one of the most important prevention interventions. Even with all the tremendous investments in HIV prevention and control, estimates indicate that approximately 40% of people infected with HIV do not know their HIV status.[20] Access to rapid, affordable, and accurate diagnosis (linked to appropriate counseling and follow-up) is essential to the long-term control and management of HIV in Africa and other low- or middle-income regions.

There are three types of HIV diagnostic tests: (1) antibody tests; (2) antigen/antibody combination tests; and (3) RNA tests. Antibody tests detect antibodies (that is, proteins that your body makes against HIV); they do not detect HIV itself. Antigen/antibody tests and RNA tests detect HIV directly. Antigen/antibody and RNA tests can detect infection in blood before antibody tests. Some newer antigen/antibody lab tests can sometimes find HIV as soon as 3 weeks after exposure to the virus. Blood tests can detect HIV infection sooner after exposure than oral fluid tests because the level of antibody in blood is higher than it is in oral fluid. No antigen/antibody or RNA tests are available for oral fluid.

In high-income countries, initial HIV tests will either be an antibody test or antigen/antibody tests. Initial HIV testing in LMICs most often is based on antibody tests because of cost, ease of use, and timeliness of results. If someone is found to have antibodies to HIV, they are then considered *seropositive* or *HIV positive*. Today, a number of rapid diagnostic tests (RDTs) exist, some of which are available as in-home test kits. Most HIV RDTs are blood-based or oral-fluid-based antibody tests that provide results on the antibody status of an individual in 30 minutes. However, the drawback of these tests is that they can only detect seropositivity 6–12 weeks after infection; this is called *the window period*. The costs of these tests vary, but they may be as low as $0.50 per test.[21]

Treatment of HIV Infection

Because HIV (and other viruses) often use the human cells' own structures and processes to replicate, it is very difficult to design drugs that specifically attack the virus and do not impair or destroy our own cells. Drugs designed against HIV have been developed to interfere with the entry and replication of HIV in the human cell. Highly active antiretroviral therapy (HAART) is a combination of drugs that must be taken each day, exactly as prescribed. HAART does not cure but reduces the viral load in the body so the immune system can recover and fight off opportunistic infections, thus promoting survival and wellness. By reducing viral load, HAART also reduces the efficiency of transmitting the virus; thus, HAART can be considered a prevention intervention as well. There are six ARV drug classes grouped according to how they fight HIV infection (**BOX 17-4**).[22] Even though these drugs are highly effective (but not without toxicity), HIV can still survive in the body, albeit at very low levels. It still has a lifelong potential to rebound, increase the viral load of the individual, and cause illness and death. Thus, compliance is essential by the individual and consistent stocks of ARVs must be on hand at the system level

BOX 17-4 HIV ARV Drug Classes

- **NNRTIs** – Non-nucleoside reverse transcriptase inhibitors
- **NRTIs** – Nucleoside reverse transcriptase inhibitors
- **PIs** – Protease inhibitors
- **FIs** – Fusion inhibitors
- **CCR5s** – CCR5 antagonists (entry inhibitors)
- **INSTIs** – Integrase strand transfer-inhibitor

Data from U.S. Food and Drug Administration. Antiretroviral drugs used in the treatment of HIV infection. U.S. Department of Health and Human Services. Available at https://www.fda.gov/forpatients/illness/hivaids/treatment/ucm118915.htm. Updated January 4, 2018. Accessed January 22, 208.

BOX 17-5 HIV Risk Factors

- Having unprotected anal or vaginal sex
- Having another sexually transmitted infection (STI) such as syphilis, herpes, chlamydia, gonorrhea, or bacterial vaginosis
- Sharing contaminated needles, syringes, and other injecting equipment and drug solutions when injecting drugs
- Receiving unsafe injections, blood transfusions, or medical procedures that involve unsterile cutting or piercing
- Experiencing accidental needle stick injuries, including those among health workers

Reproduced from World Health Organization. HIV/AIDS Fact Sheet. Available at http://who.int/mediacentre/factsheets/fs360/en/. Updated November 2017. Accessed December 18, 2017.

to ensure those on treatment have a continuous ARV supply for life.

Efforts to develop an effective and affordable vaccine to prevent or cure HIV infection continue. Although much has been learned about HIV immunobiology, a good vaccine remains elusive. Regrettably, we still do not have a clear picture of what is needed to produce a vaccine against HIV, although nonhuman primate models currently show the most promise.[23] A confounding issue rests in the fact that HIV often mutates (i.e., it changes its antigenic fingerprint), thus eluding the body's immune system. However, promise has been shown in targeting broadly neutralizing antibodies, which are powerful antibodies with the ability to fight HIV strains through binding to specific sites on the virus.[24] Further, data show that a staged immunization process may be the best hope for a vaccination strategy.[25] Efforts to find an HIV vaccine will continue; however, the virus' mutation potential and antigenic variance make finding a successful vaccine difficult. Furthermore, when an effective vaccine is developed, it must be tested, found to be effective, affordable, and then delivered. Therefore, the real key to an HIV vaccine is not only the vaccine itself, but the supply and delivery system that will be required to deliver the vaccine to all of those who need it. As of this writing, two new HIV vaccines with the potential to cover multiple strains of the virus are headed to phase II clinical trials.[26]

▶ Prevention and Control of HIV

Individuals can be exposed to, and infected with, HIV in a variety of ways. Health behaviors, socioeconomic status, substance use and abuse, sexual orientation, pregnancy, gender, occupation, religious beliefs, and many other factors can influence whether an individual becomes infected or avoids infection. HIV risk factors are clear and all are preventable (**BOX 17-5**). The prevention of HIV clearly depends on the tools and interventions we have available to prevent infection, but prevention can succeed only if those tools and interventions are applied and practiced by individuals at risk with consistency and ardor.

During the initial years of the HIV response, country epidemics were categorized as concentrated or generalized. A **concentrated epidemic** is characterized by transmission anchored in high-risk populations such as sex workers, truck drivers, prisoners, IDUs, and MSM. A **generalized epidemic** portrays a more diverse risk and spread of infection, with transmission occurring frequently beyond high-risk populations and spreading within the general population. Today, in SSA, HIV is considered a generalized epidemic. Indeed, the infection has become **endemic**, implying the population at-large is at significant risk. Thus, although high-risk groups still exist across the globe and can be a major force of infection (sub-epidemics),[27] prevention must be offered and practiced by the general population worldwide.

Condoms remain an important commodity in the prevention and control of HIV. Correct and consistent condom use of male and female condoms during vaginal or anal sex can protect against the spread of HIV and other sexually transmitted infections (STIs). Evidence shows male condoms have an 85% or greater protective effect against HIV and other STIs. Female condoms are also effective but are not as widely used as male condoms. The key to condom effectiveness and impact is correct and consistent use during sex. Factors influencing consistent use include females'

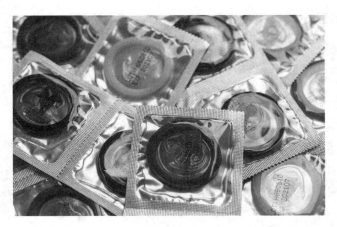

© Purple Anvil/Shutterstock

ability to negotiate male partner use, incomplete knowledge of STIs, condom use skills, motivation, access/availability,[28] and cultural beliefs (e.g., that contact with vaginal fluids during sex will promote wound healing).[29]

The WHO strongly advises voluntary testing and counseling (VTC) for all people exposed to any HIV (and other STI) risk factors. People who know their status usually seek treatment and practice safe sex. Thus, those who know their status can contribute to HIV prevention. The WHO also recommends testing and counseling for couples, especially in high prevalence countries. VTC for couples is especially important because if couples are discordant (that is, one person is HIV-positive, the other HIV-negative), it is important to know their respective status in order to eliminate or reduce the risk of infection.

Given the interface between HIV and tuberculosis (TB), the early detection and treatment of TB and linkage of TB treatment to HAART can prevent HIV and TB deaths. The WHO recommends HIV testing services integrate screening for TB, and that all individuals diagnosed with HIV and active TB begin ARV therapy.

VMMC is a cost-effective intervention with long-lasting benefits that when safely conducted by skilled providers can reduce the risk of heterosexually acquired HIV infection by approximately 60%. VMMC is a key intervention in generalized epidemics where HIV prevalence is high and rates of male circumcision are low. The 2016–2021 UNAIDS Strategy includes a target goal that 27 million more males will undergo VMMC in high-prevalence areas by 2020.[30]

If an HIV-positive pregnant woman is provided with ARV drugs throughout pregnancy, labor, delivery, and breastfeeding (when infection can occur), HIV transmission can be nearly fully prevented. The WHO recommends providing ARVs to mothers and infants during pregnancy, labor, and the postnatal period. The

WHO also recommends lifelong treatment be offered to HIV-positive pregnant women regardless of their CD4 count. Many countries are adopting this strategy to prevent MTCT. In 2014, the WHO estimated 1.1 million (approximately 73%) of the 1.5 million pregnant women living with HIV globally received effective ARV drugs to prevent MTCT. Challenges to this approach include women with limited access to family planning services, low rates of testing and treatment coverage for children, and nonadherence to treatment throughout the breastfeeding period (with some data showing higher end-of-breastfeeding transmission rates than at the 6-week breastfeeding marker).[31] Another challenge involves the influence of partner dynamics—specifically, intimate partner violence (IPV). The control asserted by a violent partner can reduce a woman's access to the support needed to maintain treatment. Further, IPV-related depression may lead some women to intentionally stop their treatment. For other women, nondisclosure of their serostatus to their partner may be a safety strategy (i.e., withholding the information to avoid violence). This creates significant complications for a woman trying to adhere to treatment, as she may need to hide medications from her partner.[32]

ARV treatment as prevention is another effective strategy. If an HIV-positive person adheres to effective ARV therapy, the risk of transmitting the virus can be reduced by 96%. For discordant couples, the WHO recommends offering ARV drugs to the HIV-positive partner, regardless of his or her CD4 count.

Oral pre-exposure prophylaxis (PrEP) is the daily use of ARV drugs by HIV-negative people to prevent HIV infection. A number of randomized controlled studies have demonstrated the efficacy of PrEP in reducing HIV transmission among a range of populations, including discordant heterosexual couples, MSM, transgender women, high-risk heterosexual couples, prisoners, and IDUs. Given the costs and difficulties of implementing PrEP globally, at this time, the WHO recommends PrEP as an additional HIV prevention choice within a comprehensive HIV prevention package for MSM. Broadening the delivery of PrEP may be considered in the future, and under specific circumstances, but costs, adherence, access, availability, and other systemic issues need to be considered.

Post-exposure prophylaxis (PEP) is the use of ARV drugs within 72 hours of exposure to HIV to prevent infection. PEP treatment includes counseling, care, HIV testing, and administering a 28-day course of ARV drugs with follow-up care. First and foremost, the individual must recognize/perceive a risky sexual act and seek PEP in order for this prevention strategy to be effective. In 2014, the WHO recommended PEP use for both occupational and nonoccupational exposures for adults and children. Simpler ARV drug regimens for PEP include ARVs already being used in treatment and imply easier prescribing, better adherence and increased completion rates. Again, this prevention strategy depends on the individual's recognition of a high-risk situation where HIV could be transmitted either by occupational exposure, unprotected sexual exposure, or sexual assault.

The prevention of HIV transmission for injecting drug users includes using sterile injecting equipment (including needles and syringes) for each injection (i.e., harm reduction). The WHO recommends a comprehensive IDU prevention package for HIV prevention and treatment. This package includes needle and syringe programs; opioid substitution therapy; HIV testing and counseling; HIV treatment and care; access to condoms; and management of STIs, TB, and viral hepatitis. Politically, harm reduction is controversial but nonetheless remains an important prevention strategy for IDUs and their partners.

Behavior Change/Behavior Formulation/Communication

The technical prevention interventions already mentioned require an understanding of the interventions, the risks associated with HIV exposure, and a willingness by individuals and communities to practice preventive behaviors and seek counseling and treatment when potential exposure occurs. Targeted and general information is required to reach high-risk groups and the general population respectively. Monogamy, delay of sexual debut, correct and consistent condom use, prevention of MTCT, and perceiving/recognizing a risky act depend on the individuals' desire and capacity to prevent transmission. Focusing on younger age groups can establish behavioral norms that will continue through adulthood. Information and education for high-risk groups will contribute to transmission-reduction behaviors. However, behavior change takes time and requires ongoing attention and effort customized to address regional and cultural norms, and the social and economic determinants of HIV transmission.

Significant challenges to HIV prevention and control remain and they run the gamut from system strengthening to cultural attitudes toward sex, survival, and faith (**BOX 17-6**). These challenges are realized in the fact that although the new annual number of HIV infections has declined by approximately 37% from 2001–2015 (3.15 million to 2 million), 2 million new infections still occur worldwide, and 1.1 million

---

> **BOX 17-6** Selected Challenges to HIV Prevention and Control
>
> - Limited health infrastructure (both physical and human)
> - Perception of risk by individuals and communities
> - Cultural norms associated with sexual behavior and HIV transmission
> - The technical and outreach capacity of public and private sectors
> - Community preparedness, mobilization, and ownership of HIV prevention programs
> - Recurrent costs to governments and patients
> - Overcoming stigma associated with testing, drug adherence, and community perceptions
> - The need for objective, compassionate, and non-judgmental, skilled providers
> - Going to scale including building the capacity in local health systems and reducing drug prices to affordable levels for governments
> - Expanding testing and counseling to better understand HIV status by the individual and at the national level
> - More appropriate technology for diagnosis and treatment in LMICs
> - Lifetime treatment incorporated into government health plans and appropriate financial support for decades-long treatment horizons

---

people die from HIV annually, a decline of approximately 41% from 2001. Perhaps the greatest challenge is the perception of risk by at-risk populations including the risks of concurrent sexual partnerships, and the risks associated with the acute stage of HIV infection. Stigma associated with testing and counseling, adherence to drug regimens, and conduct of safe behavior for discordant couples and the general population also contribute to sustaining transmission and death rates. The prevention and control of HIV are anchored in the social determinants of health, as well as the delivery system requirements for treatment and control.

▶ The Global Architecture for HIV/AIDS Prevention and Control

In 2015, a projected $21.7 billion will be made available to combat HIV/AIDS in LMICs. Pursuing an "AIDS-Free Generation" will require more resources over the next 15–20 years. In 2014, LMIC domestic resources (including many elements of the local health systems) accounted for approximately 57% of HIV global funding. For example, South Africa funds almost its entire HIV/AIDS program and spent over $1 billion in 2014. However, many low-income countries still depend on significant external bilateral and multilateral donor resources to finance their HIV programs. In 2014, bilateral funding totaled $8.64 billion. Five countries accounted for approximately 80% of the bilateral and multilateral funding from donor governments: the United States, through the President's Emergency Fund for AIDS Relief, accounted for the majority with 64.5%; followed by the United Kingdom (12.9%); France (3.7%); Germany (3.2%); and the Netherlands (2.5%) (**FIGURE 17-5**).[33]

Multilateral organizations provide approximately 25–30% of international HIV assistance. The Global Fund to Fight AIDS, TB and Malaria (GFATM) is the world's largest financier of HIV/AIDS prevention and control. Approximately 55% of the GFATM went to HIV/AIDS programs. The United States is the largest GFATM contributor followed by the United Kingdom, France, Germany, and Japan. The World Bank also finances HIV/AIDS prevention and control efforts totaling $2.1 billion in 2015. The Bank's loans provide program support for prevention and control, as well as technical assistance to increase effectiveness and sustainability for national response to the epidemic. UNAIDS is an executive coordinating body that is charged with developing strategies and policies to help countries reduce the HIV/AIDS burdens. Their annual budget is approximately $500 million per year. UNAIDS projects that by 2030, annual investments required to end the HIV epidemic as a public health threat will approach $30 billion annually. The result will be an AIDS-free generation in a world where equitable access to, and use of, ARVs and prevention interventions will be the norm. Although UNAIDS does not provide direct support to country programs, their coordination, policy, and data management efforts help set the trajectory for an AIDS-free generation.

In addition to bi- and multilateral support, the private sector provides significant support to HIV prevention and control (and indeed a number of other global health efforts). Private philanthropic organizations provided approximately $592 million for global HIV prevention and control in 2013; 73% from U.S.-based organizations and 22% from European organizations. These organizations include foundations, corporations, faith-based organizations, nongovernmental organizations (NGOs), and individuals. They provide direct support as well as nonfinancial support such as price reductions for ARVs and other commodities. The Bill & Melinda Gates foundation (BMG) is the leading philanthropic funder of global HIV efforts and provides approximately 49% of the total U.S. HIV philanthropic giving. The BMG supports country programs plus provides support to the GFATM.

Since the mid-2000s, about half of all spending on HIV has focused on treatment, care, and support programs. However, the programmatic balance of spending varies among countries and differs according to the country's economic situation and epidemic profile. For example, higher income countries spend more on treatment, and lower income countries spend less on drugs and more on prevention, information, and program implementation (**FIGURE 17-6**).

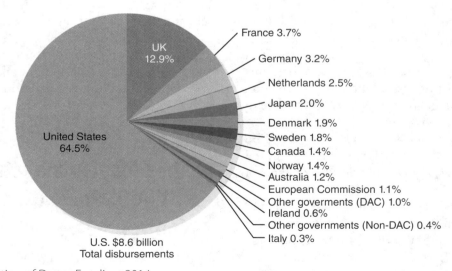

FIGURE 17-5 Proportion of Donor Funding, 2014

Note: DAC, Development Assistance Committee.

Kaiser Family Foundation. Financing the Response to HIV in Low- and Middle-Income Countries - International Assistance from Donor Governments 2014. Available at http://files.kff.org/attachment/report-financing-the-response-to-aids-in-low-and-middle-income-countries-international-assistance-from-donor-governments-in-2014. Published 2015. Accessed December 13, 2017.

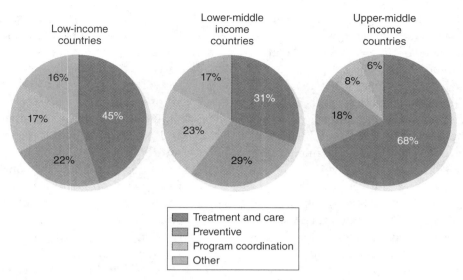

FIGURE 17-6 HIV Spending by Country Income, 2013

Reproduced from AVERT. Funding for HIV and AIDS: Global Information of HIV and AIDS. Available at http://www.avert.org/professionals/hiv-around-world/global-response/funding. http://www.avert.org /sites/default/files/Funding-page-donut.png. © Avert 2018.

▶ Conclusion

HIV remains an important pandemic disease. Integrating HIV into local health systems and ensuring appropriate and affordable treatment and control interventions are essential to realizing an AIDS-free generation. Ubiquitous treatment to all people living with AIDS will not alone reduce HIV incidence. HIV prevention and control must be pursued through "diagonal programming"[34] and horizontal, system-based interventions. HIV, although an infectious disease, is simultaneously a chronic disease that requires lifelong management and generational approaches to prevention and control. The public sector cannot alone address HIV prevention;

a trustful and functioning public-private sector alliance is required, especially in LMICs, to control HIV (and other public health problems). ARVs, an HIV vaccine, VMMC, PrEP, opportunistic infection management, system strengthening, and other interventions are all part of a holistic approach to HIV control. Working smarter to utilize the vast amount of annual HIV global resources and recognizing programmatic system synergies therein will help to sustain and fully integrate HIV prevention and control into national health systems. Ultimately, human behavior (including individual perception of HIV risk) is the key to reducing HIV incidence to a level where it no longer represents a public health problem.

Key Terms

Acquired immune deficiency syndrome (AIDS)
Acute phase of HIV infection
Budding
Capsid
Clinical latency (asymptomatic stage)
Concentrated epidemic

Endemic
Generalized epidemic
Harm reduction
Human immunodeficiency virus (HIV)
Integrase
Intracellular
Long-term non-progressors

Memory cells
Opportunistic infections
Receptors
Reverse transcriptase
Ribonucleic acid (RNA)
Vaccine
Viral load

Discussion Questions

1. How can acute transmission be prevented in LMICs? What are the technical, political, social, behavioral, and systemic challenges and opportunities to reduce the risk of HIV infection within the first 3–6 weeks of infection?

2. Name the ways HIV can be transmitted. Discuss major prevention strategies for HIV prevention and control. Discuss the challenges and opportunities associated with each approach.

3. What are some of the ways HIV can be prevented in youth? What should youth interventions focus on? What are some of the key behavior change/formulation interventions that can be applied to address younger populations? What are some of the challenges in implementing youth interventions for HIV prevention and control?

4. Describe the biology and immunobiology of HIV infection. Describe how ARVs might interrupt transmission.

5. Worldwide, HIV resources totaled over $21 billion in 2015. The U.S. government allocates approximately $6 billion to HIV while other health issues such as maternal and child health and reproductive health and family planning receive a total of approximately $2 billion annually. How might HIV resources be used in a more horizontal way to spread the wealth and promote integrated service delivery to address HIV prevention, care and treatment, <u>and</u> maternal and child deaths?

6. What is the incidence and prevalence of HIV globally? Approximately how many deaths occur annually in adults and children?

7. Name five risk factors for HIV infection. What interventions can be implemented to reduce transmission and mitigate risk?

8. Review the web for the latest World AIDS Day. Discuss what you think are the most important successes and challenges over the coming year and over the next five years.

9. Do you think that all countries should pay for all of their ARVs from their own budget? Or should the wealthy countries, foundations, and NGOs pay for ARVs for the foreseeable future?

10. What do you think of the concept of "an AIDS-free generation"? Is it feasible? Affordable? Do you see any opportunity costs associated with an AIDS-free generation strategy and policy in relation to other global health issues? If so what are they; if not, why not?

11. Should HIV/AIDS prevention and control be fully integrated into national healthcare systems, or should they remain quasi-vertical programs? Justify your answer.

12. How would you characterize the differences between the HIV epidemic in San Francisco; Washington, DC; and Nairobi, Kenya? What types of interventions should be respective priorities in each city? What are some of the social, cultural, and economic challenges that might be encountered in mitigating HIV transmission and ensuring treatment in each city?

References

1. World Health Organization. Global Health Observatory data: HIV/AIDS. Available at http://www.who.int/gho/hiv/en/. Accessed July 14, 2017.

2. Centers for Disease Control and Prevention. CDC Fact Sheet: Today's HIV/AIDS Epidemic. https://www.cdc.gov/nchhstp/newsroom/docs/factsheets/todaysepidemic-508.pdf. Published August 2016. Accessed July 14, 2017.

3. UNAIDS. Fact Sheet – Latest Statistics on the Status of the AIDS Epidemic. Available at http://www.unaids.org/en/resources/fact-sheet. Published 2016. Accessed July 14, 2017.

4. Global Burden of Disease 2015 HIV Collaborators. Estimates of global, regional, and national incidence, prevalence, and mortality of HIV, 1980–2015: The Global Burden of Disease Study 2015. *Lancet HIV.* 2016;3:e361-e387.

5. UNAIDS. AIDS by the Numbers. Available at http://www.unaids.org/sites/default/files/media_asset/AIDS-by-the-numbers-2016_en.pdf. Published 2016. Accessed July 15, 2017.

6. Mathers BM, Degenhardt L, Phillips B, et al. Global epidemiology of injecting drug use and HIV among people who inject drugs. *Lancet.* 2008;372(9651):1733-1745.

7. UNAIDS. Fact sheet - World AIDS Day 2017. http://www.unaids.org/sites/default/files/media_asset/UNAIDS_FactSheet_en.pdf. Accessed January 30, 2018.

8. Pantaleo G, Graziosi C, Fauci AS. The immunopathogenesis of human immunodeficiency virus infection. *N Engl J Med.* 1993;328:327-335.

9. Bennett NJ. HIV Disease. Medscape News and Perspective. Available at http://emedicine.medscape.com/article/211316-overview#a3. Updated November 14, 2017. Accessed November 21, 2017.

10. Cohen MS, Shaw GM, McMichael AJ, Haynes BF. Acute HIV-1 infection. *N Engl J Med.* 2011;364:1943-1954.

11. Kumar P. Long-term non-progressor (LTNP) HIV infection. *Indian J Med Res.* 2013;138(3):291-293.

12. Patel P, Borkowf CB, Brooks JT, Lasry A, Lansky A, Mermin J. Estimating per-act HIV transmission risk: a systematic review. *AIDS.* 2014;28(10):1509-1519.

13. Germain M, Robillard P, Delage G, Goldman M. Allowing blood donation from men who had sex with men more than 5 years ago: a model to evaluate the impact on transfusion safety in Canada. *Vox Sanguinis.* 2014;106(4):372-375.

14. Morar MM, Pitman JP, McFarland W, Bloch EM. The contribution of unsafe blood transfusion to human immunodeficiency virus incidence in sub-Saharan Africa: reexamination of the 5% to 10% convention. *Transfusion.* 2016;56(12):3121-3132.

15. Bernard CL, Owens DK, Goldhaber-Fiebert JD, Brandeau ML. Estimation of the cost-effectiveness of HIV prevention portfolios for people who inject drugs in the United States: a model-based analysis. *PLoS Med.* 2017;14(5):e1002312. doi: 10.1371/journal.pmed.1002312.

16. Harm Reduction Coalitions (Blog). Principles of Harm Reduction. Available at http://harmreduction.org/about-us

/principles-of-harm-reduction/. Published 2015. Accessed November 21, 2017.

17. World Health Organization. HIV – Mother-to-Child Transmission of HIV. Available at http://www.who.int/hiv/topics/mtct/en/. Accessed July 17, 2017.

18. World Health Organization. Mother-to-child transmission of HIV. Available at http://www.who.int/hiv/topics/mtct/about/en/. Accessed July 17, 2017.

19. Avert. Prevention of Mother-to-Child Transmission of HIV. Available at https://www.avert.org/professionals/hiv-programming/prevention/prevention-mother-child. Updated August 29, 2017. Accessed November 21, 2017.

20. Henry J. Kaiser Family Foundation. The global HIV/AIDS epidemic. Available at http://www.kff.org/global-health-policy/fact-sheet/the-global-hivaids-epidemic/. Published January 19, 2017. Accessed July 17, 2017.

21. UNAIDS. A Short Technical Update on Self-Testing for HIV. Available at http://www.unaids.org/sites/default/files/media_asset/JC2603_self-testing_en_0.pdf. Published 2013. Accessed November 21, 2017.

22. U.S. Food and Drug Administration. Antiretroviral drugs used in the treatment of HIV infection. U.S. Department of Health and Human Services. Available at https://www.fda.gov/forpatients/illness/hivaids/treatment/ucm118915.htm. Updated January 4, 2018. Accessed January 22, 208.

23. Evans DT, Silvestri G. Non-human primate models in AIDS research. *Curr Opin HIV AIDS*. 2013;8(4):255-261.

24. Fauci AS, Dieffenbach CW. NIH statement on HIV Vaccine Awareness Day – 2017. Available at https://www.nih.gov/news-events/news-releases/nih-statement-hiv-vaccine-awareness-day-2017. Published May 18, 2017. Accessed July 17, 2017.

25. Sze YuanLow M, Tarlinton D. HIV vaccines: one step closer. *Trends Mol. Med.* 2017;23(1):1-3.

26. MacDonald F. 2016. A first-of-its-kind HIV vaccine will move to phase II trials in 2017. *Science Alert*. Available at https://www.sciencealert.com/one-of-the-first-hiv-vaccines-will-move-onto-phase-ii-trials-in-2017. Published December 5, 2016. Accessed July 17, 2017.

27. Tanser F, de Oliveira T, Maheu-Giroux M, Bärnighausen T. Concentrated HIV sub-epidemics in generalized epidemic settings. *Curr Opin HIV AIDS*. 2014;9(2):115-125.

28. Campbell AN, Brooks AJ, Pavlicova M, et al. Barriers to condom use: results for men and women enrolled in HIV risk reduction trials in outpatient drug treatment. *J HIV/AIDS Soc Serv*. 2016;15(2):130-146.

29. Mbonye M, Kuteesa M, Seeley J, Levin J, Weiss H, Kamali A. Voluntary medical male circumcision for HIV prevention in fishing communities in Uganda: the influence of local beliefs and practice. *African J AIDS Res*. 2016;15(3):211-218.

30. Hankins C, Warren M, Njeuhmeli E. Voluntary medical male circumcision for HIV prevention: new mathematical models for strategic demand creation prioritizing subpopulations by age and geography. *PLoS One*. 2016;11(12): e0169499.

31. UNAIDS. On the Fast Track to an AIDS-Free Generation. Available at http://www.unaids.org/sites/default/files/media_asset/GlobalPlan2016_en.pdf. Published 2016. Accessed July 17, 2017.

32. Hatcher AM, Stöckl H, Christofides N, Pallitto CC, Garcia-Moreno C, Turan JM. Mechanisms linking intimate partner violence and prevention of mother-to-child transmission of HIV: a qualitative study in South Africa. *Soc Sci Med*. 2016;168:130-139.

33. Kaiser Family Foundation. Financing the Response to HIV in Low- and Middle-Income Countries - International Assistance from Donor Governments 2014. Available at http://files.kff.org/attachment/report-financing-the-response-to-aids-in-low-and-middle-income-countries-international-assistance-from-donor-governments-in-2014. Published 2015. Accessed December 13, 2017.

34. Ooms G, Van Damme W, Baker BK, Zeitz P, Schrecker T. The "diagonal" approach to global fund financing: a cure for the broader malaise of health systems. *Globalization and Health* 2008;4(6). Available at http://globalizationandhealth.biomedcentral.com/articles/10.1186/1744-8603-4-6. Accessed November 21, 2017.

Glossary

Acquired immune deficiency syndrome (AIDS) A condition of the immune system caused by the human immunodeficiency virus (HIV); characterized by having a CD4 cell count of less than 200 cells per cubic millimeter of blood, thus rendering the subject highly vulnerable to opportunistic infections such as tuberculosis, *Pneumocystis carinii*, and Kaposi sarcoma.

Active immunity Adaptive immunity developed after exposure to an infection with a microorganism or following vaccination.

Active strategies for injury control These strategies involve the individual in decision making about his or her own behavior.

Active tuberculosis State of people infected with *Mycobacterium tuberculosis* whose infection is not contained by the immune system and who are sick, frequently symptomatic, and very often contagious.

Activities of daily living (ADLs) Activities such as walking, bathing, dressing, grooming, and eating.

Acute phase of HIV infection This is the earliest stage of HIV infection, which develops 2 to 4 weeks after infection and is characterized by flu-like symptoms. During this stage, HIV multiplies rapidly in the body.

Adaptive immunity An immune response developed following exposure to a foreign agent that results in antigen recognition by T and B lymphocytes with subsequent development of specificity and memory.

Adjuvants Substances that enhance an immune response by prolonging exposure to the antigen within the body.

Aerobes Organisms that require oxygen for their metabolic activities.

Aerobic Energy production using oxygen.

Aging in place Remaining within one's home (rather than transferring to a nursing home, assisted living, or senior housing) for as long as possible in older age.

Alleles An alternative form of a genetic locus; a single allele for each locus is inherited from each parent (e.g., at a locus for eye color, the allele might result in blue or brown eyes).

Anaerobes Organisms that do not require oxygen for their metabolic activities.

Anaerobic Energy production without oxygen.

Androgens A group of hormones that include testosterone and serve as precursors to estrogen production.

Aneuploidy Abnormal number of chromosomes in a cell or organism.

Angiogenesis Formation of new blood vessels.

Anterior pituitary A small endocrine organ located just below the hypothalamus.

Anthropophilic Preference of a parasite for a human host.

Antibodies Proteins made in response to exposure to a foreign antigen that can bind to the antigen to facilitate its elimination.

Antigens Foreign agents that can stimulate an immune response and bind to antibodies and T cells.

Apoptosis Programmed cell death.

Asymptomatic stage (clinical latency) During this phase of HIV/AIDS, the person is asymptomatic; however, the immune system continues to deteriorate.

Attenuation Weakening (dilution) of the concentration, as of an antigen or a vaccine, or the decreased virulence of a virus, bacteria, or other pathogen caused by point mutations.

Autotrophs Microorganisms and plants that are capable of utilizing the energy of the sun or derive energy from the metabolism of inorganic compounds.

Bacilli Rod-shaped bacteria.

Bacteria Unicellular microbes with distinct properties; one of the five distinct types of microbes.

Binary fission An asexual mode of reproduction in which a cell splits into two new cells.

Bioactive food components The constituents in foods or dietary supplements, other than those needed to meet basic human nutritional needs, that are responsible for changes in health status.

Biogeochemical cycles Processes such as the carbon and nitrogen cycles in which bacteria play a critical role.

Bioinformatics An interdisciplinary scientific field that develops mathematical and computational tools for the retrieval and analysis of biochemical and biologic data.

Biosphere All the organisms and environments found on Earth.

Bipolar Major depression with alternating episodes of mania.

Blastocyst Term used to describe an early phase of the embryo as it migrates into the uterus and begins the implantation process.

Blood-stage vaccine A vaccine that blocks merozoite replication.

Breakpoint transmission The critical population level of an organism and host where the reproductive potential is too low to maintain the species.

Budding Budding enables a virus to exit the host cell. Budding is most common in enveloped viruses like HIV, which must acquire a host-derived membrane to form the external envelope.

Calorie The amount of energy required to increase the temperature of one gram of water by one degree Celsius.

Capsid A protein shell that covers the nucleic acid component of a virus.

Capsule A component of the bacterial envelope that may contribute to virulence; it is not present in all species of bacteria.

Carcinogenic Can either directly or indirectly lead to cancer (e.g., a substance or radiation).

Carcinoma An invasive malignant tumor, derived from epithelial tissue, which can metastasize to other areas of the body.

Cardiac output The volume of blood pumped by each ventricle per minute (CO = SV × heart rate).

Caretakers Genes involved in repair pathways that help maintain the integrity DNA through replication cycles. Inactivation of these genes results in genetic instabilities.

Case A person in the population or study group identified as being infected and as having the particular disease, health disorder, or condition (i.e., exhibiting symptoms of the specific disease).

Case fatality rate The number of deaths from a disease (in a given period) divided by the number of diagnosed cases of that disease (in the same period) and multiplied by 100.

Cell wall A component of the bacterial envelope that gives the cell its characteristic shape and confers structural integrity.

Cell-mediated immunity Immunity mediated by antigen-specific T lymphocytes and other cells that are involved in protecting against challenges such as intracellular organisms, viruses, and tumor cells.

Cervix The "neck" of the uterus; cylindrical tissue that connects the lowermost portion of the uterus to the vagina. The inner tube of the cervix, known as the endocervical canal, serves as a passageway between the internal uterus and vagina.

Chemosynthetic Organisms that derive energy from the metabolism of inorganic compounds.

Chemotaxis The process of moving toward or away from a chemical stimulus.

Child and Adult Care Food Program One of four nutrition assistance programs existing as a social safety net for food security in the United States. *See also* Supplemental Nutrition Assistance Program, Special Supplemental Nutrition Program for Women, Infants, and Children, and The Emergency Food Assistance Program.

Clinical latency (asymptomatic stage) The stage when HIV disease process has begun but the person is not yet symptomatic.

Cocci Spherical bacteria.

Commensals The two organisms in a relationship in which one organism benefits from the other, but does no harm to the host organism.

Common source epidemics Outbreaks of disease arising from contact with a single contaminated source, typically associated with fecally contaminated food or water.

Compression of morbidity Refers to the delay of chronic disease and frailty until the end of life or as close to the end of life as possible.

Concentrated epidemic HIV prevalence is high enough in one or more subpopulations, such as men who have sex with men, injecting drug users, or sex workers and their clients to maintain the epidemic in that subpopulation, but the virus is not circulating in the general population. The future course of a concentrated epidemic is determined by the size of the subpopulation(s) and interaction between a subpopulation(s) and the general population.

Conjugation A recombination process resulting in the transfer of DNA from donor to recipient during physical contact.

Contraception The deliberate use of natural or artificial methods to prevent pregnancy.

Corpus luteum A temporary ovarian structure with a yellowish appearance from the cellular uptake of lutein pigment and steroid hormones after release of the ovum. Its principal function is the production of progesterone, which switches the menstrual cycle from an estrogen-high process in the follicular phase to a progesterone-high process in the luteal phase.

Cortisol A hormone that is stimulated by chronic stress and performs in a manner similar to epinephrine in that it increases circulating levels of substrates and ensures the mobilization of fuels necessary to adapt to long-term stress.

Cristae The inner membrane of the mitochondria that forms a series of folds. The cristae project into an inner cavity containing a gel-like solution called the matrix. These two structures of the mitochondria are essential for energy production.

Cultures Growths of an organism in a laboratory for the purposes of propagation and study.

Cytoskeleton An intricate network of proteins within the cytosol that gives the cell its shape, provides for its internal organization, and regulates its movements.

Cytosol A complex, gel-like mass inside the cytoplasm that contains a number of highly organized structures called organelles.

$D = nV/R$ An equation representing the struggle between disease-producing microbes and host resistance. D is the severity of the infection; n is the number of organisms; V is the virulence factors; R is for resistance factors.

Decomposers Microbes that break down compounds into simpler constituents.

Diagnostic and Statistical Manual of Mental Disorders (DSM) A manual published by the American Psychiatric Association (APA) that offers a common language and standard criteria for the classification of mental disorders.

Dietary Guidelines for Americans (DGAs) Guidelines intended to provide science-based advice on food and nutrition choices to help all Americans aged 2 years or older meet nutritional needs, achieve and maintain a healthy weight, and minimize risk of chronic diseases.

Dietary Reference Intake (DRI) Recommendations for macro- and micronutrients. For each macro- and micronutrient, the DRI report provides four reference values that can be used in evaluating and planning to meet the nutrient needs for healthy individuals in a population: Estimated Average Requirement (EAR), the Recommended Dietary Allowance (RDA), the Adequate Intake (AI), and the Tolerable Upper Intake Level (UL).

Directly observed therapy, short-course (DOTS) The World Health Organization recommended strategy for delivering the basics of TB cure. It combines a clinical approach (patient's drug intake is monitored daily by a nurse or a trained healthcare worker to ensure patient compliance) and a management strategy for public health systems that includes political commitment, maintenance of adequate drug supply, and sound recording and reporting systems.

Disability-adjusted life year (DALY) A measure of overall disease burden, expressed as the number of years lost due to ill-health, injury, disability, or early death.

Disease A possible outcome of infection in which health is impaired in some fashion.

Dominant Describes an allele that determines a trait, even if only one copy is present.

Dopamine Part of the catecholamine family, it plays a major role in reward-motivated behavior. Most types of reward increase the level of dopamine in the brain, and most addictive drugs increase dopamine neuronal activity.

Dose–response assessment The graded relation between increasing the dose of a given agent and the magnitude of biologic or psychosocial response.

Duffy blood group An antigen located on the surface of red blood, endothelial, and epithelial cells. Characterized by the presence of Fy antigens.

Dyslipidemia High blood concentrations of cholesterol, triglycerides, or free fatty acids and a risk factor for the metabolic syndrome and cardiovascular disease.

Dysplastic Describes cells that look abnormal under the microscope. They may or may not progress to cancer.

Elective abortion Induced abortion performed at the request of the mother.

Elimination Reduction of the incidence of infection caused by a specific agent to zero in a defined geographic area; no transmission occurs; continued measures are required to prevent reestablishment of transmission (e.g., polio elimination).

Embryo Term used to describe developing human cells from time of implantation to 8 weeks of pregnancy.

Endemic According to the *Dictionary of Epidemiology, Fifth Edition*, "the constant occurrence of a disease, disorder, or noxious infectious agent in a geographic area or population group; it may also refer to the chronic high prevalence of a disease in such area or group."[(p92)]

Endocrine disruptor Chemicals that have a structure similar to hormones and, as such, are able to interfere with normal hormone function. Endocrine disruptors have been implicated in cancers and developmental defects.

Endometrial cycle The cyclical growth of the endometrial lining of the uterus; includes the proliferative, secretory, and menstrual phases.

Endoplasmic reticulum (ER) An organelle that synthesizes proteins.

Endorphins Endogenous opioid neuropeptides produced by the central nervous system and the pituitary gland.

Envelope A bacterial structure consisting of a capsule, cell wall, and cell membrane.

Epidemiologic transition The Epidemiologic Transition is defined by three phases: (1) the age of pestilence; (2) the age of receding pandemics; and, (3) the age of degenerative and manmade diseases. Basically, it is a shift from infectious to chronic disease morbidity and mortality.

Epidemiology The study of the sources, causes, and distribution of diseases and disorders that produce illness and death in humans.

Epigenetic modification Heritable changes in gene expression not accompanied by changes in DNA sequence.

Epigenome A record of the chemical changes to the DNA and histone proteins of an organism, which can be passed down to an organism's offspring.

Epinephrine Part of the catecholamine family, it functions in the human brain and body as a hormone and neurotransmitter in fight or flight responses.

Epitopes Small portions of an antigen that can stimulate an immune response and serve as a binding site for antibody.

Eradication The achievement and status whereby no further infections with a pathogen occur anywhere, and continued control measures are unnecessary (i.e., the incidence of infection caused by a specific agent globally is permanently reduced to zero).

Erythrocytic schizogony An asexual cycle of merozoites once they have invaded the red blood cells.

Essential nutrients Nutrients that are required for human health, but cannot be synthesized *in vivo*, and thus must be obtained through the diet.

Etiology Proposed origin or cause of a disease or illness.

Eukaryotes Cells possessing a nuclear membrane and other membrane-bound organelles.

Exoerythrocytic schizogony The stage of malaria infection in which the malaria parasite is found in liver cells.

Exome All of the protein-coding genes in a genome. A representation of gene expression in a cell or tissue.

Exposure assessment The determination of the prominence of a given hazard experienced within a population under different conditions.

Extensively drug-resistant tuberculosis (XDR-TB) Strain of TB that is at least MDR-TB and includes resistance to a fluoroquinolone (one class of second-line drugs) and at least one of the second-line injectable drugs. XDR-TB strains are virtually untreatable.

Extrapulmonary tuberculosis Active tuberculosis that is localized in an organ other than the lungs.

Facultative aging Determinants of aging that we do have control over, such as lifestyle.

Facultative anaerobes Organisms that grow best in the presence of oxygen but are capable of survival in its absence.

Fetal viability The developmental age at which a fetus can survive the extra-uterine environment. The exact timing is open to debate as it depends on a variety of medical, technologic, social, and ethical considerations. In the United States, fetal viability is generally defined as 24 weeks' gestation, as technologic capabilities for supporting a fetus before that time are currently unavailable.

Fetus Term used to describe developing human cells from 9 weeks of pregnancy to birth. On average, full fetal development occurs over 266 days, from the time of fertilization to birth.

Fibroblasts Immature fiber-producing cells of connective tissue capable of differentiating into a chondroblast, collagenoblast, or osteoblast.

First-line drugs Group of five antibiotics (rifampicin, isoniazid, ethambutol, pyrazinamide, and streptomycin) used against tuberculosis that are the most effective and potent for TB treatment.

Flagella Structures composed of the protein flagellin that provide motility to certain species of bacilli and cocci.

Follicle A structural and functional group of cells on the ovary responsible for housing a single oocyte and releasing gonadal hormones.

Fomites Inanimate objects that serve as means of transmission of infectious material.

Food insecurity A situation in which the availability of nutritionally adequate and safe foods or the ability to acquire acceptable food in socially acceptable ways is limited or uncertain.

Fungi A category of eukaryotic organisms including mushrooms and yeast.

Gain of function mutations Mutations that cause a functional change in the gene product.

Gametocytes Cells responsible for the transmission from human host to mosquito.

Gatekeepers The cell's internal system of checks and balances that monitor cell division. These genes can directly regulate cell growth and promote cell death.

Gene The fundamental physical and functional unit of heredity. A gene is an ordered sequence of nucleotides located in a particular position on a particular chromosome that encodes a specific functional product (i.e., a protein or RNA molecule).

Generalized epidemic HIV prevalence between 1% and 5% in the general population and/or pregnant women attending antenatal clinics; indicates that HIV frequently exists in the general population and prevalence is sufficient for sexual networking to drive the epidemic. In a generalized epidemic with more than 5% adult prevalence, no sexually active person is at low risk.

Generation time The length of time between rounds of binary fission.

Genetic variation Diversity in gene frequencies. Genetic variation can refer to differences between individuals or to differences between populations. The two major contributors to genetic variation are sexual reproduction and exchange of genetic material on homologous chromosomes during meiosis.

Genome The complete set of human DNA and contains approximately 3 billion base pairs.

Genomic imprinting Phenomenon whereby certain genes are expressed dependent upon the parent-of-origin. The allele that is imprinted is transcriptionally silent.

Genotype The genetic makeup of an organism; the sum of genes transmitted from parent to offspring.

Genus A category in the binomial system of nomenclature above the species level.

Germline mutations DNA mutations that exist within germ cells and, as such, may be inherited by the next generation.

Gluconeogenesis The breakdown of amino acids and conversion to glucose by the liver.

Glucose 6-phosphate-dehydrogenase (G6PD) deficiency A condition that causes red blood cells to break down prematurely when exposed to stress, infection, or certain drugs.

Glycogenesis The conversion of glucose to glycogen by the liver.

Glycogenolysis The breakdown of stored glycogen and conversion to glucose by the liver.

Golgi complex A set of flattened curved membrane-enclosed sacs that are stacked in layers. Proteins coming from the endoplasmic reticulum travel through the layers of the complex to be modified, sorted, and delivered to their final destination.

Gonadotropin-releasing hormone (GnRH) A neurohormone that travels to the anterior pituitary and signals the secretion of follicle-stimulating hormone and luteinizing hormone.

Gonadotropins Glycoprotein polypeptide hormones that target the gonads and serve important endocrine roles in sexual development and reproductive function.

Gram stain A cell wall staining procedure done in bacteria to determine if bacteria are Gram positive or Gram negative.

Haddon's Matrix A framework to help public health practitioners organize the opportunities and strategies for injury prevention and control pertaining to a given issue.

Harm reduction Harm reduction is a set of practical strategies and ideas aimed at reducing negative consequences associated with drug use. Harm reduction is also a movement for social justice built on a belief in, and respect for, the rights of people who use drugs. For HIV, harm reduction often entails needle-exchange programs and other interventions to reduce the risks of injecting drug abuse.

Hazard Any agent (biologic, chemical, thermal, mechanical, psychosocial) that has the potential to do harm.

Hazard identification The determination of whether or not a given agent causes an adverse effect at the biologic level based on laboratory and field studies.

Health communication The use of communication strategies to inform and influence individual and collective decisions that promote health and prevent disease.

Health literacy A measure of how well health communication messages are understood by their intended audiences.

Hemizygous Having only one copy of a particular gene. For example, in humans, males are hemizygous for genes found on the X chromosome.

Hemozoin Malarial pigment found in malaria-infected red blood cells.

Herd immunity Widespread immunity in a population to a specific pathogen sequestering the pathogen so it cannot spread rapidly, if at all; sustainable herd immunity usually requires at least 85% coverage of a vaccine in a population.

Heterogeneity of response Variation in human response to a uniform exposure due to host factors such as age, sex, disease status, or body mass.

Heterotrophs Organisms that require organic compounds as an energy source.

Heterozygous Describes an organism that has different alleles at a gene locus.

Homozygous Describes an organism that has two identical alleles of a gene.

Horizontal gene transfer A process by which genes are transferred from one organism to another.

Human chorionic growth hormone (hCG) A hormone secreted by the blastocyst to help prepare the endometrial lining for implantation. In the early pregnancy, hCG is responsible for maintaining the corpus luteum to ensure continued progesterone production until the placenta can take over production, around 6–8 weeks.

Human immunodeficiency virus (HIV) A member of the *Retroviridae* family that causes AIDS by infecting and destroying T-helper cells, which are the major types of cells dedicated to maintaining immunity and immunologic memory. Loss of the T-helper cells makes the body vulnerable to infection.

Humoral immunity Immunity that involves antibody-mediated responses.

Hyperplasia The growth of tissue due to cell proliferation, or an increased number of cells.

Hypnozoite The latent hepatic life cycle stage of a sporozoite.

Hypothalamic–pituitary–ovarian (HPO) axis A set of interactions involving the hypothalamus of the brain, the pituitary organ, and the ovaries to coordinate two concurrent cycles of growth in women's reproductive tract via negative feedback loops.

Hypothalamus A portion of the brain that secretes gonadatropin-releasing hormones.

Immunity A state of protection from disease created by innate and specific mechanisms.

Immunization Protection of individuals against disease by vaccination.

Incidence Number of specified new events during a specified period on a specified population.

Indoor residual spraying (IRS) A malaria control measure that involves the spraying of insecticide on the interior walls and surface of homes and other dwellings.

Induced abortion Termination of a pregnancy by medical or surgical means before the point of fetal viability.

Industrialized food system The modern-day food system in developed countries characterized by large farming operations, food-processing facilities, and food retail establishments.

Infection The presence of microbes in the body without definitive symptoms. According to the *Dictionary of Epidemiology, Fifth Edition,* "the entry and development or multiplication of an infectious agent in an organism, including the body of humans and animals. . . . The presence of living infectious agents upon exterior surfaces of the body is called 'infestation.'"[p147] Asymptomatic infections exist; thus, a person can be infected and infectious, but does not show symptoms.

Infection-blocking vaccine A vaccine aimed at the sporozoite.

Infectious agents Plasmids capable of exchanging genetic material from one microbe to another; some confer antibiotic resistance.

Innate immunity Nonspecific mechanisms involved in the early response to pathogens that lack specificity and involve anatomic, physiologic, phagocytic, and inflammatory mechanisms.

Insecticide-treated bed net (ITN) A mosquito net of fiber that has been treated with insecticide. Bed nets can be treated by dipping in an insecticide mixture (traditional ITN) or the insecticide can be bound to the fabric, allowing it to remain on the netting for periods of three to five years.

Instrumental activities of daily living (IADLs) Activities of cooking, shopping, and house/yard work.

Insulin resistance Impaired insulin action in the muscle, liver, or fat cells.

Integrase An enzyme characteristic to retroviruses that allows the viral genetic material to integrate into the host DNA.

Integrated malaria control An approach to malaria control that combines multiple approaches.

Intentional injuries Pre-contemplated and planned intent to harm oneself or another.

Intermittent preventive treatment for pregnant women (IPTp) A public health intervention aimed to prevent malaria infection in pregnant women, involving the administration of sulfadoxine-pyrimethamine.

Interstitial fluid Fluid surrounding the cells.

Intracellular Existing within a cell.

K-strategists Organisms that produce a few, fairly large offspring, invest in parental care, maximize reproductive opportunities in stable environments, and depend on small numbers of nurtured offspring for continuation of the species.

Kinetic energy The kinetic energy of an object is the energy that it possesses due to its motion.

Koch's postulates A set of rules used to establish that a particular organism is the cause of a particular disease.

Labor The occurrence of regular, effective contractions that are accompanied by progressive cervical change.

Latent TB infection The state of people infected with *Mycobacterium tuberculosis* whose infection is contained by the immune system and who are not sick (and therefore not symptomatic) and not contagious.

Lipolysis The breakdown of stored fat for use as fuel.

Long-term non-progressors Sometimes called "elite controllers," these are individuals infected with HIV who maintain a CD4 count greater than 500 without antiretroviral therapy with a detectable viral load.

Loss-of-function mutations Mutations that result in a loss or diminished amount of the gene product.

Lysosomes Membrane-enclosed sacs that contain hydrolytic acid. They are responsible for digesting and eliminating cellular waste products.

Macrogametes The larger of two gametes; usually female.

Macronutrients The nutrients we consume in the largest quantities as the source of calories in our food. These are carbohydrates, proteins, and fats.

Mandatory aging True biologic aging that is outside of our control.

Maternal mortality rate (MMR) The number of direct and indirect maternal deaths per 100,000 live births during pregnancy or up to and including 42 days after the end of pregnancy.

Matrix The interior of the mitochondria.

Medication abortion Induced abortion performed using two medications, mifepristone and misoprostol, administered 24–48 hours apart. This method is FDA-approved for the first 10 weeks of pregnancy in the United States.

Memory cells B-cells and T-cells that create an immunologic memory to a certain antigen after an initial exposure to the antigen; if that antigen invades the body a second time, there is a faster immune response to kill it.

Menarche The first menstruation.

Menopause The cessation of menstruation that typically occurs in midlife; onset is marked by the absence of menstrual cycle for one year.

Merozoites Small trophozoites capable of sexual or asexual development.

Metabolic flexibility The ability of the cell to switch rapidly from one fuel source to another in response to various challenges.

Methylation The installation of a methyl group onto a substrate.

Microgametes The smaller of two gametes; usually male.

Micromort A unit of risk measuring a one-in-a-million probability of death.

Miliary tuberculosis A strain of tuberculosis common in children. It is characterized by its spread to multiple organs and the small size of the lesions.

Mitochondrion The power plant of the cell, responsible for deriving energy from ingested nutrients and converting that energy to a usable form.

Monoallelic expression As a result of imprinting, occurs when only one of the two alleles present is expressed.

Monozygotic Derived from a single zygote, which split into two very early after fertilization. The result is twins with identical genes.

Mosaics Individuals composed of two genetically different cell populations derived from a single zygote.

Multidrug-resistant tuberculosis (MDR-TB) Strain of tuberculosis that is resistant to at least isoniazid and rifampicin, the two most potent first-line drugs. MDR-TB strains are more difficult to treat and require the use of second-line drugs.

Multifactorial A complex disease caused by the interaction of multiple genes and environmental factors. Examples of multifactorial diseases include cancer and heart disease.

Mutation A change in DNA that is transferred to subsequent generations.

Mutuals The two organisms in a relationship in which both organisms (mutually) benefit from one another.

Negative feedback loop A feedback loop that works by decreasing the secretion of one substance in response to the rise of another.

Neoplastic Describes an abnormal growth or cell division. A neoplasm can be benign, potentially malignant (pre-cancerous) or malignant (cancer).

Neurotoxin A substance that is toxic to the nervous system and impairs physiologic and cognitive function.

Noradrenergic function Functional capacity of parts of the body that produce the neurotransmitter noradrenaline (also called norepinephrine) or are affected by it.

Norepinephrine Part of the catecholamine family, it functions in the human brain and body as a hormone and neurotransmitter in fight or flight responses.

Nosocomial infections These kinds of infection occur as a result of being in a healthcare setting, separate from the reason an individual went to that setting.

Nucleoid The DNA-rich area in prokaryotic cells; it is not surrounded by a membrane.

Nucleus The largest single organized unit in the cell. It provides storage for the cell's genetic material.

Obesogenic environment Characteristics of the built environment that promote obesity either by providing cheap, calorically dense food or by limiting options for daily physical activity.

Obligate anaerobes Organisms to which oxygen is toxic.

Obligate intracellular parasites Microbes that can only replicate within cells.

Oncogenes Result from the mutation of cellular proto-oncogenes that normally functions to regulate cell growth and differentiation. Once de-regulated or mutated, oncogenes participate in the onset and development of cancer in a gain-of-function manner.

Oocyst An encapsulated ookinete formed by the malaria parasite.

Ookinete A motile and elongated zygote.

Opportunistic infections Infections caused by pathogens (bacteria, viruses, fungi, or protozoa) that take advantage of opportunities not normally available, such as a host with a weakened immune system.

Organic Generally, a chemical compound that contains carbon.

Organisms Living entities composed of cells.

Organogenesis The period of embryo development from weeks 3-8 after fertilization, during which the major organ structures form.

Osteoblasts A cell from which bone develops.

Osteopontin A glycoprotein that lies in the mechanistic pathway between chronic hyperglycemia, chronic inflammation, and cardiovascular disease.

Osteoporosis Low bone density.

Ovarian cycle A three-phase cycle for maturation of ova.

Oxytocin A hormone produced in the hypothalamus of the brain and secreted by the posterior pituitary organ.

Parasitemia Presence of parasites in blood.

Parasites A relationship between two organisms in which one organism benefits at the expense of the other.

Passive immunity Immunity acquired by natural or acquired transfer of preformed antibodies.

Passive strategies for injury control These strategies bypass individual choice because the protective mechanism is already in place.

Pathogens Microbes capable of producing disease.

Penetrance The probability of a gene or genetic trait being expressed. "Complete" penetrance means the gene or genes for a trait are expressed in all the population who have the genes. "Incomplete" penetrance means the genetic trait is expressed in only part of the population. The percentage of penetrance also may change with the age range of the population.

Peroxisomes Smaller than lysosomes, these organelles contain powerful oxidative enzymes that can detoxify the cell.

Phenotype The physical characteristics of an organism or the presence of a disease that may or may not be genetic.

Photosynthetic Organisms that utilize the energy of the sun and that use carbon dioxide as a carbon source.

Pili Bacterial appendages in gram negative bacteria that act as adhesions; some serve as a bridge allowing genetic exchange in the form of conjugation.

Placenta accreta The growth of placental tissue into one or more layers of the uterine muscle (versus decidua). The condition interferes with complete placental separation after birth, and subsequently results in a significantly higher risk of hemorrhage, large blood volume transfusion, intensive care unit admission, and hysterectomy.

Placenta previa A condition in which the placenta grows in front of, or immediately next to, the cervical os, which is incompatible with safe vaginal delivery and requires a planned cesarean delivery before spontaneous onset of labor.

Plasmids Small molecules of nonchromosomal DNA found in some bacteria.

Polymerase chain reaction (PCR) assay A test used to detect the presence of parasites in human blood.

Population attributable fraction The proportion of disease attributable to the presence of a given risk factor, based on the formula:

$$\text{PAF (\%)} = [\text{Pe (RR} - 1)/\text{RR}] \times 100$$

Where P_e is the proportion of exposed people among the cases of the disease and RR is the relative risk of the disease, comparing exposed people to unexposed people and adjusted for confounders.

Post-traumatic stress disorder (PTSD) A type of anxiety disorder that is triggered by a terrifying event that the person either experiences or witnesses.

Pregnancy-related mortality ratio The number of deaths directly attributable to pregnancy, or caused by a condition aggravated by pregnancy that occur during pregnancy or within the first year after pregnancy, per 100,000 live births.

Primary tuberculosis A person's first infection with *Mycobacterium tuberculosis*. Often in children but may occur in adults as well.

Prokaryotes Not having the genetic material contained within a membrane in the cell.

Propagated epidemics Epidemics resulting from direct person-to-person contact.

Prostaglandins A group of physiologically active substances made from fatty acids. They are present in tissue throughout the body and assume numerous hormone-like functions, including dilation of blood vessels, inflammation, and smooth muscle contraction.

Proto-oncogenes Normal cellular genes that become oncogenes when mutated. They are often involved in cell division or programmed cell death.

Protozoans A category of unicellular eukaryotic microbes.

Pulmonary TB Active tuberculosis that is localized in the lungs.

R-strategists Organisms that produce many offspring, offer little parental care, maximize reproductive opportunities, and depend on large numbers of offspring for continuation of the species.

R_0 (R-nought) An epidemiologic term used as a measure of the potential for transmission.

Rapid diagnostic test (RDT) A screening test that can detect the presence of malaria antigens in human blood.

Reactivated Starting again (e.g., tuberculosis infection that becomes activated again).

Reactive oxygen species (ROS) The products of aerobic metabolism (oxygen ions, free radicals, and peroxides). They are small and highly reactive molecules with important cell-signaling roles.

Receptors Cells that receive stimuli.

Recessive Describes a genetic trait that will be expressed only if there are two identical copies or, for a male, if one copy is present on the X chromosome.

Recrudesce Recur; become active again.

Recrudescent malaria This type of malaria occurs when the erythrocytic stages re-emerge after the infection no longer causes symptoms; the infection becomes active again and the patient becomes symptomatic.

Redox The cellular balance of reducing (gain of electrons) and oxidizing (loss of electrons) equivalents (a molecule, atom, or ion) in response to environmental stressors.

Relapse A second condition (e.g., infection) after the first one has occurred.

Relapsing malaria *Plasmodium* can re-emerge from liver stages after the blood stage merozoites have disappeared; this occurs because certain *Plasmodium* form quiescent liver stages called hypnozoites in addition to the erythrocytic stage

Resistant malaria A strain of malaria that is resistant to artemisinin and other drugs.

Retrotransposons DNA elements that can amplify their copy numbers in a genome by using an RNA intermediate to move around the genome.

Reverse transcriptase A viral enzyme that helps convert the RNA of a virus into double-stranded DNA.

Ribonucleic acid (RNA) A group of nucleic acids that controls several forms of cellular activity.

Risk The probability that an individual will be affected by a particular genetic disorder. Both genes and environment influence risk. An individual's risk may be higher because he or she inherits genes that cause or increase susceptibility to a disorder. Other individuals may be at higher risk because they live or work in an environment that promotes the development of the disorder.

Risk analysis The field of public health that involves risk assessment, risk communication, and risk management.

Risk characterization An estimate of risk that characterizes the association between a given exposure and the likelihood of a disease outcome.

Sarcopenia The aging- or disease-related loss of muscle mass and muscle quality.

Schizonts Matured malaria parasite cells that divide to form merozoites.

Second-line drugs Group of antibiotics with anti-TB activity that are less potent than the first-line drugs. Treatment with second-line drugs is usually the only option for patients with MDR-TB, but treatment is expensive, very long, and has many serious side effects.

Selective survival A select sample of people who have survived the putative effects of various risk factors in late middle-age and therefore represent a healthier and more robust population compared with the general population.

Sickle cell trait The condition in which a person has inherited the sickle cell gene mutation from one of his or her parents.

Single nucleotide polymorphism (SNP) The fundamental unit of genetic variation in humans.

Social marketing Another term for health marketing. According to the CDC, it involves the creation, communication, and delivery of health information and interventions.

Somatic mutations Genetic changes arising in individual cells that are not inherited.

Special Supplemental Nutrition Program for Women, Infants, and Children One of four nutrition assistance programs existing as a social safety net for food security in the United States. *See also* Supplemental Nutrition Assistance Program, The Emergency Food Assistance Program, and the Child and Adult Care Food Program.

Species The fundamental rank in the binomial system of classification or organisms.

Spirilla Spiral-shaped bacteria.

Spontaneous abortion The demise of a pregnancy without medical or mechanical assistance; miscarriage. Among clinically established pregnancies, the prevalence of miscarriage is 15%, but the actual incidence is likely much higher, as 80% of spontaneous abortions occur before 12 weeks' gestation and may occur before the pregnancy is identified.

Sporozoites Elongated motile cells that develop during the infective stage of the malaria parasite.

Stage Description of how far cancer has spread and if it has invaded other organs.

Stroke volume The volume of blood that the heart can pump out with each heartbeat.

Subsistence efficiency ratio (SER) The optimal balance between energy intake and energy expenditure for maintaining healthy metabolic regulation.

Successful aging According to Rowe and Kahn, the three domains of this model include (1) disease risk; (2) physical or cognitive capacity; and (3) engagement with life.

Supplemental Nutrition Assistance Program Formerly known as Food Stamps. One of four nutrition assistance programs existing as a social safety net for food security in the United States. *See also* Special Supplemental Nutrition

Program for Women, Infants, and Children, The Emergency Food Assistance Program, and the Child and Adult Care Food Program.

Surgical abortion The mechanical removal of the pregnancy from the uterus.

Teratogen Agents or exposures that are associated with fetal harm; these may be chemical, physical, infectious, or environmental in nature.

The Emergency Food Assistance Program One of four nutrition assistance programs existing as a social safety net for food security in the United States. *See also* Supplemental Nutrition Assistance Program, Special Supplemental Nutrition Program for Women, Infants, and Children, and the Child and Adult Care Food Program.

Therapeutic abortion Induced abortion performed for maternal medical indications or serious fetal anomalies.

Toxoid An altered toxin capable of inducing production of antibodies.

Trans-fatty acids (trans fats) A form of fatty acids where the hydrogen atoms of the carbon molecules around a double bond are on opposite sides of the molecule, rather than the usual formation where the hydrogen atoms are on the same side of the molecule (cis-fatty acids). This conformational change makes the trans-fatty acids more rigid, and foods containing these trans-fatty acids tend to be solids at room temperature.

Transduction A recombination process characterized by bacteriophage-mediated transfer of DNA.

Transformation A recombination process characterized by the uptake of "naked" DNA into competent cells.

Transmission-blocking vaccine A vaccine that induces immunity against the gametocyte that infects the mosquito.

Transport vesicles Structures that move molecules such as proteins from the rough endoplasmic reticulum to the Golgi complex.

Traumatic brain injury (TBI) Describes the impairment in brain functioning due to impact trauma to the head.

Trophozoites The growth stage of a parasite.

Tubercles Nodular lesions found on the lung, often indicative of tuberculosis.

Tumor necrosis factor A cell-signaling protein capable of inducing tumor cell death.

Tumor suppressor genes These types of genes help prevent a step toward cancer and can be further divided into "gatekeepers" and "caretakers."

Unicellular algae Plant-like organisms that produce organic compounds.

Unintentional injuries Not pre-contemplated or planned event that results in an injury.

Unipolar depressive disorder A major depressive disorder that occurs without the manic phase that occurs in the classic form of bipolar disorder.

Vaccination Injection of a vaccine in order to establish resistance to an infectious disease.

Vaccine A biologic substance with similar characteristics to microorganisms involved in a condition that is administered to strengthen immunity to that particular condition; a preparation of antigenic material designed to induce an immune response and immunologic memory when injected.

Vaults Octagonal barrel-shaped structures that transport either messenger RNA or ribosomal units from the nucleus to the cytoplasmic reticulum.

Vector/vehicle Factors that carry or distribute the agent (i.e., uncontrolled energy) of various types of injuries (e.g., a loaded handgun or a speeding car).

Vectors Living organisms that transmit microbes from one host to another.

Vertical gene transfer The transfer of genetic information from parent to offspring.

Vertical program A program intervention that focuses on the control, elimination, or eradication of a specific pathogen such as smallpox, malaria, or polio. Usually conducted though campaigns within existing health systems. System strengthening occurs, but the focus is mostly on reducing incidence and mortality from a specific disease agent.

Viral load The concentration of a virus in the blood.

Virion A complete viral particle.

Virulence The capacity of microbes to produce disease as a result of defensive and offensive strategies.

Viruses One of the categories of microbes; characterized as subcellular obligate intracellular parasites.

Visceral adiposity Deep abdominal fat accumulation that lies underneath the abdominal wall and surrounds the organs.

Viscoelastic properties Having both a relatively high resistance to flow and being capable of resuming its original shape after stretching or compression.

X chromosome inactivation The early embryonic process by which one of the X chromosomes is rendered transcriptionally inactive. Also known as Lyonization.

Zoonotic Disease for which domestic and/or wild animals are the reservoirs and that can be transmitted to humans.

Zoophilic Preference of a parasite for an animal host.

Zygote The first cell of a human embryo; a diploid cell, indicating a complete set of 46 chromosomes and an equal contribution of 23 chromosomes from the oocyte and sperm.

Index

Page numbers followed by *b*, *f*, or *t* indicate material in boxes, figures, or tables, respectively.